ESSENTIAL CHINESE FORMULAS

225 Classical and Modern Prescriptions Organized by Clinical Category

Jake Paul Fratkin

Shya Publications

ESSENTIAL CHINESE FORMULAS

225 Classical and Modern Prescriptions Organized by Clinical Category

Jake Paul Fratkin

Page and type design: Jay J. Nelson and Jake Paul Fratkin
Cover concept and design: Dominique Paul Fratkin
Cover: Jay J. Nelson
Woodblock drawings: Mary Jonaitis
Back cover photography: Jake Paul Fratkin
Printer: CDS Publications, Medford, Oregon

Library of Congress Control Number: 2014902654
ISBN-13: 978-0-9626078-0-6

Fratkin, Jake Paul
ESSENTIAL CHINESE FORMULAS, 225 Classical and Modern Prescriptions Organized by Clinical Category

1. Traditional Chinese Medicine
2. Herbal Medicine
3. Oriental Medicine

Shya Publications
7764 Jade Court, Boulder, Colorado 80303 • USA
303-554-0722
info@drjakefratkin.com

Printed in the United States of America
First printing, February, 2014

MEDICAL DISCLAIMER

This book is written primarily for practitioners of Traditional Chinese Medicine. It is a guide to important Chinese herbal formulas and products either for clinical use or as information that may aid construction of a formula for a particular patient.

I am aware that many people will use this book for self-medication. One must use one's judgment as to when to self-medicate and when to seek professional guidance. This book is not meant to be a substitute for sound medical advice. If you have a chronic or acute health problem, please consult a professional health practitioner. Too often, untrained or under-trained individuals cannot make an accurate assessment of their own health problems.

The author and publisher cannot take responsibility for someone avoiding timely medical advice, nor can we predict the effectiveness of the products described in this volume for any individual.

In terms of seeking professional guidance for use of Chinese herbal medicine, there are different levels of expertise depending on education. The best practitioners, in my opinion, are graduates of a five-year program in Traditional Chinese Medicine from China (mainland, Hong Kong, Taiwan), Korea or Vietnam. This does not include graduates of western medical colleges in those countries, unless they have also gone through at least a three-year postgraduate training in Chinese herbal medicine.

The second best level includes practitioners in North America or abroad who have obtained the following credential: Dipl. C.H. (Chinese Herbology) or Dipl. O.M (Oriental Medicine), NCCAOM. This is an American national board exam in Chinese herbal medicine that requires three or four year training in traditional Chinese medicine.

My hope in the publication of this book is for people outside of China to gain the benefits of Chinese herbal therapy through available Chinese herbal products. It will not only benefit the management of common illnesses and injuries, but can raise the level of health in every society.

For my family

Dominique, Raphaël, Thomas

ESSENTIAL CHINESE FORMULAS

225 Classical and Modern Prescriptions Organized by Clinical Category

CHAPTER INDEX

FORMULA INDEX BY CHAPTER

Formulas are listed alphabetically on p. 629

GROUP 2: FORMULAS THAT CLEAR HEAT

GROUP 3: RESPIRATORY DISORDERS

GROUP 9. DISTURBED SHEN

GROUP 10. HEART BLOOD STASIS AND ACCUMULATION OF HEART PHLEGM

GROUP 11. UROGENITAL DISORDERS

GROUP 16. QI AND BLOOD TONICS

GROUP 18. COMBINATION AND SINGLE HERB TONICS

ESSENTIAL CHINESE FORMULAS

225 Classical and Modern Prescriptions Organized by Clinical Category

1. Exogenous Wind Disorders

1A. EXOGENOUS WIND-COLD
(Common Cold: Cold-Type)

Classical Formulas:

Chuan Xiong Cha Tiao San	*chuān xiōng chá tiáo săn* (川芎茶调)
Ge Gen Tang	*gé gēn tāng* (葛根汤)
Gui Zhi Tang	*guì zhī tāng* (桂枝汤)
Jing Fang Bai Du San	*jīng fáng bài dú săn* (荆防败毒散)
Ren Shen Bai Du San	*rén shēn bài dú săn* (人参败毒散)

Wind-cold implies an exposure of the skin to external cold and is often contracted when the pores are open, such as following exercise, with subsequent exposure to cold or damp weather or air conditioning. Cold invades the channels at certain points along the shoulders, neck and head, with the most common symptom being acute headache, or muscle aching in he neck and trapezius. Wind-cold may also invade the lung causing runny nose with clear watery discharge (failure of the lung to descend fluids). Wind-cold is often the first stage of the common cold, because it inhibits the lungs from distributing *qi* through the meridians and from distributing and descending water. As the *zōng qì* (宗气) loses its strength, *wèi qì* (卫气) also diminishes, allowing toxic pathogens such as viruses to increase, leading to subsequent wind-heat presentations. For this reason, wind-cold quickly turns to wind-heat, and formulas should be changed when appropriate (see *Chapter 1B. Pathogenic Wind-Heat*). In wind-cold, pulses tend to be tight or wiry and floating, with symptoms of runny nose with clear discharge, or cough with frothy sputum.

Herbal formulas are effective for wind-cold by using herbs that warm the channels and promote sweating; this pushes pathogenic *qi* and cold to the surface. The formulas should be administered immediately, and taken in higher doses then manufacturers imply on their labels. It is traditionally recommended to take a hot bath and drink hot tea when taking these medicines, to help eliminate the pathogenic cold through sweating. In severe cases, taking a hot bath and then getting under blankets is also recommended.

The formulas are distinguished for patients with strong *zhèng qì* (正气) versus weakened *qi*. They can be summarized as follows:

Strong or normal *zheng qi*:

Chuan Xiong Cha Tiao San
Ge Gen Tang
Jing Fang Bai Du San

Weakened *zheng qi*:

Gui Zhi Tang
Ren Shen Bai Du San

When administering products for pathogenic wind it is recommended to discontinue other herbal products that one may have been taking, particularly tonic formulas.

Classical Formulas

CHUAN XIONG CHA TIAO SAN

Formula: *chuān xiōng chá tiáo săn* (川芎茶调散)
"Ligusticum (and) Tea Blended Powder"
Author: Imperial Medical Bureau (*tài yī jú,* 太医局);
revised by Chén Shī-Wén (陈师文)
Source: *Tài Píng Huì Mín Hé Jì Jú Fāng* (太平惠民和剂局方), 1078
Literal: "(Era of) Great Peace, Benefit People Harmonious Medicines, Office (of) Formulas"

Availability:

Chuan Xiong Cha Tiao San (BP, TZ)
Chuan Xiong Cha Tiao Wan (HT, MS, PM, TL)
Cnidium & Tea Formula (EG)
Ligusticum & Tea Formula (EG)
Ligusticum Teapills (PF)
Subdue Head Wind (K)

Ingredients: (from the standardized *"Ligusticum & Tea Formula"*)

bò hé (薄荷), Herba Menthae	32.7 %	BB
chuān xiōng (川芎), Rhizoma Ligustici Chuanxiong	16.3	K
jīng jiè (荆芥), Herba Schizonepetae	16.3	BA
qiāng huó (羌活), Radix Notopterygii	8.2	BA
gān căo (甘草), Radix Glycyrrhizae	8.2	AA
bái zhĭ (白芷), Radix Angelicae Dahuricae	8.2	BA
fáng fēng (防风), Radix Saposhnikov./Ledebouriellae	6.1	BA
xì xīn (细辛), Radix/Rhizoma Asari	4.1	BA

Ingredients: (from Herbal Times *"Chuan Xiong Cha Tiao Wan"*)

bò hé (薄荷), Herba Menthae	32.6 %	BB
chuān xiōng (川芎), Rhizoma Ligustici Chuanxiong	16.3	K
jīng jiè (荆芥), Herba Schizonepetae	16.3	B
bái zhĭ (白芷), Radix Angelicae Dahuricae	8.2	BA
gān căo (甘草), Radix Glycyrrhizae	8.2	AA
qiāng huó (羌活), Radix Notopterygii	8.2	BA
fáng fēng (防风), Radix Saposhnikov./Ledebouriellae	6.1	BA
màn jīng zĭ (蔓荆子), Fructus Viticis	4.1	BB

Dispels pathogenic wind, warms the channels and collaterals, frees the collaterals, relieves pain. Use for pathogenic wind-cold causing occipital and temporal headache, dizziness, aching shoulders and neck, stuffy nose, and chills and fever. Also used for headaches in general, including those due to wind-heat (common cold and flu); blood stagnation, including migraines; nervous headache; and frontal headaches due to food poisoning, indigestion, or sinus infection.

Pulse: Floating, excess
Tongue: Normal

Comments: This is a traditional prescription for acute onset headache, particularly those due to exposure to pathogenic wind. It is also used as a headache remedy, both acute and chronic, when due to excess rather than deficiency. *Chuān xiōng*, the lead herb, moves blood to disperse pain, especially parietal, along the *shaoyang* and *jueyin* channels.

Bái zhǐ treats frontal headache (*yangming* channel), and *qiāng huó* treats occipital headache (*taiyang* channels). *Fáng fēng* and *jīng jiè* aid in the dispersing of wind-cold. The formula can also be used for sudden onset of wind-cold without headache, including stuffy nose.

Traditionally, the formula is taken with green or black tea to induce sweating; this helps push pathogenic wind out the exterior. Additional benefit is available by drinking while in a hot bath, followed by getting under bed covers to facilitate sweating.

The original formula contains *xì xīn* (细辛, Radix/Rhizoma Asari). Due to regulatory FDA concerns, this herb tends to be substituted out. Herbal Times uses *màn jīng zǐ* (蔓荆子, Fructus Viticis); Plum Flower uses *guì zhī* (桂枝, Ramulus Cinnamomi).

Caution: Not intended for headaches due to deficiency, or ascending liver *yang*.

Further Reading:

Bensky et al, p. 625
Chen & Chen, p. 973
Ellis, p. 55

GE GEN TANG

Formula: *gé gēn tāng* (葛根汤), "Pueraria Decoction"
Author: Zhāng Zhòng-Jǐng (张仲景)
Source: *Shāng Hán Lùn* (伤寒论), 220
Literal: "Injury (by) Cold, Discussion"

Availability:

Kudzu Releasing Formula (K)
Kudzu Teapills (PF)
Pueraria Combination (EG)
Pueraria Formula (GF)

Ingredients: (from the standardized *"Pueraria Combination"*)

gé gēn (葛根), Radix Puerariae Lobatae	21.4 %	BB
má huáng (麻黄), Herba Ephedrae	16.1	BA
shēng jiāng (生姜), Rhizoma Zingiberis Recens	16.1	E
dà zǎo (大枣), Fructus Jujubae	14.3	AA
bái sháo (白芍), Radix Paeoniae Alba	10.7	AB
zhì gān cǎo (炙甘草), Radix Glycyrrhizae Praep.	10.7	AA
guì zhī (桂枝), Ramulus Cinnamomi	10.7	BA

Ingredients: (from Plum Flower *"Kudzu Teapills"*)

gé gēn (葛根), Radix Puerariae Lobatae	23.0 %	BB
má huáng (麻黄), Herba Ephedrae	17.4	BA
shēng jiāng (生姜), Rhizoma Zingiberis Recens	17.4	E
guì zhī (桂枝), Ramulus Cinnamomi	11.5	BA
bái sháo (白芍), Radix Paeoniae Alba	11.5	AB
gān cǎo (炙甘草), Radix Glycyrrhizae	11.5	AA
dà zǎo (大枣), Fructus Jujubae	7.7	AA

Dispels wind, releases the exterior, diffuses lung qi, dredges and opens the channels and collaterals, relieves pain. Use for *taiyang* stage of wind-cold to the lungs, causing stiff neck, heaviness of the body, headache, and fever and chills without sweating. Use for early stage of common cold or sinusitis due to wind-cold. Can be used for torticollis, pediatric diarrhea, allergic rhinitis and stomach flu.

Pulse: Floating, tight
Tongue: Thin white coat

***Comments*:** This formula is applied in the *taiyang* stage of pathogenic cold, with the key symptoms of stiff upper back and neck or headache. There may be mild fever with chills, but without sweating. The formula hopes to release the exterior by inducing sweating, using *gé gēn, má huáng* and *guì zhī*. It is also used for pediatric diarrhea with abdominal pain, with or without external cold invasion, due to the synergistic effect of *gé gēn, bái sháo* and *gān cǎo*.

***Caution**:* The original formula calls for *má huáng* (麻黄, Herba Ephedrae), which may cause agitation or insomnia in certain patients with deficiency of *qi*. Caution during pregnancy or with hypertension; also, do not take in the evening.

Further Reading:

Bensky et al, p. 19
Chen & Chen, p. 59
Ellis, p. 108

GUI ZHI TANG

Formula: *guì zhī tāng* (桂枝汤), "Cinnamomum Decoction"
Author: Zhāng Zhòng-Jǐng (张仲景)
Source: *Shāng Hán Lùn* (伤寒论), 220
Literal: "Injury (by) Cold, Discussion"

Availability:

Cinnamon Combination (EG)
Cinnamon Twig Decoction (K)
Cinnamon Twig Formula (GF, HS)
Gui Zhi Tang Teapills (PF)

Ingredients: (from the standardized *"Cinnamon Combination"*)

guì zhī (桂枝), Ramulus Cinnamomi	22.2 %	BA
bái sháo (白芍), Radix Paeoniae Alba	22.2	AB
shēng jiāng (生姜), Rhizoma Zingiberis Recens	22.2	BA
dà zǎo (大枣), Fructus Jujubae	18.5	AA
zhì gān cǎo (炙甘草), Radix Glycyrrhizae Praep	14.9	AA

Dispels wind-cold, releases the exterior, relieves muscles, harmonizes the ying and wei levels. Use for wind-cold working its way from the exterior into the muscle layer, with symptoms of low-grade fever with chills, stuffy nose and mild sweating; also, headache and stiff neck. Can also be used for stomach cramping due to cold causing dry retching.

Pulse: Floating, weak, slow
Tongue: Thin white or moist coat

***Comments*:** This formula is applied in *taiyang* stage pathogenic cold where an underlying deficiency already exists. Symptoms include slight fever with chills, mild sweating, and contractures in the muscle layer affecting the neck, occiput and upper back, or generalized aching. In this case the pathogen has worked its way slightly deeper into the body, due to pre-existing deficiency of *wei* and *ying qi*.

The formula tonifies and harmonizes *ying* and *wei qi*, and is more tonifying than other diaphoretic-type formulas. *Guì zhī* activates the dispelling of wind and cold, and when combined with *bái sháo*, it supports and harmonizes the *ying* and *wei*. The combination of *guì zhī* and *bái sháo* also relax muscle contraction. *Shēng jiāng* supports *guì zhī* in dispelling wind and cold, and *dà zăo* supports tonification of the *ying qi*.

Further Reading:

Bensky et al, p. 13
Chen & Chen, p. 51
Ellis, p. 128

JING FANG BAI DU SAN

Formula: *jīng fáng bài dú sǎn* (荆防败毒散)
"Schizonepeta, Saposhnikovia Defeat Toxin Powder"
Author: Zhāng Shí-Chè (张时彻)
Source: *Shè Shēng Zhòng Miào Fāng* (摄生众妙方), 1550
Literal: "Conserve Life Multitude (of) Marvelous Formulas"

Availability:

Release The Exterior Teapills (PF)
Schizonepeta & Siler Formula (EG)
* Dispel Invasion (K)

Ingredients: (From the standardized *"Schizonepeta & Siler Formula"*)

fáng fēng (防风), Radix Saposhnikoviae/Ledebouriellae	8.5 %	BA
jīng jiè (荆芥), Herba Schizonepetae	8.5	BA
qiāng huó (羌活), Radix Notopterygii	8.5	BA
dú huó (独活), Radix Angelicae Pubescentis	8.5	BA
chái hú (柴胡), Radix Bupleuri	8.5	BB
qián hú (前胡), Radix Peucedani	8.5	CB
jié gěng (桔梗), Radix Platycodonis	8.5	CA
zhǐ ké (枳壳), Fructus Aurantii	8.5	G
chuān xiōng (川芎), Rhizoma Chuanxiong	8.5	K
fú ling (茯苓), Poria	8.5	FC
shēng jiāng (生姜) Rhizoma Zingiberis Recens	8.5	BA
gān cǎo (甘草), Radix Glycyrrhizae	4.0	AA
bò hé (薄荷), Herba Menthae	2.5	BB

* Throughout the text, asterisks (*) indicate that the listed formula is based on the orginal, but with significant modifications or additions.

Dispels wind-cold and damp, promotes sweating, warms the channels and the collaterals, stops cough, heals sores and relieves pain. Use for wind-cold exterior pattern causing stiff neck and shoulders, body aches, headache, nasal congestion or runny nose, and early cough. It is also used in abscesses and sores, including mastitis, when there is an absence of heat symptoms.

Pulse: Floating and tight, might be rapid
Tongue: Normal, or with greasy or thin white coat

Comments: *Jing Fang Bai Du San* is used in acute wind-cold causing shivering, runny or congested nose, cough and headache. It combines wind-dispersing herbs (*fáng fēng* and *jīng jiè*) with herbs for wind-damp (*qiāng huó* and *dú huó*). *Chuān xiōng* relieves headache. *Zhǐ ké, jié gěng* and *qián hú* remove phlegm, stop cough, and descend lung *qi*. It is also used for early presentations affecting the skin, including sores and abscesses, urticaria and mastitis.

Jing Fang Bai Du San is a variation the 12th century formula *Ren Shen Bai Du San* (below). It is more appropriate for patients with normal *zheng qi*, whereas *Ren Shen Bai Du San* is preferred for patients with weakened *zheng qi*.

Although early authors consider this formula appropriate for wind-heat or heat-toxins, its composition does not readily lend itself towards this direction. It is a mix of warming herbs (57.5%) and cooling herbs (19.5%), and the overall affect is warming. Because it does not contain any herbs that clear heat-toxins, it should be combined with formulas from Chapters 1B or 2A in the presence of viral heat toxins.

Further Reading:

Bensky et al, p. 49
Chen & Chen, p. 1334
Ellis, p. 169

REN SHEN BAI DU SAN

Formula: *rén shēn bài dú sǎn* (人参败毒散), "Ginseng Defeat Pathogen Powder"
aka: *bài dú sǎn* (败毒散), "Defeat Pathogen Powder"
Author: Qián Yǐ (钱乙)
Source: *Qián Shì Xiǎo Ér Yào Zhèng Zhí Jué* (钱氏小儿药证直), 1119
Literal: "Qian's Key (to) Children's Medicines (and) Patterns, Straight Secrets"

Availability:

Ginseng & Mentha Formula (EG)
Resilient Warrior Teapills (PF)

Ingredients: (from the standardized *"Ginseng & Mentha Formula"*)

rén shēn (人参), Radix Ginseng	10. %	AA
qiāng huó (羌活), Rhizoma et Radix Notopterygii	10	BA
dú huó (独活), Radix Angelicae Pubescentis	10	BA
chái hú (柴胡), Radix Bupleuri	10	BB
qián hú (前胡), Radix Peucedani	10	CB
chuān xiōng (川芎), Rhizoma Ligustici Chuanxiong	10	K
zhǐ ké (枳壳), Fructus Aurantii	10	G
jié gěng (桔梗), Radix Platycodonis	10	CA
fú ling (茯苓), Poria	10	FC
gān cǎo (甘草), Radix Glycyrrhizae	5	AA
shēng jiāng (生姜) Rhizoma Zingiberis Recens	5	BA

Dispels wind-cold-damp, resolves the exterior, tonifies qi. Use for wind-cold damp causing low fever with chills, headache, stiffness in neck and shoulders and body aches. Also for wind-cold leading to acute watery stool. Use for common cold, sinus congestion, early stage of flu, and early stage of chicken pox in weakened patients.

Pulse: Floating, and either tight, weak or soft
Tongue: Normal, or with thin white coat

Comments: *Ren Shen Bai Du San* was originally formulated for infants catching a common cold with symptoms of nasal discharge, shivering, or sudden loose stools, and was also given during the early stage of measles and chicken pox. It was felt that infants have fragile *zheng qi*, and the use of a small amount of *rén shēn* would be of benefit. Now it is commonly used for common cold in weak patients with a pre-existing deficiency of *qi*, including post-partum women, the elderly, and following surgery or illness.

Qiāng huó is the main herb for dispelling wind-camp; *chái hú* to dispel wind and relieve muscle spasm; and *qián hú* to benefit the lung and nose and eliminate phlegm.

Because it does not contain any herbs that clear heat-toxins, it can be combined with formulas from Chapters 1B or 2A in the presence of viral infection.

Further Reading:

Bensky et al, p. 47
Chen & Chen, p. 126
Ellis, p. 237

OTHER FORMULAS APPROPRIATE FOR THIS CHAPTER:

Classical Formulas:

Gui Zhi Jia Shao Yao Tang
Cinnamon & Peony Combination (EG, HS)

Gui Zhi Ren Shen Tang
Cinnamon & Ginseng Combination (EG)

Qiang Huo Sheng Shi Tang
Notopterygium & Tuhuo Combination (EG)

Shen Su Yin
Ginseng & Perilla Combination (EG)

Xiao Qing Long Wan
Blue Green Lung Formula (K)
Minor Blue Dragon Formula (CC)
Minor Blue Dragon Combination (EG)
Xiao Qing Long Tang (GC)
* Blue Earth Dragon (SF)

Modern Formulas:

Children's Herbal Sentinel (TT)
Herbal Sentinel Yang (TT)
Minor Blue Perilla (HC)
Purge External Wind (CMS)
Respitrol-Cold (EV)

1. EXOGENOUS WIND DISORDERS

1B. PATHOGENIC WIND-HEAT
(Common Cold – Mild Heat Type)

Classical Formulas:

Chai Ge Jie Ji Tang	*chái gé jiě jī tāng* (柴葛解肌汤)
Sang Ju Yin	*sāng jú yǐn* (桑菊饮)
Yin Qiao San	*yín qiào sǎn* (银翘散)

Pathogenic wind-heat, like pathogenic wind-cold, causes the common cold (*gǎn mào,* 感冒). Unlike wind-cold, which implies an etiology, wind-heat refers to an array of heat symptoms including sore throat, low grade fever, yellow phlegm, dry cough, dry nose or eyes, stuffy nose and, occasionally, yellow nasal discharge. Pulses are floating, wiry and slightly rapid. The tongue may be red in the distal third (the tip), or the whole body.

Contrary to the *caveat* in modern medicine that "there is no real cure for the common cold", viral colds can be effectively and quickly treated with Chinese herbal formulas if administered early and at frequent intervals of every three hours. The formulas in this chapter address early stage common cold, marked by sore throat, stuffy nose, headache, aching and early cough. They use cool wind-expelling herbs that take internal heat to the surface. In this regard, they are useful for pediatric diseases such as measles, chicken pox and roseola; they can also be used, adjunctively, in skin conditions marked by redness or itching. In these cases, we recommend combining with formulas for heat toxins (Chapter 2A) or skin conditions (Chapter 13A).

Chapter 2A. Heat Toxins and Damp-Heat Toxins contains stronger formulas for colds and flu, such as *Gan Mao Ling*. That chapter also addresses viral or bacterial infections of the lymphatics or throat, and other infections. If the common cold has progressed to a cough, refer to *Group 3. Respiratory Disorders.*

When administering products for pathogenic wind, it is best to discontinue any tonic formulas that can pull wind and toxins into the interior. It is best to take these formulas every three hours until symptoms are alleviated.

CHAI GE JIE JI TANG

Formula: *chái gé jiě jī tāng* (柴葛解肌汤)
"Bupleurum, Pueraria Resolve Muscle Decoction"
Author: Táo Huá (陶华)
Source: *Shāng Hán Liù Shū* (伤寒六书), 1445
Literal: "Injury (by) Cold, Six Books"

Availability:

Bupleurum & Pueraria Combination (EG)
Chai Ge Jie Ji Wan (HT)

Ingredients: (from the standardized *"Bupleurum & Pueraria Combination"*)

gé gēn (葛根), Radix Puerariae Lobatae	9.8 %	BB
chái hú (柴胡), Radix Bupleuri	9.8	BB
shí gāo (石膏), Gypsum Fibrosum	9.8	DA
qiāng huó (羌活), Rhizoma et Radix Notopterygii	9.8	BA
bái zhǐ (白芷), Radix Angelicae Dahuricae	9.8	BA
huáng qín (黄芩), Radix Scutellariae	9.8	DB
bái sháo (白芍), Radix Paeoniae Alba	9.8	AB
jié gěng (桔梗), Radix Platycodonis	9.8	CA
shēng jiāng (生姜), Rhizoma Zingiberis Recens	7.8	BA
dà zǎo (大枣), Fructus Jujubae	7.8	AA
gān cǎo (甘草), Radix Glycyrrhizae	6.0	AA

Ingredients: (from Herbal Times *"Chai Ge Jie Ji Wan"*)

gé gēn (葛根), Radix Puerariae Lobatae	20. %	BB
chái hú (柴胡), Radix Bupleuri	16	BB
bái zhǐ (白芷), Radix Angelicae Dahuricae	11	BA
bái sháo (白芍), Radix Paeoniae Alba	11	AB
huáng qín (黄芩), Radix Scutellariae	11	DB
qiāng huó (羌活), Rhizoma et Radix Notopterygii	11	BA
dà zǎo (大枣), Fructus Jujubae	5	AA
gān cǎo (甘草), Radix Glycyrrhizae	5	AA
jié gěng (桔梗), Radix Platycodonis	5	CA
shēng jiāng (生姜), Rhizoma Zingiberis Recens	5	BA

Dispels pathogenic wind and cold, clears heat in the interior, harmonizes and resolves half-exterior, half-interior, relieves muscles. Use for pathogenic wind-cold moving into the interior and transforming into heat, causing muscle aching, low-grade fever or alternating fever and chills, headache, dry nose, slight sore throat, and irritability. Use in common cold, influenza, and sinus congestion without discharge. Also used in tooth pain.

Pulse: Floating, forceful, occasionally flooding and slightly rapid
Tongue: Normal

Comments: This formula is intended for wind-cold that is moving into the interior and turning to heat, with symptoms of stiff neck and shoulders, headache, eye pain and swollen glands. *Gé gēn*, the lead herb, is particularly useful for stiff neck and shoulder muscles. Both *gé gēn* and *chái hú* help trapped wind-heat release back to the surface. *Shí gāo* reduces fever and heat in the channels, and also releases heat trapped in the muscle layer. *Bái zhǐ, qiāng huó* and *bái sháo* reduce pain and achiness.

The version by Herbal Times contains 20% *gé gēn*, the lead herb, but lacks *shí gāo.*

Further Reading:

Bensky et al, p. 39
Chen and Chen, p. 107
Ellis, p. 39

SANG JU YIN

Formula: *sāng jú yǐn* (桑菊饮), "Morus, Chrysanthemum Cool-Decoction"
Author: Wú Táng (吴瑭) *aka* Wú Jū-Tōng (吴鞠通)
Source: *Wēn Bìng Tiáo Biàn* (温病条辨), 1798
Literal: "Warm Diseases Systematic Differentiation"

Availability:

Clear Wind-Heat Teapills (PF)
Initial Defense (K)
Mulberry & Chrysanthemum Combination (EG)
Sang Ju Wan (HT)
Sang Ju Yin (BP)
Sang Ju Yin Wan (TL)

Ingredients: (from the standardized *"Mulberry & Chrysanthemum Combination"*)

sāng yè (桑叶), Folium Mori	19.7 %	BB
xìng rén (杏仁), Semen Armeniacae Amarum	15.9	CC
jié gěng (桔梗), Radix Platycodonis	15.9	CA
lú gēn (芦根), Rhizoma Phragmitis	15.9	DA
lián qiào (连翘), Fructus Forsythiae	11.9	DD
jú huā (菊花), Flos Chrysanthemi	7.9	BB
bò hé (薄荷), Herba Menthae	6.4	BB
gān cǎo (甘草), Radix Glycyrrhizae	6.4	AA

Releases the exterior to dispel pathogenic wind, clears heat-toxin, diffuses lung qi, relieves cough. Use for early stage of common cold or influenza with symptoms of dry cough, slight fever, dry or sore throat with watery or red eyes. Can be used in very early presentation of heat-toxins causing tonsillitis, influenza, bronchitis, conjunctivitis, chicken pox and measles, especially when accompanied by cough.

Pulse: Floating, slightly rapid
Tongue: Normal, or thin yellow coat

Comments: Formulated by Wu Ju-Tong, the creator of *Yin Qiao San* (below), this prescription is a *wēn bìng* (温病) formula of the late 18th century. It is effective for early stage of pathogenic wind-heat marked by dry cough, with difficulty for the lung to descend and circulate *qi*. It uses spicy-cool herbs to release the exterior, including *sāng yè*, *bò hé* and *jú huā*. *Lián qiào* clears heat toxins, while *jié gěng* and *xìng rén* descends lung *qi* and stops cough.

The formula can be used for early dry cough before lung fire develops; it is not effective once phlegm develops. It is considered a light formula, because the formulator, Wu Ju-Tong, felt that the lungs should be dealt with gently when attacked by heat. So said, the Chinese promoted the use of this formula, with additions of herbs for heat-toxins, in the treatment of the SARS epidemic of 2003 and avian fu in 2006.

Further Reading:

Bensky et al, p. 35
Chen & Chen, p. 89
Ellis, p. 253

YIN QIAO SAN

Formula: *yín qiào săn* (银翘散), "Lonicera, Forsythia Powder"
aka: *yín qiào jiě dú săn* (银翘解毒散)
"Lonicera, Forsythia Resolve Toxin Pills"
Author: Wú Táng (吴瑭) *aka* Wú Jū-Tōng (吴鞠通)
Source: *Wēn Bìng Tiáo Biàn* (温病条辨), 1798
Literal: "Warm Diseases Systematic Differentiation"

Availability:

Dr. Shen's Yin Chiao (DS)
Lonicera & Forsythia Formula (EG)
Yin Chiao Chieh Tu Pien (PF, PM)
Yin Chiao Formula (GF)
Yin Chiao Jin (HC)
Yin Chiao Junior (HC)
Yin Qiao (K)
Yin Qiao Formula (CC, HS)
Yin Qiao Jie Du Pian (PIM, PM)
Yin Qiao Jie Du Wan (HT, MS, TL)
* Initial Defense (K)
* Lonicera Complex (EC)
* Yin Qiao-Echinacea Plus (PH)

Ingredients: (from the standardized *"Lonicera & Forsythia Formula"*)

jīn yín huā (金银花), Flos Lonicerae Japonicae	18.0 %	DD
lián qiào (连翘), Fructus Forsythiae	17.9	DD
jié gěng (桔梗), Radix Platycodonis	10.7	CA
niú bàng zǐ (牛蒡子), Fructus Arctii	10.7	BB
bò hé (薄荷), Herba Menthae	10.7	BB
dàn dòu chǐ (淡豆豉), Semen Sojae Praep.	8.9	BB
gān căo (甘草), Radix Glycyrrhizae	8.9	AA
dàn zhú yè (淡竹叶), Herba Lophatheri	7.1	DA
jīng jiè (荆芥), Herba Schizonepetae	7.1	BA

Releases the exterior to dispel pathogenic wind, clears heat-toxin, benefits the throat, relieves thirst, diffuses lung qi. Use for early stage of common cold with symptoms of sore throat, low fever, thirst, aching shoulders and neck, headache or dry cough. Helpful for pediatric ear infection, tonsillitis and influenza. Also useful in early presentations of childhood viral diseases, including chicken pox, rubella, roseola and measles. May have beneficial effects in hives or skin itching with heat.

Pulse: Floating, rapid, excess or tight
Tongue: Normal, or with red tongue tip

Comments: This is an effective medicine for common cold when taken within the first twelve hours of the earliest symptoms of sore throat or general aching. Like other formulas for early wind-heat invasion, it should be given every 3 to 4 hours. The herbs *jīn yín huā* and *lián qiào* (which define the name *Yin Qiao*) are effective against viruses causing upper respiratory infections; *niú bàng zǐ* addresses sore throat. Once the viral pathogen works its way into the interior with more pronounced symptoms, switch to, or combine with, formulas in *Chapter 2A. Heat-Toxins and Damp-Heat Toxins.*

Yin Qiao San is an important formula for pushing heat toxins to the surface and is used as a foundation for treating pediatric chicken pox, measles, and roseola. It is usually combined with a formula from Chapter 2A.

Yin Qiao is not appropriate once the pathogen has entered the lungs and is producing cough. For cough, look at formulas in *Group 3. Respiratory Disorders.*

Further Reading:

Bensky et al, p. 35.
Chen & Chen, p. 94
Ellis, p. 386

OTHER FORMULAS APPROPRIATE FOR THIS CHAPTER:

See *Chapter 2A. Heat-Toxins & Damp-Heat Toxins*

Modern Formulas:

Chrysanthemum 9 (SF)
Children's Free And Clear Formula (GF)
Cold Quell (BP)
Gan Mao Ling Wan (HT)

1. EXOGENOUS WIND DISORDERS

1C. NASAL AND EAR CONGESTION

Classical Formulas:

Cang Er Zi San	*cāng ěr zǐ sǎn* (苍耳子散)
Xin Yi Wan	*xīn yí wán* (辛夷丸)

Modern Formulas:

Bi Min Gan Wan	*bí mǐn gǎn wán* (鼻敏感丸)
Bi Yan Pian	*bí yán piān* (鼻炎片)
Children's Ear Formula (GF)	

The formulas in this chapter are indicated for nasal and ear congestion. These events can be due to exogenous wind-cold, exogenous pathogenic heat (including viral or bacteria) associated with the common cold, or due to pollen or food allergies. Some formulas are appropriate for sneezing, watery or itchy eyes and runny nose associated with allergies or the common cold; other products are directed towards thick congestion.

The *materia medica* used in the formulas include herbs to dispel wind, herbs to dissolve phlegm-turbidity, and herbs that transport the formula to the sinus area.

Acute sinus and ear congestion is often due to an invasion of external pathogen, including viral or bacterial. In those cases, the formulas in this chapter may be combined with formulas for wind-heat (Chapter 1B), heat-toxins or damp-heat toxins (Chapter 2A). In many cases, Chinese herbal combinations offer faster results than antibiotics, and without the consequences of disrupting intestinal flora. In chronic and stubborn presentations, lab culture for fungal infection may be helpful. Bacterial infections are rare, even in acute episodes, and should be confirmed by lab analysis.

Pollen allergies that cause runny nose and itchy eyes also respond to the included formulas. Chronic sinusitis may be due to food allergies, particularly gluten or dairy. Both chronic sinusitis and food allergies may have an underlying deficiency of spleen *qi* or *yang* at its root – the inability to digest pollen protein. In modern functional medicine, this is often seen as a deficiency of hydrochloric acid production. Boosting spleen *qi* or *yang* at the same time as using these formulas may be beneficial. Also, during hay fever season, additional supplementation with *Yu Ping Feng* (Chapter 16A) is helpful.

Classical Formulas:

CANG ER ZI SAN

Formula: *cāng ěr zǐ sǎn* (苍耳子散), "Xanthium Powder"
Author: Yán Yòng-Hé (严用和)
Source: *Jì Shēng Fāng* (济生方), 1253
Literal: "Aid (the) Living Formulas"

Availability:

Upper Chamber Teapills (PF)
Xanthium Formula (EG)
Xanthium Powder (BP)
* Fragrant Jade (K)

Ingredients: (from the standardized *"Xanthium Formula"*)

bái zhǐ (白芷), Radix Angelicae Dahuricae	40.8 %	BA
bò hé (薄荷), Herba Menthae	20.4	BB
xīn yí huā (辛夷花), Flos Magnoliae	20.4	BA
cāng ěr zǐ (苍耳子), Fructus Xanthii	10.2	FA
cōng bái (葱白), Bulbus Allii Fistulosi	4.1	BA
chá yè (茶叶), Herba Camelliae	4.1	

Ingredients: (Plum Flower *"Upper Chamber Teapills"*)

cāng ěr zǐ (苍耳子), Fructus Xanthii	34.9 %	FA
bái zhǐ (白芷), Radix Angelicae Dahuricae	34.9	BA
xīn yí huā (辛夷花), Flos Magnoliae	20.0	BA
bò hé (薄荷), Herba Menthae	10.2	BB

Dispels pathogenic wind, eliminates heat, dispels turbidity, opens the nasal passages, relieves pain. Use for nasal discharge with accompanying symptoms of sneezing, red, itchy eyes, nasal obstruction and frontal headache. Applicable for acute and chronic sinusitis and rhinitis, and for nasal symptoms due to the common cold.

Pulse: Tight
Tongue: Normal, or thin white or yellow coat

Comments: This small formula for sinus congestion and runny nose, like *Xin Yi Wan*, below, was developed by Yan Yong-He. Often, congested nose manifests during a common cold due to wind-heat attacking the lungs, impairing its ability to descend fluid. The formula can be applied with either cold or heat conditions; it can be used alone or adjunctively to reinforce other formulas. With bacterial infections, combine with products from Chapter 2A. In common cold due to wind-heat of pathogenic heat, combine with products from Chapters 1B or 2A.

Caution: *Cāng ěr zǐ* is drying. Use in sinus cases with watery or thick phlegm.

Further Reading:

Bensky et al, p. 628
Chen & Chen, p. 82

XIN YI WAN

Formula: *xīn yí wán* (辛夷丸) "Magnolia Flower Pills")
Author: Yán Yòng-Hé (严用和)
Source: *Jì Shēng Fāng* (济生方), 1253
Literal: "Aid (the) Living Formulas"

Availability:

Magnolia Flower Formula (EG)
Magnolia Flower Teapills (PF)
Xanthium & Magnolia Formula (GF)
Xin Yi San (TL)

Ingredients: (from the standardized *"Magnolia Flower Formula"*)

xīn yí huā (辛夷花), Flos Magnoliae	11.2 %	BA
bái zhǐ (白芷), Radix Angelicae Dahuricae	11.1	BA
fáng fēng (防风), Radix Saposhnikov./Ledebouriellae	11.1	BA
gǎo běn (藁本), Rhizoma Ligustici	11.1	BA
shēng má (升麻), Rhizoma Cimicifugae	11.1	BB
mù tōng (木通), Caulis Akebiae	11.1	FC
chuān xiōng (川芎), Rhizoma Ligustici Chuanxiong	11.1	K
gān cǎo (甘草), Radix Glycyrrhizae	11.1	AA
chá yè (茶叶), Herba Camelliae	11.1	

Ingredients: (from Plum Flower's *"Magnolia Flower Teapills"*)

xīn yí huā (辛夷花), Flos Magnoliae	15.2 %	BA
bái zhǐ (白芷), Radix Angelicae Dahuricae	13.1	BA
fáng fēng (防风), Radix Saposhnikov./Ledebouriellae	10.9	BA
gǎo běn (藁本), Rhizoma Ligustici	10.9	BA
shēng má (升麻), Rhizoma Cimicifugae	10.9	BB
mù tōng (木通), Caulis Akebiae	10.9	FC
chuān xiōng (川芎), Rhizoma Ligustici Chuanxiong	10.9	K
qiāng huó (羌活), Radix Notopterygii	8.6	BA
gān cǎo (甘草), Radix Glycyrrhizae	8.6	AA

Dispels pathogenic wind and cold, transforms phlegm and dispels turbidity, opens the nasal passages. Use for nasal congestion or watery nasal discharge with accompanying symptoms of frontal headache or orbital pain, sneezing, and loss of smell. Applicable for acute onset of wind-cold sneezing or sinusitis; also for nasal allergy.

Pulse: Floating, tight
Tongue: Normal

Comments: This formula is an elaboration of *Cang Er Zi San* (above), also formulated by Yan Yong-He. Six of the herbs used in this formula dispel pathogenic wind-cold. It is a warming formula, and is suitable for sneezing or clear runny nose at the start of a cold or due to allergies. It is also useful for sinus pain and headache. The combination of *xīn yí huā* and *bái zhǐ* is helpful in cases of stubborn sinus mucus congestion with accompanying pain. Combining *gǎo běn* and *chuān xiōng* addresses frontal and orbital headache.

The original formula contained *xì xīn* (细辛, Radix et Rhizoma Asari), which is no longer available in North American, and the formula has been adjusted. The Plum Flower version has substituted *qiāng huó.*

Further Reading:

Bensky et al, p. 629
Chen & Chen, p. 84
Ellis, p. 364

Modern Formulas:

BI MIN GAN WAN
(PE MIN KAN WAN)

Formula: *bí mǐn gǎn wán* (鼻敏感丸),"Nasal Susceptibility Pill"
Source: Modern Chinese patent medicine

Availability:

Bi Min Gan Wan (PM, TL)
Nasal Allergy Pills (BP)
Pe Min Gan Wan (HT)
Pe Min Kan Wan (PM, PF)
Seasonal Allergies (JD)
Te Xiao Bi Min Gan Pian (GC)

Ingredients: (from Herbal Times *"Pe Min Gan Wan"*)

xīn yí huā (辛夷花), Flos Magnoliae	14. %	BA
qiāng huó (羌活), Radix Notopterygii	12	BA
bái zhǐ (白芷), Radix Angelicae Dahuricae	9	BA
cāng ěr zǐ (苍耳子), Fructus Xanthii	9	FA
chuān xiōng (川芎), Rhizoma Ligustici Chuanxiong	9	K
fáng fēng (防风), Radix Saposhnikov./Ledebouriellae	9	BA
gǎo běn (藁本), Rhizoma Ligustici	9	BA
màn jīng zǐ (蔓荆子), Fructus Viticis	9	BB
shēng má (升麻), Rhizoma Cimicifugae	9	BB
gān cǎo (甘草), Radix Glycyrrhizae	6	AA
guì zhī (桂枝), Ramulus Cinnamomi	5	BA

Ingredients: (from Plum Flower *"Pe Min Kan Wan"*. Ingredient percentages are not given.)

xīn yí huā (辛夷花), Flos Magnoliae	BA
cāng ěr zǐ (苍耳子), Fructus Xanthii	FA
bǎn lán gēn (板蓝根), Radix Isatidis	DD
huò xiāng (藿香), Herba Agastachis	FB
yě jú huā (野菊花), Flos Chrysanthemi Indici	BB
fáng fēng (防风), Radix Saposhnikov./Ledebouriellae	BA
é bù shí cǎo (鹅不食草), Herba Centipedae	CA
bò hé (薄荷), Herba Menthae	BB
zǐ sū yè (紫苏叶), Folium Perillae	BA

Dispels pathogenic wind, clears heat, resolves toxin, transforms phlegm, dispels turbidity, diffuses the lung, opens the nasal passages, dispels damp. Use for acute and chronic sinus congestion marked by thick yellow nasal discharge, heat and redness around the sinus cavities, and sinus pain or headache. Also useful for earache or congestion, and common cold marked by nasal congestion.

Pulse: Floating, possibly slippery
Tongue: Normal, or red in tip

Comments: There are many versions of *Bi Min Gan* (*Pe Min Kan*) formulas available. Although ingredients and dosages vary, the applications of the various products are consistent, namely for nasal congestion due to common cold or allergy. Here we present two versions. In the first by Herbal Times, *xīn yí huā, bái zhǐ* and *cāng ěr zǐ* bring the formula to the nasal area, open the nasal passages, and control sneezing. *Qiāng huó, gǎo běn* and *chuān xiōng* counter sinus headache and pain.

The version from Plum Flower uses *cāng ěr zǐ* and *é bù shí cǎo* to open the nasal passages. *Huò xiāng* drains phlegm and damp, and *bǎn lán gēn* clears toxic pathogen. Ingredient percentages are not provided by the manufacturer.

BI YAN PIAN

Formula: *bí yán piān* (鼻炎片),"Nasal Inflammation Tablet"
Source: Modern patent medicine

Availability:

Bi Yan Pian/Wan (HT, K, PF, PIM, PM, TZ)
Nasal Clearing Formula (HS)
Nasal Formula (BP)

Ingredients: (from Herbal Times *"Bi Yan Wan"*)

xīn yí huā (辛夷花), Flos Magnoliae	24. %	BA
cāng ěr zǐ (苍耳子), Fructus Xanthii	20	FA
huáng bǎi (黄柏), Cortex Phellodendri	7	DB
lián qiào (连翘), Fructus Forsythiae	7	DD
gān cǎo (甘草), Radix Glycyrrhizae	6	AA
wǔ wèi zǐ (五味子), Fructus Schisandrae Chinensis	6	L
bái zhǐ (白芷), Radix Angelicae Dahuricae	5	BA
fáng fēng (防风), Radix Saposhnikov./Ledebouriellae	5	BA
jié gěng (桔梗), Radix Platycodonis	5	CA
jīng jiè (荆芥), Herba Schizonepetae	5	BA
jú huā (菊花), Flos Chrysanthemi	5	BB
zhī mǔ (知母), Rhizoma Anemarrhenae	5	DA

Dispels pathogenic wind, eliminates heat, resolves toxin, transforms phlegm, dispels turbidity, benefits the eyes, opens the nasal passages. Use for nasal congestion or rhinitis with thick yellow discharge, sneezing, and red, itchy eyes. Useful for sinus infection, nasal congestion due to common cold, and hay fever allergies. Can be used in pediatric ear infection.

Pulse: Floating, possibly slippery, rapid
Tongue: Normal, or red in tip

Comments: The *Bi Yan Pian* formulas are effective for sinus congestion marked by heat: yellow nasal discharge and red, watery itchy eyes. They can be used for sinus symptoms due to the common cold or pollen allergies. *Cāng ěr zǐ, xīn yí huā,* and *jú huā* bring the formula to the sinus area, *huáng bǎi* and *lián qiào* clear heat-toxins, and *zhī mǔ* moistens sticky-phlegm in the sinus.

In the Herbal Times version, presented here, large amounts of *xīn yí huā* and *cāng ěr zǐ* are used, comprising 44% of the formula.

CHILDREN'S EAR FORMULA

Source: Golden Flower
Author: Jake Paul Fratkin

Ingredients:

huò xiāng (藿香), Herba Agastachis	10. %	FB
fú líng (茯苓), Poria	10	FC
jú huā (菊花), Flos Chrysanthemi	8	BB
huáng lián (黄连), Rhizoma Coptidis	8	DB
lián qiào (连翘), Fructus Forsythiae	8	DD
chì sháo (赤芍), Radix Paeoniae Rubra	8	K
qián hú (前胡), Radix Peucedani	8	CB
bái zhǐ (白芷), Radix Angelicae Dahuricae	7	BA
chái hú (柴胡), Radix Bupleuri	7	BB
zhè bèi mǔ (浙贝母), Bulbus Fritillariae Thunbergii	7	CB
bàn xià (半夏), Rhizoma Pinelliae	7	CA
màn jīng zǐ (蔓荆子), Fructus Viticis	7	FA
shēng jiāng (生姜), Rhizoma Zingiberis Recens	5	BB

Dispels pathogenic wind, clears heat-toxins, dissolves phlegm, dispels dampness, relieves pain. Use for acute ear pain in children with accompanying symptoms of nasal congestion, fever, and malaise. Recommended for children under the age of three.

Comments: This formula, which comes as a flavored syrup, was specifically developed for acute ear infection in children, especially under 3 years. The pain of ear infection is from accumulation of fluid and phlegm behind the eardrum, and the key to the formula is to clear phlegm and turbid dampness. The formula dissolves phlegm (*qián hú, zhè bèi mǔ, bàn xià*), clears turbid dampness (*huò xiāng, fú líng*), clears heat toxins (*huáng lián, lián qiào,* dispels wind (*jú huā, bái zhǐ*), and targets the affected area (*màn jīng zǐ*). *Chái hú* and *chì sháo* circulate *qi* and blood and clear the lymphatics.

OTHER FORMULAS APPROPRIATE FOR THIS CHAPTER:

Classical Formulas:

Qing Bi Tang
Pueraria "N" Formula (CC)
Pueraria Nasal Combination (EG)

Su Zi Jiang Qi Tang
See Chapter 3C

Modern Formulas:

For sinus infection:

Huang Lian Shang Qing Pian
See Chapter 3A

Qing Fei Yi Huo Pian
See Chapter 3A

Other:

Allerease (BP)
Bupleurum & Angelica (BP)
Dr. Shen's Allergy Pills (DS)
Dr. Shen's Sinus & Nose Pills (DS)
Fragrant Passage (BP)
Golden Pearls (CP)
Jade Screen & Xanthium Formula (GF)
Herbal ENT (EV)
Magnolia Clear Sinus (EV)
Nasal Tabs 2 (HC)
Perilla Pearls (CP)
Platycodon 14 (SF)
Pueraria Clear Sinus (EV)
Serramend (HC)
Wind Pearls (CP)
Xanthium 12 (SF)
Xanthium Nasal Formula (GF)
Xanthium Relieve Surface (HC)

2. FORMULAS THAT CLEAR HEAT

2A. HEAT-TOXINS AND DAMP-HEAT TOXINS (Viral and Bacterial Infections; Severe Common Cold; Influenza)

Classical Formulas:

Da Huang Mu Dan Pi Tang	*dà huáng mŭ dān pí tāng* (大黄牡丹皮汤)
Huang Lian Jie Du Tang	*huáng lián jiě dú tāng* (黄连解毒汤)
Nei Xiao Luo Li Wan	*nèi xiāo luŏ lì wán* (内消瘰沥丸)
Pu Ji Xiao Du Yin	*pŭ jì xiāo dú yĭn* (普济消毒饮)
Wu Wei Xiao Du Yin	*wŭ wèi xiāo dú yĭn* (五味消毒饮)
Watermelon Frost	*xī guā shuāng* (西瓜霜)

Modern Formulas:

Chuan Xin Lian Wan	*chuān xīn lián wán* (穿心莲丸)
Gan Mao Ling	*gǎn mào líng* (感冒灵)
Zhong Gan Ling	*zhòng gǎn ling* (重 感灵)

The concept of heat-toxins (*rè dú,* 热毒) is as old as the history of Chinese medicine. Originally used to describe a group of symptoms due to a specific etiology, we know from modern clinical application that heat-toxins include pathogenic viruses and bacteria. The numerous herbs that make up the two categories "Clear Heat, Resolve Toxin" (*qīng rè jiě dú,* 清热解毒) and "Clear Heat and Drain Dampness" (*qīng rè lì shī,* 清热利湿) have been shown in modern times to have strong anti-viral and anti-bacterial effect.

Pathogenic virus and bacteria present with different symptoms, and require different formulas. How do we tell the difference between a viral infection and a bacterial infection? Viral infections often follow specific patterns that are described by their modern diagnoses (herpes zoster, influenza, West Nile fever, etc). In bacterial infections, fever is usually higher (above 103.0° f; 39.4° c). In either case, a definite diagnosis can be made with blood tests. Bacterial infections have elevated neutrophils in the acute stage, while viral infections have elevated lymphocytes in the acute or chronic stages, with normal neutrophil counts.

In terms of viruses, Chinese herbs and formulas can control both mild and serious infections. Besides killing viruses directly, many of the herbs also boost the body's innate immune system. Herbal formulas for viral heat-toxins can be directed to the blood and lymphatic system, or to specific organs such as the heart and liver. Viral infections include the common cold as well as the more severe influenza; also, herpes simplex, herpes zoster (shingles), mononucleosis and West Nile fever. They are also used for pediatric viral diseases such as chicken pox and roseola, and the less common measles, mumps or rubella.

Formulas are also used for acute and chronic viral infections of the heart and pericardium, as well as elevated viral loads in Hepatitis B and C. Pharmaceutical doctors are quick to prescribe antibiotics for viral infections because they lack awareness of effective alternatives. The Chinese herbal antiviral formulas are a great contribution to managing common infections.

Herbal formulas are also effective for common bacterial infections affecting epithelial tissue of the nose, mouth, ear, throat, lungs, bladder, urethra and intestines. The infections usually resolve within three days with herbal treatment. Antibacterial formulas utilize herbs with strong antibacterial properties. Many contain the chemical berberine, giving the yellow color (*huáng*, 黄) to *huáng lián, huáng qín, huáng bǎi* and *zhī zǐ*.

The advantage of herbal antibacterials for epithelial infections is that therapeutic courses can be kept short, posing less disruption to the body's beneficial bacteria in the digestive tract. Common bacterial infections that are treatable include strep throat, ear infection, abscess, impetigo, sinus and lung infections, and infections of the urethra, bladder and prostate. Chinese herbal prescriptions are also effective for early stage appendicitis, and for pelvic or gynecological inflammation due to infection. For wounds or deep surgery affecting the blood or organs, pharmaceutical antibiotics are preferred and recommended.

All formulas listed in this chapter contain herbs that clear or drain fire. These herbs are cooling and drying, and can damage stomach fluids and digestive function if taken for long periods of time. Administer only as long as fire and heat symptoms are evident, and then discontinue.

This chapter covers formulas for general viral and bacterial infections, and can be taken alone, or combined with site-specific formulas. Other formulas that treat heat-toxins and infection, or to combine with site-specific formulas, can be found in the following chapters:

1C. Nasal and Ear Congestion
3A. Lung Heat or Fire
5A. Traumatic Injury
8C. Uterine Blood Stasis
7C. Liver-Gallbladder Damp-Heat and Fire
11B. Bladder or Prostate Infection
13A. Skin Rashes
14. Eye and Vision Disorders

FORMULA DIFFERENTIATION:

Classical Formulas:

Da Huang Mu Dan Pi Tang	Appendicitis, intestinal abscess
Huang Lian Jie Du Tang	Any and all bacterial infections
Nei Xiao Luo Li Wan	Swollen tonsils or lymph glands
Pu Ji Xiao Du Yin	Swollen tonsils or lymph glands
Wu Wei Xiao Du Yin	Viral infection
Xi Gua Shuang	Sore throat (topical spray)

Modern Formulas:

Chuan Xin Lian Wan	Sore throat, herpes, viral infection
Gan Mao Ling	Common cold
Zhong Gan Ling	Common cold or influenza

Classical Formulas:

DA HUANG MU DAN PI TANG

Formula: *dà huáng mŭ dān pí tāng* (大黄牡丹皮汤)
"Rheum, Moutan Decoction"

Author: Zhāng Zhòng-Jĭng (张仲景)

Source: *Jīn Guì Yào Lüè* (金匮要略), 220
Literal: "Golden Cabinet Essential Summary"

Availability:

Da Huang Mu Dan Pi Wan (HT)
Rhubarb & Moutan Combination (EG)

Ingredients: (from the standardized *"Rhubarb & Moutan Combination"*)

dōng guā zĭ (冬瓜子), Semen Benincasae	26.1 %	F
dà huáng (大黄), Radix/Rhizoma Rhei	26.1	PA
táo rén (桃仁), Semen Persicae	17.4	K
máng xiāo (芒硝), Natrii Sulfa/Mirabilitum	17.4	PA
mŭ dān pí (牡丹皮), Cortex Moutan	13.0	DC

Ingredients: (from Herbal Times *"Da Huang Mu Dan Pi Wan"*)

dōng guā zĭ (冬瓜子), Semen Benincasae	43.5 %	FC
dà huáng (大黄), Radix/Rhizoma Rhei	17.4	PA
táo rén (桃仁), Semen Persicae	13.0	K
máng xiāo (芒硝), Natrii Sulfa/Mirabilitum	13.0	PA
mŭ dān pí (牡丹皮), Cortex Moutan	13.0	DC

Clears heat, resolves toxin, breaks blood stasis, cools blood, discharges pus, reduces swelling, frees the stool. Use for early stage intestinal abscess and appendicitis with symptoms of lower abdominal pain and distension in the lower right quadrant, and fever with intermittent chills. Indicated for acute appendicitis, pelvic inflammatory disease, and post-surgical infection. Can also be used for constipation.

Pulse: Excess, rapid, possibly slippery
Tongue: Yellow greasy coat, possibly red

Comments: This is an effective formula for early-stage acute appendicitis before perforation. It is also effective for other infections in the lower abdomen, including pelvic inflammatory disease and post-surgical infection. In acute cases, increase the dosage, and monitor for improvement. If no significant improvement within twelve hours, refer to a hospital. It is also helpful for chronic ileocecal valve syndrome.

Dōng guā zǐ, the lead herb, clears heat and drains phlegm and infected pus. *Dà huáng* has strong antibacterial effects, and helps to target the lower burner. The combination of *dà huáng* and *máng xiāo* also makes the formula an effective choice for constipation due to heat, forming small hard stool.

The Herbal Times version contains a high amount of Benincasa *dōng guā zǐ*, the lead herb (43.5%).

Caution 1: Suspected cases of appendicitis should be treated and monitored by qualified practitioners. Also, this formula can cause loose stools. In those cases, reduce dosage.

Caution 2: Due to the inclusion of *dà huáng, táo rén* and *máng xiāo,* this formula is contraindicated during pregnancy. Also, *táo rén* is contraindicated in patients taking blood thinners, including Coumadin.

Further Reading:

Bensky et al, p. 880
Chen & Chen, p. 1378

HUANG LIAN JIE DU TANG

Formula: *huáng lián jiě dú tāng* (黄连解毒汤),"Coptis Resolve Toxin Decoction"
Author: Wáng Tāo (王焘)
Source: *Wài Tái Mì Yào* (外台秘要), 752
Literal: "Outer Platform (Imperial Library) Secret Essentials"

Availability:

Coptis & Scute Combination (KP/EG)
Coptis Detoxifying Formula (HS)
Coptis Relieve Toxicity Formula (GF)
Huang Lian Jie Du Teapills (PF)
Huang Lian Jie Du Tang (BP)
Huang Lian Jie Du Wan (HT, TL)
* Coptidetox (K)
* Coptis Purge Fire Formula (HC)

Ingredients: (from the standardized *"Coptis & Scute Combination"*)

huáng lián (黄连), Rhizoma Coptidis	30. %	DB
zhī zǐ (栀子), Fructus Gardeniae	30	DA
huáng qín (黄芩), Radix Scutellariae	20	DB
huáng bǎi (黄柏), Cortex Phellodendri	20	DB

Drains fire, clears heat, resolves toxin. Use for heat-toxins causing fever, sore throat, swollen glands, or high fever with delirium. Also for nosebleed due to heat, insomnia due to heart fire, jaundice due to damp-heat, and urinary tract infection. Can be applied to sinus infection, conjunctivitis, boils and abscesses, septicemia and infected wounds. Effective against strep and staph bacterial infections. Use in lung-fire pneumonia, bacterial meningitis and dysentery.

Pulse: Rapid, excess
Tongue: Red, sometimes with yellow coat

Comments: This formula contains four herbs with strong antibacterial properties. They are known as the "four yellows" because of the yellow color (*huáng*, 黄) associated with berberine alkaloids. The product offers a successful alternative to pharmaceutical antibiotics, especially for epithelial infections of the skin, throat, sinus, or lungs. For infections of the eye, skin, sinus, etc, it is often combined with site-specific formulas. If the infection shows no improvement within 24 hours of using this formula, consider pharmaceutical antibiotics.

This formula clears damp-heat from all three *jiao*. Coptis *huáng lián* cools heat in the heart, and the formula can be used for heart-fire causing insomnia, mania or delirium, as well as spontaneous nosebleed. Scutellaria *huáng qín* and Gardenia *zhī zǐ* clears heat from the middle *jiao*. Phellodendron *huáng bǎi* clears heat from the lower burner, making it useful for pelvic inflammation, urinary tract infections, and dysentery.

Caution: This is a cold formula. Discontinue if loose stools or epigastric pain become uncomfortable. Discontinue once signs of heat or infection normalize.

Further Reading:

Bensky et al, p. 167
Chen & Chen, p. 341
Ellis, p. 142

NEI XIAO LUO LI WAN

Formula: *nèi xiāo luǒ lì wán* (内消瘰沥丸), "Internal Disperse Scrofula Pills"
Author: Gù Shì-Chéng (顾世澄)
Source: *Yáng Yī Dà Quán* (疡医大全), 1760
Literal: "Sores Medicine Great Compendium"

Availability:

Nei Xiao Luo Li Teapills (PF)
Nei Xiao Luo Li Wan (GC, HT, PM, TL)

Ingredients: (from Herbal Times *"Nei Xiao Luo Li Wan"*)

xià kū cǎo (夏枯草), Spica Prunellae	25.0 %	DA
dà qīng yán (大青盐), Halitum	15.8	R
xuán shēn (玄参), Radix Scrophulariae	15.8	DD
bái liǎn (白蔹), Radix Ampelopsis	3.1	DD
bò hé (薄荷), Herba Menthae	3.1	BB
dà huáng (大黄), Radix/Rhizoma Rhei	3.1	PA
dāng guī (当归), Radix Angelicae Sinensis	3.1	AB
shēng dì huáng (生地黄), Radix Rehmanniae	3.1	DC
gān cǎo (甘草), Radix Glycyrrhizae	3.1	AA
hǎi gé ké (海蛤壳), Concha Meretricis/Cyclinae	3.1	CB
hǎi zǎo (海藻), Sargassum	3.1	CB
jié gěng (桔梗), Radix Platycodonis	3.1	CA
lián qiào (连翘), Fructus Forsythiae	3.1	DD
máng xiāo (芒硝), Natrii Sulfas/Mirabilitum	3.1	PA
tiān huā fěn (天花粉), Radix Trichosanthis	3.1	CB
zhè bèi mǔ (浙贝母), Bulbus Fritillariae Thunbergii	3.1	CB
zhǐ ké (枳壳), Fructus Aurantii	3.1	G

Clears heat, resolves toxins, disperses swelling, transforms phlegm, softens hardness, dissipates nodules. Use for scrofulous swellings in the skin, marked by soreness with either red or blue discoloration. Also for chronic carbuncle, boils and abscesses marked by heat and swelling, and chronic lymphadenitis. Can be used for swollen glands in mononucleosis or tonsillitis, chronic lymphatic swelling, goitre due to phlegm-fire, and breast mastitis.

Pulse: Rapid, slippery or wiry
Tongue: Yellow greasy coat

Comments: This large 17-herb formula was originally created for scrofula, large painless masses in the lymph glands due to tuberculosis infection. Although bacterial scrofula is rare in modern clinical practice, the formula is available from numerous manufacturers, where it is an important medicine for infected or swollen lymph glands (lymphadenitis). It can be used for lymphadenitis found in acute mononucleosis, tonsillitis and other infections, and also can be used for impetigo, boils and carbuncles and mastitis. It is also useful for treating goitre in phlegm-fire presentations of hyperthyroid.

75% of the formula uses cold herbs to bring down heat and infection. In the Herbal Times version, three lead herbs comprise 57% of the formula. *Xià kū cǎo* (25%) is a cool herb that clears liver fire, *dà qīng yán* (15.8%) is a hard rock salt that cools and breaks up masses, and *xuán shēn* (15.8%) clears heat toxins in the lymphatics.

The author of this formula, Gu Shi-Cheng, also created *Xi Gua Shuang* (Watermelon Frost), below.

Caution: *Dà huáng, dà qīng yán, máng xiāo* and *xuán míng fěn* are prohibited during pregnancy.

PU JI XIAO DU YIN

Formula: *pŭ jì xiāo dú yĭn* (普济消毒饮)
"Universal Benefit Disperse Toxin Cool-Decoction"
Author: Lĭ Găo (李杲) *aka* Lĭ Dōng-Yuán (李东垣), edited by Luō Tān-Yì (罗天益)
Source: *Dōng Yuán Shì Xiào Fāng* (东垣试效方), 1266
Literal: "Dong-Yuan's Tested, Effective Formulas"

Availability:

Pu Ji Xiao Du Wan (HT)
Pu Ji Xiao Du Yin (BP)
Scute & Cimicifuga Combination (EG)
Universal Benefit Teapills (PF)

Ingredients: (from the standardized *"Scute & Cimicifuga Combination"*)

huáng qín (黄芩), Radix Scutellariae	18.9 %	DB
huáng lián (黄连), Rhizoma Coptidis	18.9	DB
chén pí (陈皮), Pericarpium Citri Reticulatae	7.6	G
gān căo (甘草), Radix Glycyrrhizae	7.6	AA
xuán shēn (玄参), Radix Scrophulariae	7.6	DC
chái hú (柴胡), Radix Bupleuri	7.6	BB
jié gěng (桔梗), Radix Platycodonis	7.6	CA
lián qiào (连翘), Fructus Forsythiae	3.8	DD
băn lán gēn (板蓝根), Radix Isatidis	3.8	DD
mă bó (马勃), Lasiosphaera seu Calvatia	3.8	D
niú bàng zĭ (牛蒡子), Fructus Arctii	3.8	BB
bò hé (薄荷), Herba Menthae	3.8	BB
jiāng cán (僵蚕), Bombyx Batryticatus	2.6	O
shēng má (升麻), Rhizoma Cimicifugae	2.6	BB

Ingredients: (from Herbal Times *"Pu Ji Xiao Du Wan"*)

lián qiào (连翘), Fructus Forsythiae	11.4 %	DD
băn lán gēn (板蓝根), Radix Isatidis	8.6	DD
chái hú (柴胡), Radix Bupleuri	8.6	BB
jié gěng (桔梗), Radix Platycodonis	8.6	CA
mă bó (马勃), Lasiosphaera seu Calvatia	8.6	DD
huáng qín (黄芩), Radix Scutellariae	8.6	DB
niú bàng zĭ (牛蒡子), Fructus Arctii	8.6	BB
xuán shēn (玄参), Radix Scrophulariae	8.6	DC

bò hé (薄荷), Herba Menthae	5.7	BB
chén pí (陈皮), Pericarpium Citri Reticulatae	5.7	G
huáng lián (黄连), Rhizoma Coptidis	5.7	DB
shēng má (升麻), Rhizoma Cimicifugae	5.7	BB
gān cǎo (甘草), Radix Glycyrrhizae	2.8	AA
jiāng cán (僵蚕), Bombyx Batryticatus	2.8	O

Clears heat, resolves toxins, dispels pathogenic wind, cools the blood, moistens the throat. Use for acute sore throat or tonsillitis with fever, chills, thirst, headache, and swollen lymph nodes in the neck region. Also for fever with difficulty swallowing. Applicable for strep throat, mumps, tonsillitis and swollen glands due to infectious mononucleosis.

Pulse: Floating, rapid, excess
Tongue: Red with yellow coating, or red tongue tip

Comments: Having both antiviral and antibacterial effects, this is one of the best formulas for strep throat, tonsillitis and swollen lymph glands in the neck. Historically, it was used during diphtheria epidemics and for treating mumps. *Pu Ji Xiao Du Yin* can be combined with *Watermelon Frost* (below) for topical application in strep throat and tonsillitis.

The two representative versions differ in ingredient percentages. *Huáng lián* and *huáng qín* are the main herbs to clear heat-toxins. The standardized Taiwan granule extract contains 38% combined *huáng lián* and *huáng qín,* while the version offered by Herbal Times contains only 14%. However, the Herbal times version is stronger in antiviral herbs (Categories DD and DC, 28% versus 19%). Both formulas contain significant percentage of herbs to clear pathogenic wind-heat (25-28%).

Chái hú helps take the formula into the lymphatic level, and the synergistic combination of *chái hú, mǎ bó* and *xuán shēn* addresses swollen lymph glands. Both *chái hú* and *shēng má* guide the formula upwards to the neck and head. *Niú bàng zǐ* is specific for sore throat.

Caution: This formula contains several cold or cool herbs. Prolonged use may cause stomach upset or loose stools.

Further Reading:

Bensky et al, p. 173
Chen & Chen, p. 355
Ellis, p. 208

WU WEI XIAO DU WAN

Formula: *wǔ wèi xiāo dú yǐn* (五味消毒饮)
"Five Flavor Disperse Toxin Cool-Decoction"
Author: Wú Qiān (吴谦)
Source: *Yī Zōng Jīn Jiàn* (医宗金鉴), 1742
Literal: "Medical Tradition Golden Mirror"
Availability:

Dandelion & Wild Chrysanthemum Combination (EG)
Five Flavor Teapills (PF)
Wu Wei Xiao Du Yin (BP, TL)
Wu Wei Xiao Du Yin (EG)
* Patrinia 7 (SF)

Ingredients: (from Plum Flower *"Five Flavor Teapill"*)

jīn yín huā (金银花), Flos Lonicerae Japonicae	22.7%	DD
yě jú huā (野菊花), Flos Chrysanthemi Indici	22.7	BB
zǐ huā dì dīng (紫花地丁), Herba Violae	22.7	DD
pú gōng yīng (蒲公英), Herba Taraxaci	22.7	DD
zǐ bèi tiān kuí (紫背天葵), Herba Begoniae Fimbris.	9.2	DD

Clears fire, resolves toxins, cools blood, disperses swelling. Use for fire-toxins causing boils and carbuncles with fever, especially with deep hard lesions, and for infected wounds. Applicable in scrofula, abscess, mastitis, and lymphatic swelling. Can be used for various viral infections including tonsillitis, measles, chicken pox, mumps, hepatitis, and influenza.

Pulse: Rapid, possibly slippery or excess
Tongue: Red, or with red on the tip and sides

Comments: *Wu Wei Xiao Du Yin* was originally formulated to treat blood poisoning, infected wounds, and hardened skin boils or carbuncles with fever. *Jīn yín huā* and *jú huā* are the chief herbs, and help guide the formula to the surface. *Zǐ bèi tiān kuí* is an uncommon herb used for infected and hardened sores.

Besides boils and abscesses, the antimicrobial nature of the formula lends itself to a variety of infections, including upper respiratory, throat, mastitis and urinary tract infections, and acute viruses of unknown origin. The formula can be reinforced by combining with *Huang Lian Jie Du Tang* (above).

Caution: This is a cold formula intended for short-term use, until the infection has cleared. Caution to guard patients with weakened spleen *qi*.

Further Reading:

Bensky et al, p. 863
Chen & Chen, p. 1337
Ellis, p. 329

XI GUA SHUANG

Formula: *xī guā shuāng* (西瓜霜), "Watermelon Frost"
Author: *Gù Shì-Chéng* (顾世澄)
Source: *Yáng Yī Dà Quán* (疡医大全), 1760
Literal: "Sores Medicine Great Compendium"

Availability:

Guilin Watermelon Frost (PM)
Watermelon Frost (PM)

Ingredients: (from Guilin Chinese Medicine Factory *"Guilin Watermelon Frost"*)

xī guā shuāng (西瓜霜), Exoc.Citrulli/Mirab Prep.	50. %	DB
chuān bèi mǔ (川贝母), Bulbus Fritillariae Cirrh.	15	CB
rén gōng bīng piàn (人工冰片), Borneolum Synth.	10	R
shān dòu gēn (山豆根), Radix/Rhizoma Sophorae Tonk.	5	DD
shè gān (射干), Rhizoma Belamcandae	5	DD
qīng dài (青黛), Indigo Naturalis	5	DD
gān cǎo (甘草), Radix Glycyrrhizae	5	AA
bò hé nǎo (薄荷脑), Mentholum	5	BB

Packing and Dosage:

Spray bottles of 3 g. Apply 1 to 2 squirts, 3 x day.

Clears heat, resolves toxin, invigorates blood, disperses swelling, relieves pain. Use topically for sore throat, laryngitis, tonsillitis, or mouth ulcers. Can be applied topically for sinus infection, external ear infection, ulcerative skin lesions, burns, and bleeding wounds.

Comments: This is an effective formula when applied topically to the throat, sinus, gum, tooth or open wound. Strong herbs to clear heat-toxins include *xī guā shuāng, shān dòu gēn, shè gān, and qīng dài,* comprising 65% of the formula. It is helpful for sore throat, and can be used to treat strep throat topically.

The "frost" (*shuāng,* 霜) is made by packing a hollowed watermelon-rind with salt. After a a period of time, a dark "frost" appears on the outside of the skin, which is scraped off. Another method uses an entire cut-up watermelon that is mixed with salt and put into a clay jar; the crystalline frost will seep to the exterior of the jar. The frost has strong antibacterial properties.

The author of this formula, Gu Shi-Cheng, also created *Nei Xiao Luo Li Wan,* above.

Note 1: Avoid *Compound Prescribed Watermelon Frost,* which contains arsenic, and is meant for topical application only. It is not safe to take internally.

Note 2: *Shè gān* and *bīng piàn* are contraindicated internally during pregnancy in large quantities. As a spray for the throat, it is safe.

Modern formulas:

CHUAN XIN LIAN

Formula: *chuān xīn lián wán* (穿心莲丸), "Andrographis Pills"
Source: Modern patent medicine

Availability:

Andrographis Formula (GF)
Antiphlogistic Formula (K)
Chuan Xin Lian Kang Yan Pian (BP)
Chuan Xin Lian Pian (PF, PM)
Chuan Xin Lian Wan (HT)
Isatis Formula (CC)
*Isatis 6 (SF)

Ingredients: (most sources)

chuān xīn lián (穿心莲), Herba Andrographis	50. %	DD
pú gōng yīng (蒲公英), Herba Taraxaci	25	DD
bǎn lán gēn (板蓝根), Radix Isatidis	25	DD

Clears heat, resolves toxin, cools blood, disperses swelling. Use for acute heat-toxin inflammation affecting the lymph, blood or organ level. Effective for viral tonsillitis, viral hepatitis, herpes simplex and zoster, common cold, influenza, mononucleosis, measles, mumps, and chicken pox. Also used for bacterial infections causing sore throat, tonsillitis, sinusitis, and skin infections and boils.

Pulse: Floating, rapid, excess
Tongue: Normal, or with red tongue tip

Comments: This small formula is a valuable treatment for heat-toxins (viral and bacterial) attacking the throat, lymph or liver. All three of the herbs used have strong antiviral properties. *Chuān xīn lián,* a recently utilized herb, is not commonly found in the classical literature. It is reinforced with *bǎn lán gēn* and *pú gōng yīng*.

Besides treatment of sore throat, the formula is good for swollen lymph glands in acute mononucleosis, and is a good adjunct in influenza. It is also effective for outbreaks of herpes simplex (oral and genital) and zoster (shingles), when combined with *Long Dan Xie Gan Tang* (Chapter 7C), which clears heat out of the liver or gallbladder channel.

The pills can be crushed and mixed with salve or vaseline and applied directly to zoster sores or infected wounds.

Caution: *Chuān xīn lián* is a cold herb. Prolonged use may lead to epigastric pain or cramping.

GAN MAO LING

Formula: *gǎn mào líng* (感冒灵), "Common Cold Effective-Remedy"
Source: Modern patent medicine

Availability:

Children's Clear and Release Formula (GF)
Dr. Shen's Gan Mao Ling (DS)
Gan Mao Ling (K, PF)
Gan Mao Ling Formula (GF)
Gan Mao Ling Jie Du Wan (HT)
Ganmaoling Tablets (PM)

Ingredients: (From Yang Cheng Brand *"Ganmaoling Tablets"*)

gǎng méi gēn (岗梅根), Radix Ilex Asprellae	32.8 %	DD
sān chā kǔ (三叉苦), Folium Evodiae Leptae	22.2	DD
mǔ jīng yè (牡荆叶), Folium Viticis Negundo	16.4	BB
yě jú huā (野菊花), Flos Chrysanthemi Indici	12.3	BB
bǎn lán gēn (板蓝根), Radix Isatidis	12.3	DD
jīn yín huā (金银花), Flos Lonicerae Japonicae	4.0	DD

Clears heat, resolves toxin, dispels wind, relieves cough, opens the nasal passages, brightens the eyes. Use for *shaoyang* and *yangming* stages of pathogenic wind with symptoms of flu, fever with chills, headache, sore throat, red eyes, stiffness of upper back and neck, nasal discharge, general aching, and swollen lymph glands. Useful in common cold, influenza and viral pneumonia.

Pulse: Floating, rapid, excess
Tongue: Normal, or with red tongue tip

Comments: This is the most effective herbal product for the treatment of common cold, especially when administered early and at every 3 hours. It is the largest-selling patent medicine in China. The two lead herbs, *gǎng méi gēn* and *sān chā kǔ*, are not referenced in classical or modern TCM source books, and are indigenous to Taiwan. It is combined with other herbs to fight heat-toxins such as *bǎn lán gēn* and *jīn yín huā*, totalling 71% of the formula. *Yě jú huā* and *mǔ jīng yè* clear wind-heat and bring the formula to the nose and eyes. (*Mǔ jīng yè* is a cousin to *màn jīng zǐ,* 蔓荆子, Fructus Viticis).

Gan Mao Ling can be taken alone or combined with *Yin Qiao San* (Chapter 1B), which reinforces the dispersal of wind-heat.

There are many versions of *Gan Mao Ling*. Both Plum Flower, and Herbal Times' *Gan Mao Jie Du Wan* follow the original Yang Cheng formula. Some providers, including Kan and Golden Flower, substitute *máo dōng qīng* (毛冬青, Radix Ilex Pubescens) for *gǎng méi gēn*. Kan and Golden Flower also substitute *wú zhū yú* (吴茱萸, Fructus Evodiae), a hot herb, for Evodia *sān chā kǔ*, a cold herb. This is probably a mistake, but it does have the benefit of warming the stomach and protecting against the coldness of the other herbs.

Note: The formula from Herbal Times using the name *Gan Mao Ling* is quite different, addressing stiffness and headache in the early stage of common cold. Herbal Times releases the traditional *Gan Mao Ling* as *Gan Mao Ling Jie Du Wan*.

Ingredients: (from Herbal Times "*Gan Mao Ling*")

gé gēn (葛根), Radix Puerariae Lobatae	20. %	BB
dà qīng yè (大青叶), Folium Isatidis	14	DD
bò hé (薄荷), Herba Menthae	11	BB
jié gěng (桔梗), Radix Platycodonis	10	CA
jú huā (菊花), Flos Chrysanthemi	10	BB
lián qiào (连翘), Fructus Forsythiae	10	DD
qián hú (前胡), Radix Peucedani	10	CA
xìng rén (杏仁), Semen Armeniacae	10	CC
gān cǎo (甘草), Radix Glycyrrhizae	5	AA

Comments: *Gé gēn*, the lead herb, dispels wind from the neck and occipital region, allowing the muscles to relax. *Dà qīng yè* and *lián qiào* clear heat-toxins (24%), while other herbs dispel wind-heat and stop cough.

ZHONG GAN LING

Formula: *zhòng gǎn líng* (重 感灵), "Severe Common-Cold Effective-Remedy"
Source: Modern patent medicine

Availability:

Cold Burst (JD)
Dr. Shen's Zong Gan Ling (DS)
Zhong Gan Ling (HT, JD, (K, PF, TL)
Zhong Gan Ling Formula (CC, GF)
Zhong Gan Ling Wan (HT)
Zhong Gan Qing Pian/Wan (GC)

Ingredients: (From both Plum Flower and Meizhou Medicine Factory *"Zhong Gan Ling"*)

máo dōng qīng (毛冬青), Radix Ilex Pubescens	27. %	DD
gé gēn (葛根), Radix Puerariae Lobatae	27	BB
mǎ biān cǎo (马鞭草), Herba Verbenae	18	K
bǎn lán gēn (板蓝根), Radix Isatidis	14	DD
qīng hāo (青蒿), Herba Artemisiae Annuae	7	DE
shí gāo (石膏), Gypsum Fibrosum	4	DA
qiāng huó (羌活), Rhizoma et Radix Notopterygii	3	BA

Ingredients: (from Golden Flower *"Zhong Gan Ling"*)

máo dōng qīng (毛冬青), Radix Ilex Pubescens	19.6 %	DD
gé gēn (葛根), Radix Puerariae Lobatae	19.6	BB
dà qīng yè (大青叶), Folium Isatidis	14.5	DD
mǎ biān cǎo (马鞭草), Herba Verbenae	13.0	K
bái huā shé shé cǎo (白花蛇舌草), Herba Hedyotis	13.0	DD
bǎn lán gēn (板蓝根), Radix Isatidis	9.9	DD
qīng hāo (青蒿), Herba Artemisiae Annuae	4.9	DE
shí gāo (石膏), Gypsum Fibrosum	2.9	DA
qiāng huó (羌活), Radix Notopterygii	2.2	BA

Ingredients: (From Herbal Times *"Zhong Gan Ling"*)

huáng qín (黄芩), Radix Scutellariae	10. %	DB
lián qiào (连翘), Fructus Forsythiae	10	DD
gǎng méi gēn (岗梅根), Radix Ilex Asprellae	10	DD
máo dōng qīng (毛冬青), Radix Ilex Pubescens	10	DD
bǎn lán gēn (板蓝根), Radix Isatidis	10	DD
jīng jiè (荆芥), Herba Schizonepetae	10	BA
niú bàng zǐ (牛蒡子), Fructus Arctii	10	BB
jú huā (菊花), Flos Chrysanthemi	7	BB
gé gēn (葛根), Radix Puerariae Lobatae	7	BB
xuán shēn (玄参), Radix Scrophulariae	7	DC
gān cǎo (甘草), Radix Glycyrrhizae	5	AA
dàn zhú yè (淡竹叶), Herba Lophatheri	4	DA

Dispels pathogenic wind, clears heat, resolves toxins, cools the blood, moistens the throat. Use for influenza and severe common cold with symptoms of fever, aching neck and shoulders, chills, headache, sore throat, and swollen lymph nodes.

Pulse: Floating, rapid, excess
Tongue: Normal, or with red tongue tip

Comments: Various formulas use the name *Zhong Gan Ling* ("severe common-cold remedy"); all of them are useful for influenza and severe common cold. The original formula from Meizhou Medicine Factory contains 66% herbs with strong antiviral properties (*máo dōng qīng, mǎ biān cǎo, bǎn lán gēn* and *qīng hāo*). Here, the pathogens are beginning to enter the *shaoyang* stage, with aching neck and shoulders and increased fever. *Gé gēn* in a high dose treats muscle contraction in the neck and shoulders, and helps stop shivering and chills found in flu.

The Meizhou formula is reproduced by Plum Flower. Golden Flower's version contains the original formula, adding in a large amount of *dà qīng yè* and *bái huā shé shé cǎo*. In the Herbal Times version, both *gé gēn* and *máo dōng qīng* are reduced in dosage, but *huáng qín* and *gǎng méi gēn* are added to reinforce the effect of clearing microbial heat-toxins.

Caution: These formulas contains several cold or cool herbs. Prolonged use may cause stomach cramping or loose stools. Caution in very cold patients.

OTHER FORMULAS APPROPRIATE FOR THIS CHAPTER:

Classical Formulas:

Gan Cao Xie Xin Tang
Pinellia & Licorice Combination (EG)

San Huang Xie Xin Tang
Coptis & Rhubarb Combination (EG)
Coptis, Scute and Rhubarb Formula (HS)
San Huang Wan (PM)

Sheng Ma Ge Gen Tang
Cimicifuga & Pueraria Combination (EG)

Xiang Lian Wan
Aucklandia & Coptis Teapills (PF)

Modern Formulas:

Huang Lian Shang Qing Pian
See Chapter 3A

Qing Fei Yi Huo Pian
See Chapter 3A

Other:

Astra Isatis (HC)
Bidens 6 (SF)
Children's Clear and Release Formula (GF)
Chrysanthemum 9 (SF)
Chuan Xin Lian Kang Yan Wan (HT)
Clear Heat (HC)
Cold Away (HC)
Cold Quell (BP)
Enhance (HC)
Dragon Pearls (CP)
Forsythia 18 (SF)
Ganmao Tuire Chongji (PM)
Herbal ABX (EV)
Ilex 15 (SF)
Isatis Formula (CC)
Isatis Gold (HC)
Jade Dew Ointment (BP)
Lightening Pearls (CP)
Niu Huang Chieh Tu Pien (PM)
Paris 7 (SF)
Patrinia 7 (SF)
Purge Heat (CMS)
Scrophularia 12 (SF)
Shuang Huang Lian Formula (HS)
Viola Clear Fire Formula (GF)
Windbreaker (GW)

Topical Application:

Clear Heat Ointment (BP)
Gout Ointment (BP)
Mastitis Ointment (BP)

2. FORMULAS THAT CLEAR HEAT

2B. FEVER AND STOMACH FIRE

Classical Formulas:

Bai Hu Tang	*bái hŭ tāng* (白虎汤)
Dao Chi San	*dăo chì săn* (导赤散)
Fang Feng Tong Sheng San	*fáng fēng tōng shèng săn* (防风通圣散)
Liang Ge San	*liáng gé săn* (凉膈散)
Qing Wei San	*qīng wèi săn* (清胃散)

The products in this chapter focus on the treatment of fever, and also on fire or heat in the stomach or intestines. Fever can be due to exogenous pathogenic factors, involving heat-toxins produced by bacteria or virus, or it can be due to an endogenous etiology. Normal fevers run from 99.5° to 103.4° F (37.5° to 39.7°C). High fevers are from 103.5° to 106° F (39.7° to 41.1°C), and may "obstruct the orifices", leading to delirium, spasm, convulsion or coma.

The formulas described here are effective in bringing down a fever, and are commonly used to reduce fever in children and infants. Children tend to run higher fevers than adults. The typical pharmaceutical medicine approach employs aspirin or acetaminophen to reduce fever, but does not address the cause. The fever often returns, and complete recovery is actually slowed down. TCM formulas reduce heat in the *qi* network and in certain organs, thereby limiting the amount of *qi* that is consumed. Where a child might recover from a high fever quickly and without noticeable consequence, fever in adults can lead to fatigue lasting many days after the event.

If the fever is due to a microbial heat-toxin, it is best to combine these formulas with appropriate formulas from *Chapter 2A. Heat-Toxins & Damp-Heat Toxins*. Prolonged high fevers can be life threatening, and patients may need to be hospitalized or given appropriate pharmaceuticals, including antibiotics.

Stomach fire without fever exhibits mouth ulcerations (canker sores), bleeding gums, toothache, nosebleeds, bad breath and constipation.

The formulas in this chapter contain herbs that clear, drain or expel fire. Many of the herbs are cooling and drying, and can damage stomach fluids and digestive function if taken for long periods of time. Administer only as long as fire and heat symptoms are evident, and then discontinue. This normally takes one to three days, although may be necessary for longer periods. Caution is advised in conditions with preexisting deficiency of stomach *yin* or *qi.*

This chapter addresses heat and fire in the channels, and in the stomach and large intestine. Other formulas that clear heat and fire are also found in the following chapters:

- 3A. Lung Heat or Fire
- 6E. Menopausal Disorder and Deficiency Fire
- 7C. Liver-Gallbladder Damp-Heat and Fire
- 10B. Bladder or Prostate Infection
- 13. Eye and Vision Disorders

QUICK SUMMARY FOR REFERENCE:

Bai Hu Tang	Fever, stomach fire
Dao Chi San	Fever with painful urination
Fang Feng Tong Sheng San	Fever or skin rash
Liang Ge San	Fever with constipation
Qing Wei San	Stomach fire, toothache, canker sores

Classical Formulas:

BAI HU TANG

Formula: *bái hǔ tāng* (白虎汤), "White Tiger Decoction"
Author: Zhāng Zhòng-Jǐng (张仲景)
Source: *Shāng Hán Lùn* (伤寒论), 220
Literal: "Injury (by) Cold, Discussion"

Availability:

Gypsum Combination (EG)
White Tiger Teapills (PF)
* White Tiger (K)

Ingredients: (from Plum Flower *"White Tiger Teapills"*)

shí gāo (石膏), Gypsum Fibrosum	52. %	DA
gǔ yá (谷芽), Fructus Oryzae Germinatus	26	H
zhī mǔ (知母), Rhizoma Anemarrhenae	16	DA
zhì gān cǎo (炙甘草), Radix Glycyrrhizae Praep.	6	AA

Clears heat in the qi level, clears heat in the lungs, drains stomach fire, generates fluid, relieves thirst. Use for pathogenic heat in the *qi* level (*yangming* stage) with symptoms of fever, sweating, extreme thirst, dry throat, irritability, and flushed face. Can also be used for stomach fire causing toothache, epistaxis (nosebleed), bad breath, canker sores on the gums or lips, or bleeding from the gums. Used for high fever in encephalitis, meningitis, pneumonia, heat stroke, septicemia, conjunctivitis and tooth infection.

Pulse: Large, rapid, forceful
Tongue: Red with dry yellow coat

Comments: This formula relies on a large quantity of *shí gāo*, a cold medicinal that clears heat out of the *qi* level quickly without being too drying. *Zhī mŭ* clears heat while protecting and moistening *yin*; *gŭ yá* and *zhì gān căo* nourish and replenish the *qi* that is consumed during fever. Some products may substitute *shān yào* (山药, Rhizoma Dioscoreae) for *gŭ yá*. In decoction form, three herbs are cooked with rice instead of using the sprouted rice *gŭ yá*.

Classically, the formula was prescribed for the "four greats" found in fever due to excess: great fever, great thirst, great sweating, and great (large and bounding) pulse. It is safe for most fevers, including pediatric, and can work quickly.

Further Reading:

Bensky et al, p. 150
Chen & Chen, p. 321
Ellis, p. 17

DAO CHI SAN

Formula: *dǎo chì sǎn* (导赤散), "Guide-Away (the) Red Powder"
Author: Qián Yǐ (钱乙)
Source: *Qián Shì Xiǎo Ér Yào Zhèng Zhí Jué* (钱氏小儿药证直), 1119
Literal: "Qian's Children's Medical Patterns, Straight Secrets"

Availability:

Dao Chi San (BP, PM, TL)
Red Door Teapills (PF)
Rehmannia & Akebia Formula (EG)
Rehmannia & Clematis Formula (KP)

Ingredients: (from KPC "*Rehmannia & Clematis Formula*")

shēng dì huáng (生地黄), Radix Rehmanniae	25. %	DC
chuān mù tōng (川木通), Caulis Clematidis Armandii	25	FC
gān cǎo (甘草), Radix Glycyrrhizae	25	AA
dàn zhú yè (淡竹叶), Herba Lophatheri	25	DA

Clears heat, drains fire, clear heart and blood heat, nourishes yin. Use for pathogenic heat accumulating in the heart and small intestine, marked by fever, thirst, irritability, uneasy sleep and flushed face. Useful for fever with difficult, scanty or dark urination. The formula can also be used for fever due to urinary tract infection or kidney infection. It is also effective for stomach fire causing mouth sores, swollen gums, epistaxis (nose bleed) or bad breath.

Pulse: Rapid, slippery
Tongue: Red, or red in the tip with yellow coat

Comments: This classical formula drains heart fire downwards via the small intestine channel to the urinary bladder, so that fever can be discharged through urination. *Shēng dì* huáng cools blood and heart heat while replenishing *yin; dàn zhú yè* clears heat in the *qi* level, and with *mù tōng*, leads the formula to the bladder; and *gān cǎo* replenishes *qi* consumed by the fever and calms irritation in the bladder and urethra.

Dao Chi San was recorded in a book of pediatric formulas, and is useful for fever with tonsillitis or pharyngitis, conjunctivitis, and urinary burning. In children, excessive heat in the heart can manifest as poor sleep or nightmares. The name of the prescription refers to guiding the heat (red) away, relying on the strategy to guide the fever down and out through the bladder.

The original prescription called for *mù tōng* (木通, Caulis Akebiae). Due to availability, most manufacturers are substituting *chuān mù tōng* (川木通, Caulis Clematidis Armandii).

Further Reading:

Bensky et al, p. 195
Chen & Chen, p. 365
Ellis, p. 79

FANG FENG TONG SHENG SAN

Formula: *fáng fēng tōng shèng sǎn* (防风通圣散)
"Ledebouriella Unblocking Sagely, Powder"
Author: Liú Wán-Sù (刘完素)
Source: *Huáng Dì Sù Wèn Xuán Míng Lùn Fāng* (黄帝素问宣明论方), 1172
Literal: "Yellow Emperor's Plain Questions Proclaimed Clear Discussion (of) Formulas"

Availability:

Fang Feng Tong Sheng Wan (HT, TL)
Ledebouriella Sagely Unblocks Teapill (PF)
Siler & Platycodon Formula (EG, GF)

Ingredients: (From Herbal Times, *"Fang Feng Tong Sheng Wan"*)

shí gāo (石膏), Gypsum Fibrosum	9. %	DA
huá shí (滑石), Talcum	9	FB
fáng fēng (防风), Radix Saposhnikov./Ledebouriellae	7	BA
jīng jiè (荆芥), Herba Schizonepetae	7	BA
lián qiào (连翘), Fructus Forsythiae	7	DD
dāng guī (当归), Radix Angelicae Sinensis	7	AB
jié gěng (桔梗), Radix Platycodonis	6	CA
bái zhú (白术), Rhizoma Atractylodis Macrocephalae	6	AA
bái sháo (白芍), Radix Paeoniae Alba	6	AB
shēng jiāng (生姜), Rhizoma Zingiberis Recens	5	BA
zhī zǐ (栀子), Fructus Gardeniae	5	DA
bò hé (薄荷), Herba Menthae	5	BB
gān cǎo (甘草), Radix Glycyrrhizae	5	AA
huáng qín (黄芩), Radix Scutellariae	4	DB
máng xiāo (芒硝), Natrii Sulfas/Mirabilitum	4	PA
chuān xiōng (川芎), Rhizoma Ligustici Chuanxiong	4	K
dà huáng (大黄), Radix/Rhizoma Rhei	4	PA

Dispels pathogenic wind, clears heat, resolves toxin, frees the stool. Use to clear heat from both the interior and the exterior, found in both *yangming* presentation of the common cold or flu moving to the interior, or in a common cold with pre-existing endogenous heat. Symptoms include fever, constipation, dark urine, sore throat, headache, red or sore eyes and fatigue. Useful for pediatric fevers accompanying chicken pox, roseola, measles and rubella. The formula can also be used for wind-heat skin disorders, including boils, urticaria, eczema, psoriasis and acne with redness.

Pulse: Flooding, rapid; occasionally slippery or wiry
Tongue: Red with yellow coat

Comments: *Fang Feng Tong Sheng San* is a larger elaboration of *Liang Ge San* (below), containing 7 of the original 8 herbs. It can be used for fever accompanied by constipation, and is equally good at treating skin conditions marked by redness and heat, including carbuncles, heat rash, and acne. Due to the wind-dispersing effects, it is a good formula for pediatric fever with rash, such as roseola and chicken pox.

44% of the formula clears heat (*huáng qín, shí gāo, zhī zǐ, lián qiào, huá shí* and *dà huáng*) while 19% clears the surface (*fáng fēng, jīng jiè, bò hé*). A small amount of *dà huáng* and *máng xiāo* (8%) purge the stool to reduce fever. The original formula contained *má huáng* (麻黄, Herba Ephedrae), which is unavailable due to regulatory concerns. The Plum Flower version, a bit different, contains neither *shí gāo* nor *huá shí*.

In Japan, due to the purgative effects of *máng xiāo* and *dà huáng*, this formula is being recommended for weight reduction, an inappropriate application of the prescription.

Caution: *Máng xiāo* and *dà huáng* are prohibited during pregnancy.

Further Reading:

Bensky et al, p. 290
Chen & Chen, p. 291
Ellis, p. 93

LIANG GE SAN

Formula: *liáng gé sǎn* (凉膈散), "Cool (above the) Diaphragm Powder"
Author: Imperial Medical Bureau (*tài yī jú*, 太医局);
revised by Chén Shī-Wén (陈师文)
Source: *Tài Píng Huì Mín Hé Jì Jú Fāng* (太平惠民和剂局方), 1078
Literal: "(Era of) Great Peace, Benefit People Harmonious Medicines, Office (of) Formulas"

Availability:

Cool Valley Teapills (PF)
Forsythia & Rhubarb Formula (EG)

Ingredients: (from the standardized *"Forsythia & Rhubarb Formula"*)

lián qiào (连翘), Fructus Forsythiae	28.7 %	DD
dà huáng (大黄), Radix/Rhizoma Rhei	14.3	PA
gān cǎo (甘草), Radix Glycyrrhizae	14.3	AA
máng xiāo (芒硝), Natrii Sulfas/Mirabilitum	14.3	PA
huáng qín (黄芩), Radix Scutellariae	7.1	DB
bò hé (薄荷), Herba Menthae	7.1	BB
dàn zhú yè (淡竹叶), Herba Lophatheri	7.1	DA
zhī zǐ (栀子), Fructus Gardeniae	7.1	DA

Ingredients: (from Plum Flower *"Cool Valley Teapills"*)

dàn zhú yè (淡竹叶), Herba Lophatheri	23.5 %	DA
lián qiào (连翘), Fructus Forsythiae	23.5	DD
dà huáng (大黄), Radix/Rhizoma Rhei	12.0	PA
máng xiāo (芒硝), Natrii Sulfas/Mirabilitum	12.0	PA
gān cǎo (甘草), Radix Glycyrrhizae	11.0	AA
zhī zǐ (栀子), Fructus Gardeniae	6.0	DA
huáng qín (黄芩), Radix Scutellariae	6.0	DB
bò hé (薄荷), Herba Menthae	6.0	BB

Clears heat in the qi level, drains fire, frees the stool. Use for intense heat in the upper *jiao* causing fever with delirium, constipation, thirst, dry lips, tongue sores, spitting up blood, nosebleed, and swollen throat or tonsils. It can be used for stomach fire conditions marked by mouth sores, epistaxis (nosebleed) or acute conjunctivitis. Use in high fevers with constipation due to encephalitis and meningitis, and fever accompanying gallstone or appendicitis attack.

Pulse: Rapid, excess; occasionally slippery
Tongue: Red, with yellow or dry yellow coat

Comments: *Liang Ge San* uses the purgation method to drain fire in the upper burner (lungs, throat, eye, nose) and direct it downwards to the intestines and out with the stool. In these cases, fever is accompanied by constipation, and once the stools are freed, the fever drops. It is intended for fevers due to excess with constipation, and can also be used for acute tonsillitis, pharyngitis and acute conjunctivitis.

Unlike *Fang Feng Tong Sheng San* (above) which is based on this formula, here 29% of the Taiwan EG version consists of the purgatives *dà huáng* and *máng xiāo* (24% in the Plum Flower version). Another 57% clears heat and fever (*bò hé, dàn zhú yè, zhī zǐ, huáng qín* and *lián qiào*; 65% in the Plum Flower version). The lead herbs are *dàn zhú yè* to clear heat in the *qi* level, and *lián qiào*, which clears and disperses heat in the upper *jiao*. This formula is intended for high fever with constipation, and should be used cautiously in the absence of constipation.

Caution 1: This formula can cause loose stool, which is part of the therapeutic effect and should end once the formula is discontinued. Caution in those with a weaker constitution.

Caution 2: *Máng xiāo* and *dà huáng* are prohibited during pregnancy.

Further Reading:

Bensky et al, p. 176
Chen & Chen, p. 351
Ellis, p. 180

QING WEI SAN

Formula: *qīng wèi sǎn* (清胃散), “Clear Stomach Powder”
Author: Lǐ Gǎo (李杲) *aka* Lǐ Dōng-Yuán (李东垣)
Source: *Lán Shì Mì Cáng* (兰室秘藏), date unknown, published 1276
Literal: “Orchid Chamber’s Secrets Concealed”

Availability:

Chu Kou Wei Pian (GC)
Coptis & Rehmannia Formula (EG)
Qing Wei San Teapills (PF)
Qing Wei San (BP)
Qing Wei Wan (HT)
* Cool the Stomach (K)
* Stomach Support (K)

Ingredients: (from the standardized *“Coptis & Rehmannia Formula”*)

shēng má (升麻), Rhizoma Cimicifugae	41.7 %	BB
mŭ dān pí (牡丹皮), Cortex Moutan	20.8	DC
dāng guī (当归), Radix Angelicae Sinensis	12.5	AB
huáng lián (黄连), Rhizoma Coptidis	12.5	DB
shēng dì huáng (生地黄), Radix Rehmanniae	12.5	DC

Ingredients: (from Herbal Times *“Qing Wei Wan”* and Plum Flower “*Qing Wei San Teapills*”)

shēng má (升麻), Rhizoma Cimicifugae	37. %	BB
huáng lián (黄连), Rhizoma Coptidis	22	DB
mŭ dān pí (牡丹皮), Cortex Moutan	19	DC
shēng dì huáng (生地黄), Radix Rehmanniae	11	DC
dāng guī (当归), Radix Angelicae Sinensis	11	AB

Drains fire, resolves toxins, cools blood, tonifies yin and blood. Use for stomach fire causing toothache, bleeding gums, swollen gums, nosebleed, and ulcerations on the tongue or gums, including canker sores. Accompanying symptoms may include frontal headache, flushed cheeks, swelling and pain of the lips, fever, bad breath and constipation. Can be used for trigeminal neuralgia, strep throat and acute pharyngitis.

Pulses: Rapid, large, occasionally slippery
Tongue: Red or red in the center, with dry yellow coat

Comments: Stomach fire, moving upwards as excess heat in the stomach channel, is often involved in acute onset toothache, spontaneous nosebleeds, bleeding gums, sore throat or frontal headache. This formula is also excellent for canker sores (mouth ulcers).

Qing Wei San was formulated to treat acute toothache due to an excess heat presentation; it is not suitable for toothaches due to kidney deficiency or attack of pathogenic cold. *Shēng má* is the lead herb, taking the formula upwards to the face; *huáng lián* cools stomach heat, while the other herbs cool, nourish and circulate the blood.

Further Reading:

Bensky et al, p. 191
Chen & Chen, p. 393
Ellis, p. 230

OTHER FORMULAS APPROPRIATE FOR THIS CHAPTER:

Classical Formulas:

Bai Hu Jia Ren Shen Tang
Ginseng & Gypsum Combination (EG)
White Tiger (K)

Da Chai Hu Tang
See Chapter 7C

Gan Lu Yin
Gan Lu Yin (BP)
Sweet Combination (EG)

Huang Lian Shang Qing Pian
See Chapter 3A

Qing Fei Yi Huo Pian
See Chapter 3A

Yu Nu Jian
Rehmannia & Gypsum Combination (EG)
Stomach Support (K)

Zhu Ye Shi Gao Tang
Bamboo Leaves & Gypsum Combination (EG)

Modern Formulas:

Huang Lian Shang Qing Pian
See Chapter 3A

Qing Fei Yi Huo Pian
See Chapter 3A

Other:
Resolve-AI (EV)

3. RESPIRATORY DISORDERS

3A. LUNG HEAT OR FIRE
(Barking Cough, Upper *Jiao* Inflammation)

Classical Formulas:

Qing Zao Jiu Fei Tang	*qīng zào jiù fèi tāng* (清燥救肺汤)

Modern Formulas:

Huang Lian Shang Qing Wan	*huáng lián shàng qīng wán* (黄连上清丸)
Li Fei Pian	*lì fèi piān* (利肺片)
Qing Fei Yi Huo Pian	*qīng fèi yi huǒ piān* (清肺抑火片)

Lung heat or fire and upper *jiao* inflammation appear as acute events. They are due to either exogenous wind-heat or accumulation of heat-toxins, which include infectious virus or bacteria. When in the lung, the patient feels heat in his chest, pain on inhalation and a dry, sore throat. There is a sharp and barking cough without the rattle of phlegm. Lung heat or fire causing acute cough can be present during common cold, influenza, bronchitis, viral or bacterial pneumonia, croup, pulmonary abscess or infection, and high fever affecting the lungs.

Lung heat or fire is distinguished from lung phlegm conditions by the absence of any significant amount of phlegm, although sticky and difficult to expectorate phlegm may be present. Lung fire can precede or follow an acute phlegm-heat presentation. Effective treatment may involve combining the formulas of this chapter with a cough syrup (*Chapter 3D*). Also, with significant phlegm production, the formulas in this chapter can be combined with formulas for phlegm-heat (*Chapter 3B*) or phlegm-damp (*Chapter 3C*). Dry coughs without fire are treated with products from *Chapter 3E*. In severe coughs found in flu or pneumonia, combine with formulas from *Chapter 2A*. In cases of acute bacterial pneumonia, however, pharmaceutical antibiotics are recommended.

Upper *jiao* inflammation, often due to heat-toxins, includes swollen lymph glands, toothache or infection, sinus infection, eye infections, ear infections, and mouth ulcers. They can be treated with several of the formulas in this chapter; other formulas can be found in their appropriate chapters..

Classical Formulas:

QING ZAO JIU FEI TANG

Formula: *qīng zào jiù fèi wán* (清燥救肺丸)
"Clear Dryness, Rescue Lungs Decoction"
Author: Yù Chāng (喻昌) *aka* Yù Jiā-Yán (喻嘉言)
Source: *Yī Mén Fǎ Lǜ* (医门法律), 1658
Literal: "Physicians' Door (to) Methods (and) Rules"

Availability:

Eriobotrya & Ophiopogon Combination (EG)
Qing Zao Jiu Fei Wan (HT, TL)

Ingredients: (from the standardized *"Eriobotrya & Ophiopogon Combination"*)

sāng yè (桑叶), Folium Mori	25.2 %	BB
shí gāo (石膏), Gypsum Fibrosum	21.6	DA
mài mén dōng (麦门冬), Radix Ophiopogonis	10.0	AD
gān cǎo (甘草), Radix Glycyrrhizae	8.4	AA
huǒ má rén (火麻仁), Fructus Cannabis	8.4	PA
ē jiāo (阿胶), Colla Corii Asini	6.6	AB
xìng rén (杏仁), Semen Armeniacae Amarum	6.6	CC
rén shēn (人参), Radix Ginseng	6.6	AA
pí pá yè (枇杷叶), Folium Eriobotryae	6.6	CC

Ingredients: (from Herbal Times *"Qing Zao Jiu Fei Wan"*)

shí gāo (石膏), Gypsum Fibrosum	19.1 %	DA
ē jiāo (阿胶), Colla Corii Asini	11.5	AB
mài mén dōng (麦门冬), Radix Ophiopogonis	11.5	AD
pí pá yè (枇杷叶), Folium Eriobotryae	11.5	CC
rén shēn (人参), Radix Ginseng	11.5	AA
sāng yè (桑叶), Folium Mori	11.5	BB
gān cǎo (甘草), Radix Glycyrrhizae	7.8	AA
huǒ má rén (火麻仁), Fructus Cannabis	7.8	PA
xìng rén (杏仁), Semen Armeniacae Amarum	7.8	CC

Clears lung heat, moistens lung yin, tonifies lung qi, relieves cough. Use for dry heat injuring the lungs, causing dry or hacking cough without phlegm. This can follow an attack of pathogenic wind or is due to chronic endogenous lung heat. Other signs include headache, dry throat, thirst and dry nose. The formula can be used in an acute presentation for patient with pre-existing deficiency of *qi* and *yin*, or in more chronic cases where *qi* and *yin* have been depleted. Applicable for chronic dry cough found in smoker's cough or dry-cough asthma with signs of heat.

Pulse: Weak, thin, rapid
Tongue: Dry with scanty coat

Comments: This formula is appropriate for dry cough due to heat, but without obvious heat-toxins. This may follow clearance of heat-toxins with earlier formulas. It is appropriate for chronic cough due to heat, with concurrent deficiency of lung *yin* and *qi*. In chronic cases, this may be due to age or smoking.

The formula uses moistening herbs such as *ē jiāo, mài mén dōng,* and *huǒ má rén*; *shí gāo* clears lung heat; *sāng yè, xìng rén* and *pí pá yè* to stop cough due to heat. *Rén shēn* and *gān cǎo* replenish lung *qi*. The formula avoids herbs that are too bitter or too spicy, both of which can be too drying.

The Taiwan extract granule version is more appropriate for sudden dry cough due to wind-heat, while the Herbal Times and Tanglong versions are more appropriate for lung heat presentation following successful clearance of heat-toxins.

Caution: Reduce dosage if loose stool develops.

Further Reading:

Bensky et al, p. 667
Chen & Chen, p. 1029
Ellis, p. 235

Modern Formulas:

HUANG LIAN SHANG QING WAN

Formula: *huáng lián shàng qīng wán* (黄连上清丸), "Coptis Upper Clearing Pill"
Author: Chinese Medicine Research Institute of China Academy of TCM (中国中医研究院中医研究所)
Source: *Quán Guó Zhōng Yào Chéng Yào Chù Fāng Jí* (全国中药成药处方集), 1962
Literal: "Nation-wide Chinese Medicine Manufactured Medicine Medical Prescription Collection"

Availability:

Coptis, Phellodendron & Mint Formula (EG)
Huang Lien Shang Ching Pien (PM)
Huang Lien Shang Qing Pian (BE, PM)

Ingredients: (From the standardized *"Coptis, Phellodendron & Mint Formula"*)

dà huáng (大黄), Radix/Rhizoma Rhei	15.6 %	PA
huáng lián (黄连), Rhizoma Coptidis	10.7	DB
huáng qín (黄芩), Radix Scutellariae	10.7	DB
huáng bǎi (黄柏), Cortex Phellodendri	10.7	DB
zhī zǐ (栀子), Fructus Gardeniae	10.7	DA
jiāng huáng (姜黄), Rhizoma Curcumae Longae	7.8	K
lián qiào (连翘), Fructus Forsythiae	7.8	DD
jú huā (菊花), Flos Chrysanthemi	5.2	BB
dāng guī wěi (当归尾), Radix Extemis Angelicae Sinensis	5.2	AB
jié gěng (桔梗), Radix Platycodonis	2.6	CA
gé gēn (葛根), Radix Puerariae Lobatae	2.6	BB
bò hé (薄荷), Herba Menthae	2.6	BB
xuán shēn (玄参), Radix Scrophulariae	2.6	DC
guā lóu rén (瓜蒌仁), Semen Trichosanthis	2.6	CB
chuān xiōng (川芎), Rhizoma Ligustici Chuanxiong	2.6	K

Ingredients: (From Tianjin Drug Manufactory *"Huang Lian Shang Ching Pien"*)

dà huáng (大黄), Radix/Rhizoma Rhei	25.2 %	PA
màn jīng zǐ (蔓荆子), Fructus Viticis	16.6	BB
jú huā (菊花), Flos Chrysanthemi	12.6	BB
huáng lián (黄连), Rhizoma Coptidis	7.8	DB
jié gěng (桔梗), Radix Platycodonis	6.3	CA
huáng qín (黄芩), Radix Scutellariae	6.3	DB
jīng jiè (荆芥), Herba Schizonepetae	6.3	BA
bái zhǐ (白芷), Radix Angelicae Dahuricae	6.3	BA
fáng fēng (防风), Radix Saposhnikov./Ledebouriellae	3.1	BA
shí gāo (石膏), Gypsum Fibrosum	3.1	DA
gǎo běn (藁本), Rhizoma Ligustici	3.1	BA
gān cǎo (甘草), Radix Glycyrrhizae	3.1	AA

Clears heat, drains fire, resolves toxins, dispels pathogenic wind, frees the stool, benefits the eyes, opens the orifices, relieves pain. Use for toxic heat accumulation in the upper *jiao* causing fever, headache, sore throat, red eye, eye stye, ear infection or sinus infection. Can be used for harsh cough, strep throat, tonsillitis, infectious conjunctivitis and ear infection, also for stomach and intestinal heat causing tooth infection, mouth ulcers, swollen infected gums or nosebleed. Also for infected wounds or toxic boil with redness and pain.

Pulses: Rapid, large, occasionally slippery
Tongue: Red or red in the tip, with dry yellow coat

Comments: There are two different versions of this formula that are available as products. The first, as the Taiwan-formulated extract granules, is closest to the original prescription. It contains *huáng lián, huáng qín, dà huáng, huáng bǎi,* and *zhī zǐ*, comprising 58% of the formula. These are all strong antibacterial herbs, making it most appropriate for bacterial infections in the upper burner including bacterial cough, as well as strep infections of the throat or eye. It is a large formula, with 15 herbal ingredients.

The second version, available as a popular patent medicine, uses a smaller and different formula (12 herbs). It contains only five herbs from the original formula (*dà huáng, huáng lián, jú huā, jié gěng* and *huáng qín*) and adds herbs that dispel exogenous wind and bring it to the sinus area, including *màn jīng zǐ, jīng jiè, bái zhǐ* and *gǎo běn.* That makes this formula more appropriate for sinus infection, wind headache, or conjunctivitis, but it is still effective for strep throat.

The large amount of *dà huáng* follows the principle of purging heat-toxins through the stool, but excessive amounts may be too purging for many patients. The version from Tianjin contains 25% *dà huáng.*

Caution 1: In both formulas, *dà huáng* is the largest ingredient and will cause diarrhea in many cases. Adjust dosage accordingly. The formula should be discontinued once heat symptoms subside or change.

Caution 2: Due to the inclusion of *dà huáng* and *jiāng huáng*, this formula is prohibited during pregnancy. *Jiāng huáng* is contraindicated for patients taking blood thinners such as Coumadin.

Further Reading:

Bensky et al, p. 170
Chen & Chen, p. 347
Ellis, p. 144

LI FEI PIAN

Formula: *lì fèi piān* (利肺片), "Benefit Lung Tablet"
Source: Modern patent medicine

Availability:

Li Fei Lung Support (K)
Li Fei Pian (PF)
Lifei Tangyipian (PM)

Ingredients: (from Plum Flower *"Li Fei Pian"*)

bái jí (白及), Rhizoma Bletillae	29.1 %	J
bǎi bù (百部), Radix Stemonae	16.1	CC
wǔ wèi zǐ (五味子), Fructus Schisandrae	14.0	L
mǔ lì (牡蛎), Concha Ostreae	11.8	N
pí pá yè (枇杷叶), Folium Eriobotryae	10.8	CC
bǎi hé (百合), Bulbus Lilii	8.6	AD
gān cǎo (甘草), Radix Glycyrrhizae	6.5	AA
dōng chóng xià cǎo (冬虫夏草), Cordyceps	2.9	AC
gé jiè (蛤蚧), Gecko	0.2	AC

Clears lung heat, nourishes lung yin, descends lung qi, stops bleeding, relieves cough. Indicated for harsh dry cough, especially with bits of blood, pus, or sticky pieces of yellow phlegm that is difficult to expectorate. Use for coughs due to trapped heat in the lungs, and applicable for coughs due to tuberculosis, AIDS, or pulmonary abscess. Use this formula for chronic dry cough due to deficiency of lung *yin* and *qi*.

Pulse: Thin, occasionally rapid
Tongue: Normal, or pale, or slightly red with scanty coat

Comments: This formula was originally used to treat chronic dry heat cough found in tuberculosis; thus the attention to coughing up of blood and pus, for which Bletilla *bái jí* is indicated (29% of the formula). *Bǎi bù* clears harsh cough; *bǎi hé* helps to moisten the lung; *mǔ lì* helps descend and astringe lung *qi*. Small amounts of *gé jiè* and *dōng chóng xià cǎo* are also used, both valued tonics for lung *qi* and *yin*. In spite of its original application in tuberculosis and expectoration of blood, it is commonly used for controlling heat in the lungs causing dry cough.

QING FEI YI HUO PIAN

Formula: *qīng fèi yì huǒ piān* (清肺抑火片), "Clear Lungs, Inhibit Fire Tablet"
Source: Modern patent medicine

Availability:

Ching Fei Yi Huo Tablets (PM)
Qing Fei Clearing Formula (K)
Qing Fei Yi Huo Wan (HT)

Ingredients: (from Herbal Times *"Qing Fei Yi Huo Wan"*)

huáng qín (黄芩), Radix Scutellariae	20.6 %	DB
dà huáng (大黄), Radix/Rhizoma Rhei	17.6	PA
jié gěng (桔梗), Radix Platycodonis	11.8	CA
zhī zǐ (栀子), Fructus Gardeniae	11.8	DA
tiān huā fěn (天花粉), Radix Trichosanthis	11.7	CB
kǔ shēn (苦参), Radix Sophorae Flavescentis	8.8	DB
huáng bǎi (黄柏), Cortex Phellodendri	5.9	DB
zhī mǔ (知母), Rhizoma Anemarrhenae	5.9	DA
qián hú (前胡), Radix Peucedani	5.9	CA

Clears lung heat and fire, moistens the lung and throat, dissolves phlegm, frees the stool, relieves cough. Use for lung fire conditions producing sharp, barking cough, painful lung, dry cough or cough with difficult to expectorate yellow phlegm, dry mouth, and sore throat. Use for acute and chronic bronchitis and pulmonary abscess. Also applicable for tonsillitis, pharyngitis, strep throat, mouth sores, bleeding gums, toothache, and fever.

Pulse: Excess, occasionally rapid; or thin
Tongue: Normal, or red with scanty coat

Comments: This modern formula addresses lung fire conditions, marked by a sensation of burning lungs, with dry, barking and painful cough. It can be added with other formulas for phlegm-heat, to reinforce the effect of draining fire and clearing heat. *Tiān huā fěn* and *zhī mǔ* moisten the lung, while *qián hú* addresses early development of phlegm.

Because of the inclusion of *huáng qín, dà huáng, zhī zǐ, kǔ shēn* and *huáng bǎi* (65% of the formula), it is appropriate for bacterial infections affecting the lung, sinus, ear or throat.

Caution 1: *Dà huáng* (at 17.6% of the formula) can cause loose stools or diarrhea; in that case, reduce dosage. Discontinue the medicine after heat symptoms subside, usually within three days.

Caution 2: *Dà huáng* and *tiān huā fěn* are prohibited during pregnancy.

OTHER FORMULAS APPROPRIATE FOR THIS CHAPTER:

Classical Formulas:

Sang Ju Yin

See Chapter 1B

Xie Bai San

Morus & Lycium Formula (EG)
Mulberry and Lycium Formula (GF)

Modern Formulas:

Yang Yin Qing Fei Wan

Yang Yin Qing Fei Wan (PM)
Yang Yin Qing Fei Tang Jiang (PM)

Other:

Belamcanda 15 (SF)
Stemona Tablets (SF)

3. RESPIRATORY DISORDERS

3B. LUNG PHLEGM-HEAT
(Acute Productive Cough)

Classical Formulas:

Qing Qi Hua Tan Wan	*qīng qì huà tán wán* (清气化痰丸)

Modern Formulas:

Ning Sou Wan	*níng sòu wán* (宁嗽丸)

The expectoration in lung phlegm-heat is yellow or yellow-brown in color; the viscosity can vary from sticky to thick to runny. There is a rattling cough, and there may also be yellow nasal discharge. Phlegm-heat may be accompanied by lung fire, manifesting as painful harsh cough, dry mouth or throat, and fever. Phlegm-heat can present as an acute early stage cough, or develop following the common cold or influenza, and include bronchitis and pertussis. Chronic phlegm-heat may also show with smokers, or as a stage in emphysema.

Phlegm, being a secondary pathogenic factor, is difficult to dissolve or eliminate, and treatment can take a week to several weeks. A secondary pathogenic factor means that it is created by pathology, and in turn it creates more pathology. The heat aspect can resolve quickly (within days), but phlegm can be stubborn. Herbs that address phlegm dissolve it into a fluid so that it can be eliminated in the stool. It is not uncommon, and it is a good sign, when odorous or loose stools follow the taking of these formulas. During treatment the patient should be advised to avoid greasy and oily foods, dairy products and sugar, which tend to aggravate phlegm production.

These formulas are not recommended for early stage of pathogenic wind or lung fire, but when the pathogen has settled in the lung and is producing phlegm. It is often advantageous to reinforce the formulas in this chapter with one of the cough syrups presented in *Chapter 3D.*

After taking formulas for phlegm-heat, clear or white phlegm may remain although the heat has been cleared. In those cases, change the formulas to the products in *Chapter 3C.*

Classical Formulas:

QING QI HUA TAN WAN

Formula: *qīng qì huà tán wán* (清气化痰丸),"Clear Qi, Dissolve Phlegm Pill"
Author: Wú Kūn (吴昆)
Source: *Yī Fāng Kǎo* (医方考), 1584
Literal: "Medical Formula Investigations"

Availability:

Clean Air Teapills (PF)
Pinellia & Scute Formula (EG)
Pinellia "X" Formula (CC)
Pinellia Phlegm Dispersing Formula (K)
Pinellia Root Teapills (MS)
Qing Qi Hua Tan Wan (HT, TL)

Ingredients: (from the standardized *"Pinellia & Scute Formula"*)

dǎn nán xīng (胆南星), Arisaema cum Bile	15.8 %	CB
bàn xià (半夏), Rhizoma Pinelliae	15.8	CA
guā lóu rén (瓜蒌仁), Semen Trichosanthis	10.5	CA
huáng qín (黄芩), Radix Scutellariae	10.5	DB
chén pí (陈皮), Pericarpium Citri Reticulatae	10.5	G
xìng rén (杏仁), Semen Armeniacae Amarum	10.5	CC
zhǐ shí (枳实), Fructus Aurantii Immaturus	10.5	G
fú líng (茯苓), Poria	10.5	FC
shēng jiāng (生姜), Rhizoma Zingiberis Recens	5.3	BA

Dissolves phlegm, clears heat, descends lung qi, relieves cough. Use for acute or chronic cough with accumulation of yellow phlegm, either copious or sticky, with signs of a rattling cough and difficulty in breathing. Indicated for acute bronchitis including pertussis, as well as cough due to pneumonia. Also useful in asthma and emphysema due to phlegm-heat.

Pulses: Slippery, rapid, excess
Tongue: Normal, or red with greasy yellow coat

Comments: *Qing Qi Hua Tan Wan* is the primary formula for treating phlegm-heat cough; it can also be applied to phlegm-damp cough. The use of *dǎn nán xīng*, coated in pig bile, is particularly good at emulsifying thick phlegm (as bile is with fat); being cold, it is effective at clearing heat and resolving toxin. In this regard, *huáng qín* furthers the cooling aspect of the formula. Herbs to dissolve phlegm include *bàn xià*, *guā lóu rén*, *chén pí* and *fú líng*. *Xìng rén* stops cough. Together, *chén pí* and *zhǐ shí* direct *qi* downwards as well as dissolve phlegm, allowing the lungs to circulate *qi* more freely.

Some manufacturers use *tiān nán xīng* (天南星, Rhizoma Arisaematis) instead of *dǎn nán xīng*. Less cooling, it allows the formula to be used for phlegm-damp as well as phlegm-heat; however *dǎn nán xīng* is preferred in heat presentations. In cases of pronounced heat, *Qing Qi Hua Tan Wan* can be combined with with formulas from Chapter 3A, as well as cough syrups from *Chapter 3D.*

Caution: Not for use in dry cough. Reduce dosage should loose stools develop.

Further reading:

Bensky et al, p. 790
Chen & Chen, p. 1222
Ellis, p. 225

Modern Formulas:

NING SOU WAN

Formula: *níng sòu wán* (宁嗽丸), "Quiet Cough Pills"
Author: Chinese Herbal Medicine Committee, Ministry of the Interior
Source: *Zhōng Guó Guó Yào Gù Yǒu Chéng Fāng Xuǎn* (中国国药故有成方选集), 1967
Literal: "China's Chinese Medicine Administration Selected Formulas Anthology"

Availability:

Fritillaria & Platycodon Formula (EG)
Ning Sou Wan (GF, HT, TL)
Quiet Cough Teapills (PF)

Ingredients: (from the standardized *"Fritillaria & Platycodon Formula"*)

jié gěng (桔梗), Radix Platycodonis	10.5 %	CA
shí hú (石斛), Caulis Dendrobii	10.5	AD
jiāng bàn xià (姜半夏), Rhizoma Pinelliae Praep.	10.5	CA
chuān bèi mǔ (川贝母), Bulbus Fritillariae Cirrhosae	10.5	CB
zǐ sū zǐ (紫苏子), Fructus Perillae	10.5	CC
fú líng (茯苓), Poria	10.5	FC
sāng bái pí (桑白皮), Cortex Mori	7.9	CC
bò hé (薄荷), Herba Menthae	7.9	BB
xìng rén (杏仁), Semen Armeniacae Amarum	7.9	CC
jú hóng (橘红), Exocarpium Citri Rubrum	5.3	G
gǔ yá (谷芽), Fructus Oryzae Germinatus	5.3	H
gān cǎo (甘草), Radix Glycyrrhizae	2.7	AA

Dissolves phlegm, clears heat, moistens lung yin, relieves cough. Use for a dry or rattling cough with sticky yellow phlegm found in acute and chronic bronchitis, asthma, pertussis (whooping cough) and emphysema. The cough may be dry, with small pieces of phlegm expectorated in upon waking.

Pulses: Slippery or excess, rapid; may be thin
Tongue: Red with a dry, scanty yellow coat

Comments: *Ning Sou Wan* treats lung phlegm-heat that is more sticky and difficult to expectorate, rather than profuse. There will be a harsh and rattley cough with occasional expectoration of small pieces of yellow phlegm. The formula is very useful for the stage when lung fire begins to turn to phlegm-heat.

Bàn xià, chuān bèi mŭ and *jú hóng* dissolve phlegm; *jié gĕng, zĭ sū zĭ, sāng bái pí* and *xìng rén* stop cough; and *shí hú* moistens the lung to allow release of sticky phlegm. In the version from Plum Flower, *bĕi shā shen* (北沙参, Radix Glehniae) is substituted for *shí hú*.

Further Reading:

Bensky et al, p. 30
Chen & Chen, p. 113
Ellis, p. 203

OTHER FORMULAS APPROPRIATE FOR THIS CHAPTER:

Classical Formulas:

Qing Fei Tang

Platycodon & Fritillaria Combination (EG)
Qing Fei Clearing (K)
Qing Fei Tang (BP)

Modern Formulas:

Ping Chuan Wan

See Chapter 3F

Other:

Chest Relief (GW)
Children's Clear Lung (GF)
Chuanbei Juhong Wan (PM)
Dispel Cough (K)
Fritillaria and Pinellia Tablets (GF)
Fritillaria Extract Sugar Coated Tablets (PM)
Golden Pearls (CP)
Harmonize Heart & Lung (CMS)
Harmonize Lung & Liver (CMS)
Pinellia XPT (EV)
Respitrol-Heat (EV)
Ringing Metal (TT)
San She Dan Chuan Bei Ye (PM)
Specific Cough Relieving Capsules (PM)
SVP Lung Formula (DJ)
Trichosanthes Fruit Tablets (SF)
Zhu Li Da Tan Pian/Wan (GC)

3C. PHLEGM-DAMP
(Chronic Productive Cough)

Classical Formulas:

Ban Xia Hou Po Tang	*bàn xià hòu pò tāng* (半夏厚朴汤)
Er Chen Tang	*èr chén tāng* (二陈汤)
Su Zi Jiang Qi Tang	*sū zǐ jiàng qì tāng* (苏子降气汤)
Xing Su San	*xìng sū sǎn* (杏蘇丸)

Modern Formulas:

Chuan Ke Wan	*chuǎn ké wán* (喘咳丸)
/ Qi Guan Yan Wan	*qì guǎn yán wán* (气管炎丸)

Lung phlegm-damp conditions are differentiated from phlegm-heat presentations. The expectoration is white or clear in color, whereas phlegm-heat conditions present with yellow or brown phlegm. In either case, viscosity may vary from thick to watery, and it may be confined to the lungs or include nasal discharge. Phlegm-damp often follows the stage of acute phlegm-heat, which converts to phlegm-damp either through herbal intervention or its own natural course. Once the phlegm has turned clear or white, it indicates that the heat phase is over.

Lung phlegm-damp is difficult to treat and can last for days, weeks, or even months. Chronicity is complicated when there is an underlying deficiency of vital *qi*. Despite the difficulty, Chinese herbs offer the best therapy.

Besides exogenous factors, chronic phlegm-damp in the lung can also arise from endogenous causes affecting the lung, causing cough, asthma or emphysema. Endogenous causes include deficiency of *qi* and *yang* leading to stasis of *qi* circulation. Endogenous phlegm can also originate in the stomach; this is due to deficiency of *qi* or *yang* leading to food stasis. Many formulas in this chapter can therefore address stomach phlegm in addition to lung phlegm. Many chronic cases involve accumulation of phlegm in both the lung and stomach.

Herbal formulas that address phlegm do their work by dissolving phlegm that is then eliminated in the stool. The development of loose stools shows that the phlegm is being eliminated. During recovery the patient should be advised to avoid greasy, oily or fried foods, dairy products and sugar, all of which aggravate phlegm.

Classical Formulas:

BAN XIA HOU PO TANG

Formula: *bàn xià hòu pò tāng* (半夏厚朴汤)
"Pinellia, Magnolia Bark Decoction"
Author: Zhāng Zhòng-Jǐng (张仲景)
Source: *Jīn Guì Yào Lüè* (金匮要略), 220
Literal: "Golden Cabinet Essential Summary"

Availability:

Ban Xia Hou Po Wan (HT, TL)
Pinellia & Magnolia Combination (KP/EG)
Pinellia & Magnolia Formula (CC, GF)
Pinellia & Magnolia Teapills (PF)
Pinellia And Magnolia Bark Formula (HS)
Plum Pit Qi (K)
* Augmented Plum Pit Qi (K)

Ingredients: (from the standardized *"Pinellia & Magnolia Combination"*)

bàn xià (半夏), Rhizoma Pinelliae	30. %	CA
shēng jiāng (生姜), Rhizoma Zingiberis Recens	25	BA
fú líng (茯苓), Poria	20	FC
hòu pò (厚朴), Cortex Magnoliae Officinalis	15	FB
zǐ sū yè (紫苏叶), Folium Perillae	10	BA

Dissolves phlegm, activates and descends qi, dispels wind-cold, relieves cough. Use for accumulation of phlegm-damp in the lung, stomach or esophagus, with symptoms of chest oppression, cough with white phlegm, and occasional vomiting of sputum. Also for "plum pit *qi*", the sensation of of phlegm accumulation in the throat (globus hystericus). Applicable in esophageal constriction, chronic bronchitis, asthma and emphysema. Also used for poor digestion due to food stagnation, and for fatigue, depression and lack of motivation.

Pulse: Wiry, tight, or slippery
Tongue: Moist, with a white or greasy coat

Comments: This formula from Zhang Zhong-Jing was originally intended for treating "plum-pit *qi*", the sensation of something being stuck in the throat with esophageal swelling. This is esophageal constriction due to stasis of *qi* and phlegm, which is rare in the clinic. However, the formula is useful for accumulated phlegm in the lung or stomach, including chronic cough, esophageal constriction or reflux, and chronic pharyngitis.

All of the herbs move *qi* downwards. *Bàn xià*, combined with *fú ling* and *hòu pò*, transform phlegm while allowing lung *qi* to descend. *Shēng jiāng* benefits the stomach, descends *qi*, and dispels wind-cold. *Zǐ sū yè* activates the circulation of *qi* and soothes the liver. In some versions, *zǐ sū zǐ* (紫苏子, Fructus Perillae) is used instead of *zǐ sū yè* (the seed versus the leaf).

Further Reading:

Bensky et al, p. 516
Chen & Chen, p.
Ellis, p. 23

ER CHEN TANG

Formula: *èr chén tāng* (二陈汤), "Two Aged Decoction"
Author: Imperial Medical Bureau (*tài yī jú,* 太医局);
revised by Chén Shī-Wén (陈师文)
Source: *Tài Píng Huì Mín Hé Jì Jú Fāng* (太平惠民和剂局方), 1078
Literal: "(Era of) Great Peace, Benefit People Harmonious Medicines, Office (of) Formulas"

Availability:

Citrus & Pinellia Combination (EG)
Citrus and Pinellia Formula (GF)
Er Chen Teapills (PF)
Er Chen Wan (HT, MS, PIM, TL)
Gastroquell (BP)
Two Cured Formula (HS)
* Citrus & Pinellia Plus Formula (CC)
* Lucid Channel (K)

Ingredients: (from Herbal Times *"Er Chen Wan"*)

chén pí (陈皮), Pericarpium Citri Reticulatae	32.3 %	G
bàn xià (半夏), Rhizoma Pinelliae	32.2	CA
fú líng (茯苓), Poria	19.5	FC
gān cǎo (甘草), Radix Glycyrrhizae	10.0	AA
shēng jiāng (生姜), Rhizoma Zingiberis Recens	6.0	BA

Ingredients: (from the standardized *"Citrus & Pinellia Combination"*)

chén pí (陈皮), Pericarpium Citri Reticulatae	25.0 %	G
bàn xià (半夏), Rhizoma Pinelliae	25.0	CA
fú líng (茯苓), Poria	25.0	FC
gān cǎo (甘草), Radix Glycyrrhizae	12.4	AA
shēng jiāng (生姜), Rhizoma Zingiberis Recens	6.3	BA
wū méi (乌梅), Fructus Mume	6.3	L

Dissolves and dispels phlegm, dries dampness, regulates qi, harmonizes the stomach and spleen. Use for accumulation of phlegm-damp in the lung causing chronic bronchitis, emphysema, and asthma. Use for accumulation of phlegm in the stomach leading to nausea, fullness, vomiting and poor appetite. Can be used for morning sickness due to phlegm accumulation.

Pulse: Wiry or slippery
Tongue: Moist, with a white coat

Comments: *Er Chen Tang* was influenced by *Ban Xia Hou Po Tang* (above) and is often used as a foundation formula for accumulation of phlegm-damp in the lung or stomach. It can be used alone for cough, or it can be used to reinforce other formulas.

"Two Aged" refers to *chén pí* and *bàn xià*, whose therapeutic strength is increased by aging prior to use. The two herbs dissolve phlegm and regulate *qi*. *Fú líng* helps dispel dissolved phlegm through the urine and further removes damp. *Wū méi* is used in the classical prescription, as represented by the Taiwan extracted granules, which astringes *qi* so that it will not be lost by the dispersing action of the other herbs. Many of the manufacturers, such as Herbal Times and Minshan, do not include *wū méi.*

Er Chen Tang serves as the foundation formula for *Liu Jun Zi Tang* (Chapter 6A), which adds the *qi* tonics *rén shēn* (人参, Radix Ginseng) and *bái zhú* (白术, Rhizoma Atractylodis Macrocephalae).

Further Reading:

Bensky et al, p. 775
Chen & Chen, p. 1209
Ellis, p. 88

SU ZI JIANG QI TANG

Formula: *sū zǐ jiàng qì tāng* (苏子降气汤), "Perilla Seed Descend Qi Decoction"
Author: Imperial Medical Bureau (*tài yī jú,* 太医局);
revised by Chén Shī-Wén (陈师文)
Source: *Tài Píng Huì Mín Hé Jì Jú Fāng* (太平惠民和剂局方), 1078
Literal: "(Era of) Great Peace, Benefit People Harmonious Medicines, Office (of) Formulas"

based on:

Formula: *zǐ sū zǐ tāng* (紫苏子汤), "Perilla Fruit Decoction"
Author: Sūn Sī-Miǎo (孙思邈)
Source: *Qiān Jīn Yào Fāng* (千金要方), 652
Literal: "Thousand Gold (Pieces) Important Formulas"

Availability:

Perilla Seed Combination (EG)
Su Zi Jiang Qi Tang (BP, TZ)
Su Zi Jiang Qi Pian/Wan (GC)

Ingredients: (from the standardized *"Perilla Seed Combination"*)

zǐ sū zǐ (紫苏子), Fructus Perillae	18.5 %	CC
bàn xià (姜半夏), Rhizoma Pinelliae	18.5	CA
chén pí (陈皮), Pericarpium Citri Reticulatae	11.1	G
ròu guì (肉桂), Cortex Cinnamomi	11.1	E
qián hú (前胡), Radix Peucedani	7.4	CB
hòu pò (厚朴), Cortex Magnoliae Officinalis	7.4	FB
gān cǎo (甘草), Radix Glycyrrhizae	7.4	AA
dāng guī (当归), Radix Angelicae Sinensis	7.4	AB
shēng jiāng (生姜), Rhizoma Zingiberis Recens	7.4	BA
dà zǎo (大枣), Fructus Jujubae	3.8	AA

Dissolves and dispels phlegm-cold, descends lung and stomach qi, regulates qi, relieves cough, stops wheezing. Use for accumulation of copious lung phlegm with cough and labored breathing or wheezing. Applicable in chronic bronchitis, emphysema, smoker's cough, and asthma with phlegm. Can also be used for nasal discharge due to wind-cold or chronic sinusitis.

Pulse: Slippery, wide
Tongue: White coat

Comments: This formula addresses accumulation of loose phlegm-damp, with difficulty breathing, wheezing or chronic cough. An elaboration of Zhang Zhong-Jing's *Ban Xia Hou Po Tang* (above), it adds *zǐ sū zǐ* as the principal herb to descend *qi* and eliminate phlegm. *Qián hú* further transforms phlegm, *chén pí* and *chén xiāng* downbear lung and stomach *qi* and phlegm, and *dà zǎo* and *dāng guī* support *qi* and blood. It can be used for phlegm-damp bronchitis following the common cold, prolonged cough, phlegm-damp asthma, and cough in the elderly. It is also appropriate for nasal disorders including common cold and chronic sinusitis.

Further Reading:

Bensky et al, p. 537
Chen & Chen, 842
Ellis, p. 299

XING SU SAN

Formula: *xìng sū săn* (杏蘇丸), "Armeniaca, Perilla Leaf Powder"
Author: Wú Táng (吴瑭) *aka* Wú Jū-Tōng (吴鞠通)
Source: *Wēn Bìng Tiáo Biàn* (温病条辨), 1798
Literal: "Warm Diseases Systematic Differentiation"

Availability:

Apricot Seed & Perilla Formula (EG)
Armenica AndPerilla Powder (BP)
Xing Su Wan (HT)

Ingredients: (from the standardized *"Apricot Seed & Perilla Formula"*)

xìng rén (杏仁), Semen Armeniacae Amarum	13.3 %	CC
zĭ sū yè (紫苏叶), Folium Perillae	13.3	BA
qián hú (前胡), Radix Peucedani	13.3	CA
fú líng (茯苓), Poria	13.3	FC
bàn xià (半夏), Rhizoma Pinelliae	13.3	CA
jié gĕng (桔梗), Radix Platycodonis	6.6	CA
zhĭ ké (枳壳), Fructus Aurantii	6.6	G
gé gēn (葛根), Radix Puerariae Lobatae	6.6	BB
chén pí (陈皮), Pericarpium Citri Reticulatae	6.6	G
gān căo (甘草), Radix Glycyrrhizae	3.6	AA
shēng jiāng (生姜), Rhizoma Zingiberis Recens	3.5	BA

Ingredients: (from Herbal Times *"Xing Su Wan"*)

fú líng (茯苓), Poria	12. %	FC
bàn xià (半夏), Rhizoma Pinelliae	9	CA
jié gĕng (桔梗), Radix Platycodonis	9	CA
qián hú (前胡), Radix Peucedani	9	CA
qiāng huó (羌活), Radix Notopterygii	9	BA
xìng rén (杏仁), Semen Armeniacae Amarum	9	CC
zhĭ ké (枳壳), Fructus Aurantii	9	G
zĭ sū yè (紫苏叶), Folium Perillae	9	BA
dà zăo (大枣), Fructus Jujubae	7	AA
gān căo (甘草), Radix Glycyrrhizae	6	AA
jú hóng pí (橘红皮), Pericarpium Citri Rubrum	6	G
shēng jiāng (生姜), Rhizoma Zingiberis Recens	6	BA

Dispels wind-cold-dryness, disperses and descends lung qi to resolve phlegm, relieves cough. Use for wind-cold entering the lungs and interfering with the descent of lung *qi*, creating stagnation and phlegm. Other symptoms include body chills, or aches, slight headache and nasal congestion. Phlegm production is mild. Use for cough with common cold, chronic cough, emphysema and asthma aggravated by wind-cold.

Pulse: Floating, slightly wiry
Tongue: Dry or normal with white coat

Comments: *Xing Su San* treats cough due to wind-cold attack, either dry, or with early signs of phlegm-damp. It addresses wind-cold inhibiting the lung's ability to downbear *qi*, resulting in cough and phlegm production. The formula is appropriate for early cough in a wind-cold presentation, without signs of heat. Wu Ju-Tong felt that wind-induced cough was common, with resulting stagnation leading to production of phlegm.

Xìng rén is one of the principal herbs; it disperses the lung to stop cough and dissolve phlegm. It is assisted by *jié gěng* and *zhǐ ké. Zǐ sū yè* dispels wind cool-dryness, aided by *qián hú.* They promote slight sweating to release the exterior. *Bàn xià, chén pí* (or *jú hóng pí*) and *fú líng* dispel phlegm.

The Herbal Times version uses *qiāng huó* to help dispel wind, while the Taiwan extract granules use *gé gēn.* Both are additions to the original formula.

Further Reading:

Bensky et al, p. 663
Chen & Chen, p. 1025
Ellis, p. 365

Modern Formulas:

CHUAN KE WAN / QI GUAN YAN WAN

Formula: *chuăn ké wán* (喘咳丸), "Asthma Cough Pills"
Source: Modern patent medicine
also available as:
Formula: *qì guăn yán wán* (气管炎丸), "Bronchitis Pills"
Source: Modern patent medicine

Availability:

Chuan Ke Wan (HT)
Qi Guan Yan Wan (PF)

Ingredients: (From Herbal Times *"Chuan Ke Wan"*)

pí pá yè (枇杷叶), Folium Eriobotryae	28. %	CC
dăng shēn (党参), Radix Codonopsis	16	AA
dà zăo (大枣), Fructus Jujubae	12	AA
sāng yè (桑叶), Folium Mori	8	BB
shēng jiāng (生姜), Rhizoma Zingiberis Recens	8	BA
chuān bèi mŭ (川贝母), Bulbus Fritillariae Cirrhosae	6	CB
xìng rén (杏仁), Semen Armeniacae Amarum	6	CC
qián hú (前胡), Radix Peucedani	4	CA
yuăn zhì (远志), Radix Polygalae	4	N
jú hóng huā (橘红花), Flos Citri Rubrum	2	G
kuăn dōng huā (款冬花), Flos Tussilaginis Farfarae	2	CC
wŭ wèi zĭ (五味子), Fructus Schisandrae	2	L
zĭ wăn (紫菀), Radix/Rhizoma Asteris	2	CC

Ingredients: (From Plum Flower *"Qi Guan Yan Wan"*)

pí pá yè (枇杷叶), Folium Eriobotryae	28. %	CC
dǎng shēn (党参), Radix Codonopsis	16	AA
dà zǎo (大枣), Fructus Jujubae	12	AA
sāng yè (桑叶), Folium Mori	8	BB
shēng jiāng (生姜), Rhizoma Zingiberis Recens	8	BA
chuān bèi mǔ (川贝母), Bulbus Fritillariae Cirrhosae	6	CB
xìng rén (杏仁), Semen Armeniacae Amarum	6	CC
qián hú (前胡), Radix Peucedani	4	CA
yuǎn zhì (远志), Radix Polygalae	4	N
jú hóng (橘红), Fructus Citri Rubrum	2	G
kuǎn dōng huā (款冬花), Flos Tussilaginis Farfarae	2	CC
sāng bái pí (桑白皮), Cortex Mori	2	CC
wǔ wèi zǐ (五味子), Fructus Schisandrae	2	L

Dissolves and dispels phlegm, diffuses lung qi, benefits qi, regulates and harmonizes ying and wei, relieves cough. Use for accumulation of loose or thick phlegm with rattle-like cough and labored breathing. Applicable in bronchitis, smoker's cough, and the phlegm-damp stage of pertussis or emphysema. Helpful for chronic cough aggravated by depleted *qi*, particularly in the elderly or in cases of prolonged cough.

Pulse: Slippery, soft
Tongue: White coat, possibly wet

Comments: *Qi Guan Yan Wan* from Plum Flower is identical to Herbal Times' *Chuan Ke Wan*, except that Plum Flower uses *jú hóng* (橘红, Exocarpium Citri Rubrum) and *sāng bái pí* (桑白皮, Cortex Mori) instead of *jú hóng huā* and *zǐ wǎn*.

The formula treat cough with copious or thick phlegm-damp. This may follow a pathogenic wind invasion, or it may occur as a phlegm-heat cough cools and changes, due to herbal intervention or natural progression. *Pí pá yè, sāng yè* and *xìng rén* stop cough; *chuān bèi mǔ, qián hú, yuǎn zhì* and *kuǎn dōng huā* resolve phlegm. *Dǎng shēn* and *dà zǎo* support and boost *qi*.

OTHER FORMULAS APPROPRIATE FOR THIS CATEGORY:

Classical Formulas:

jie geng tang

Jie Geng Wan (PM)
Platycodon Combination (EG)
Platycodon Teapills (MS)

qing qi hua tan wan

See Chapter 3C.

Modern Formulas:

Ping Chuan Wan

See *Chapter 3F*

Zhi Sou San

Citrus & Aster Formula (EG)
Zhi Sou San (PF, TZ)

Other:

Breathe Easy (TT)
Clear Qi (TT)
Deep Breath (GW)
Dispel Cough (K)
Er Chen He San Zi Yang Qin Pian/Wan (GC)
Glacier Pearls (CP)
Golden Qi (BP)
Ke Chuan Pian/Wan (GC)
Lung Qi Jr (BP)
Open Air (GW)
Pinellia 16 (SF)
Pipe Cleaner (GW)
Purge Phlegm (CMS)

3. RESPIRATORY DISORDERS

3D. COUGH SYRUPS

Modern Formulas:

Chuan Bei Pi Pa Lu — *chuān bèi pí pá lù* (川贝枇杷露)
San She Dan Chuan Bei Ye — *sān shé dǎn chuān bèi yè* (三蛇胆川贝液)
Xiao Ke Chuan (Hsiao Keh Chuan) — *xiāo ké chuǎn* (消咳喘)

Chinese herbal cough syrups are a convenient way to administer herbal medicines, and often provide a solution for children too young to swallow pills. The syrups described here are used for lung fire, phlegm-heat, and/or phlegm-damp, and are applied to bronchitis, emphysema, pertussis and asthma, smoker's cough. All of the syrups are soothing to the throat, and are helpful for sore throat and laryngitis.

Cough syrups on their own do not seem to be strong enough to handle cough and phlegm. It is best to combine them with pills in order to reinforce the therapeutic effect. Most contain sugar or honey, which may be a concern to certain patients, although it helps compliance when administering to children.

Modern Formulas:

CHUAN BEI PI PA LU
LOQUAT & FRITILLARY EXTRACT

Formula: *chuān bèi pí pá lù* (川贝枇杷露), "Fritillaria, Eriobotrya Liquid"
Source: Modern patent medicine

Availability:

Fritillaria & Pinellia Syrup (GF)
Loquat Fritillary Extract Syrup (PF)
Loquat & Fritillary Extract (PM)
Natural Herb Loquat Extract (PM)
Nim Jiom Pei Pa Koa (PM)

Ingredients: (from Pangaoshou Pharmaceutical; Guangzhou *"Loquat & Fritillary Extract"*. Ingredient percentages are not given.)

chuān bèi mŭ (川贝母), Bulbus Fritillariae Cirrh.	CB
jié gĕng (桔梗), Radix Platycodonis	CA
xìng rén (杏仁), Semen Armeniacae Amarum	CC
pí pá yè (枇杷叶), Folium Eriobotryae	CC
băi bù (百部), Radix Stemonae	CC
bò hé (薄荷), Herba Menthae	BB
yí táng (饴糖), Saccharum Granorum (sugar)	
Water	

Packing and Dosage: Bottles of 5 fluid oz. (150 ml.) Take 1tsp to 1 tablespoon, 3 x day. Children: 1 teaspoon, 3 x day.

Ingredients: (from Golden Flower "Fritillaria and Pinellia Syrup")

bàn xià (半夏), Rhizoma Pinelliae	11.6 %	CA
zhè bèi mǔ (浙贝母), Bulbus Fritillariae Thunbergii	11.5	CB
luó hàn guǒ (罗汉果), Fructus Momordicae	11.5	AD
yú xīng cǎo (鱼腥草), Herba Houttuyniae	11.5	DD
tiān zhú huáng (天竹黄), Concretio Silicea Bambusae	7.7	CB
huáng qín (黄芩), Radix Scutellariae	7.7	DB
chén pí (陈皮), Pericarpium Citri Reticulatae	7.7	G
xìng rén (杏仁), Semen Armeniacae	7.7	CC
zhǐ shí (枳实), Fructus Aurantii Immaturus	7.7	G
fú líng (茯苓), Poria	7.7	FC
fú líng (甘草), Radix Glycyrrhizae	7.7	AA

Dissolves phlegm, clears heat, relieves cough, calms wheezing. Use for acute or chronic cough with phlegm including bronchitis, asthma, pertussis, emphysema and smoker's cough. Can also be used for dry or sore throat, thirst and laryngitis.

Pulse: Excess and floating, or submerged, slippery or wide
Tongue: Red in tip, possible yellow coat

Comments: The *Loquat and Fritillaria* syrups are good for hacking coughs with phlegm expectoration, and are especially useful with children. They can be used for heat presentations with dry sore throat and hoarse voice, and can also be used for chronic cough due to phlegm-damp. The formulas tend to be neutral in temperature, or only slightly cooling.

The two syrups described here have quite different formulations. In the Pangaoshou version, *chuān bèi mǔ* is the principal herb to reduce phlegm; *xìng rén, pí pá yè* and *bǎi bù* stop cough; *bò hé* clears heat from the lung. "Loquat" actually refers to the fruit of the Eriobotrya tree and is a commonly used folk medicine for cough, and it is the fruit that often appears on the product box. The formulas, however, rely on the leaf (*pí pá yè*), not the fruit.

The version from Golden Flower uses *Er Chen Tang* as a foundation to dissolve phlegm (*bàn xià, chén pí, fú líng,* and *fú líng*), supported by *zhè bèi mǔ* and *tiān zhú huáng*. *Luó hàn guǒ* and *xìng rén* moisten the lung to stop cough; and *huáng qín* and *yú xīng cǎo* clear heat and toxic heat.

The prescription from Golden Flower is also available in tablet form.

SAN SHE DAN CHUAN BEI YE

Formula: *sān shé dǎn chuān bèi yè* (三蛇胆川贝液)
"Three Snake Gallbladder Fritillaria Liquid"
Source: Modern patent medicine

Availability:

San She Dan Chuan Bei Ye (PM)

Ingredients: (from United Pharmaceutical Manufactory; Guangzhou)

chuān bèi mǔ (川贝母), Bulbus Fritillariae Cirrh.	51.7 %	CB
xìng rén (杏仁), Semen Armeniacae Amarum	34.5	CC
shé dǎn (蛇胆), Fel Serpentis	13.8	CB
Honey and sugar		

Dissolves phlegm, clears heat, resolves toxins, descends lung qi, moistens the throat, relieves cough. Use for acute or chronic phlegm-heat causing cough, lung congestion, or yellow nasal discharge. Useful in heat conditions with stubborn sticky phlegm and a barking cough. Can be used alone, or adjunctively with pills for cough due to phlegm-heat.

Pulse: Excess and floating, or submerged
Tongue: Red in tip, possible yellow coat

Comments: This cough remedy for acute phlegm-heat in the lungs comes in small glass vials with straws. It is particularly useful for stubborn sticky phlegm, but can be used in any phlegm-heat presentation. Due to its sweet taste, children enjoy taking it. The formula uses *xìng rén* and *chuān bèi mǔ* to relieve cough and dissolve phlegm. Snake gallbladder (*shé dǎn*) relies on bile to dissolve phlegm, similarly to how it emulsifies fat. Also, bile is cold, making it useful for lung heat or fire.

Snakes from southern China are commonly raised in captivity or wild crafted for food or medicine, and include the Chinese rat snake, Ptyos Korros, (*guò shù lóng shé*, 过树龙蛇); the banded krait, Bungarus fasciatus (*jīn huán shé*, 金环蛇); and the Chinese cobra, Naja atra (*yǎn jing shé*, 眼镜蛇).

Caution: Caution during pregnancy. Bile is contraindicated during pregnancy.

Packing and Dosage: Box of 6 glass vials, each with 10 cc. of liquid. Take 1 to 3 vials per day.

XIAO KE CHUAN
HSIAO KEH CHUAN

Formula: *xiāo ké chuǎn* (消咳喘), "Disperse Cough, Panting"
also as: *xiāo ké chuǎn zhuān zhī qì guǎn yán* (消咳喘专支气管炎)
"Disperse Cough, Panting, Special Bronchitis"
Author: Modern patent medicine

Availability:

Hsiao Keh Chuan: Special Medicine For Bronchitis (PM)
Sooth Herb Tea Extract (Xiao Ke Chuan) (PM)

Ingredients: (from Harbin Second Chinese Medicine Factory *"Hsiao Keh Chuan"*)

mǎn shān hóng (满山红), Folium Rhododendri Daurici — CB
Sugar, distilled water

Dissolves phlegm, clears heat, relieves cough, calms panting. Use for acute cough due to phlegm-heat or lung fire, including bronchitis, pertussis and pneumonia. Can be used alone, or adjunctively with pills for cough due to phlegm-heat.

Pulse: Excess and floating, or submerged
Tongue: Red in tip, possible yellow coat

Comments: Rhododendron root is a folk medicine from northeast China for treatment of cough. It has been shown to have strong antitussive and expectorant effects, stopping cough and relieving bronchial spasm. It also has significant antibacterial properties. It is best for harsh barking cough due to lung fire or heat in the early stage of a phlegm-heat cough. The product here is a single herb extract in syrup form.

Packing and dosage:

Bottles of 100 or 200 ml.
Take 1 tablespoon, 3 x day. Children: 1 teaspoon, 3 x day.

3E. LUNG YIN DEFICIENCY
(Dry Nonproductive Cough)

Classical Formulas:

Ba Xian Chang Shou Wan	*bā xīan cháng shōu wán* (八仙长寿丸)
/ Mai Wei Di Huang Wan	*mài wèi dì huáng wán* (麦味地黄丸)
Bai He Gu Jin Tang	*băi hé gù jīn tang* (百合固金汤)
Sha Shen Mai Dong Tang	*shā shēn mài dōng tāng* (沙参麦冬汤)
Sheng Mai San	*shēng mài săn* (生脉散)

Modern Formulas:

Gu Ben Wan	*gù běn wán* (固本丸)

Dry cough manifests in several different patterns. The first is due to exogenous wind-heat and dryness, and is seen as an early stage of the common cold. For this we use *Sang Ju Yin*, discussed in Chapter 1B. The second is a dry harsh cough due to acute lung fire. For this, we choose formulas from Chapter 3A.

This chapter address lung dryness due to deficiency of lung *yin*. This can have an exogenous etiology, due to dryness or heat that slowly depletes lung *yin*. Exogenous factors include chronic exposure to smoking, airborne pollutants, or an overly dry and hot environment. More likely, deficiency of lung *yin* is a chronic condition with an endogenous etiology, due to an underlying deficiency of kidney *yin* affecting lung *yin*.

Besides a history of dry cough and weak breathing, there may be other *yin* deficiency symptoms such as dry eyes and nose, or dizziness, ringing of the ears, and heart palpitation. The nose may be dry, with small pieces of blood on discharge. The pulse will be weak and thready, and the tongue reddish with a dry coat. In lung *yin* deficiency, the cough is weak, not harsh, and is indicative of a deficiency pattern: the patient's *qi* is usually also weak. In these cases, the formulas in this chapter are appropriate, but may need to be combined with kidney *yin* tonics (*Chapter 15A*) or *qi* tonics (*Chapters 14A* or *16A*).

Due to their lung moistening properties, the formulas in this chapter can benefit lungs, mouth and throat made dry by oral steroid use or radiation therapy. They may offer some benefit for Sjögren's syndrome (autoimmune damage to the saliva glands).

Some cases of dry cough, following an an initial exogenous event, may persist stubbornly for months. These cases could be due to infection with mycobacteria, virus or fungi, and require concomitant treatment with formulas from Chapter 2A or 3A.

QUICK SUMMATION:

Ba Xian Chang Shou Wan	Chronic dry cough due to kidney *yin* deficiency
Bai He Gu Jin Tang	*Yin* deficient cough with slight phlegm
Sha Shen Mai Men Dong Tang	*Yin* deficient cough following heat or fever
Sheng Mai San	*Qi* and *yin* deficiency of lung and heart
Gu Ben Wan	Very dry lung or mouth

BA XIAN CHANG SHOU WAN

Formula: *bā xīan cháng shōu wán* (八仙长寿丸)
"Eight Immortals Long Life Pill"
aka: *mài wèi dì huáng wán* (麦味地黄丸)
"Ophiopogon, Schisandra, Rehmannia Pill"
Author: Gōng Tíng-Xián (龚廷贤)
Source: *Shòu Shì Bǎo Yuán* (寿世保元), 1615
Literal: "Long Life Protect (the) Source"

Availability:

Eight Immortals Formula (GF)
Eight Immortals Teapills (PF)
Mai Wei Di Huang Wan (BP, MS, TL)
Schizandra & Rehmannia Formula (EG)
Yin Fountain (K)

Ingredients: (from Minshan *"Mai Wei Di Huang Wan"*)

shú dì huáng (熟地黄), Radix Rehmanniae Praep.	26.7 %	AB
shān zhū yú (山茱萸), Fructus Corni	13.3	L
shān yào (山药), Rhizoma Dioscoreae	13.3	AA
mǔ dān pí (牡丹皮), Cortex Moutan	10.0	DC
zé xiè (泽泻), Rhizoma Alismatis	10.0	FC
fú líng (茯苓), Poria	10.0	FC
mài mén dōng (麦门冬), Radix Ophiopogonis	10.0	AD
wǔ wèi zǐ (五味子), Fructus Schisandrae	6.7	L

Nourishes and consolidates lung yin, moistens the lung, benefits kidney yin. Use for underlying deficiency of kidney *yin* leading to deficiency of lung *yin*, with symptoms of dry cough, dry throat and dry nasal passages. Secondary symptoms can include dizziness, night sweats, tidal fever, ringing of the ears, weakness, or palpitation. Applicable in chronic dry cough following infection with tuberculosis, mycobacteria, and HIV; also for deficiency asthma with dryness.

Pulse: Thready and rapid
Tongue: Normal, or reddish, with a dry coat

Comments: This formula is for chronic lung *yin* deficiency due to an underlying kidney *yin* deficiency, and is commonly used in lung-kidney deficiency in the aged. It is a elaboration of *Liu Wei Di Huang Wan* (*Chapter 17A*), adding *mài mén dōng* to moisten the lung, and *wǔ wèi zǐ* to astringe the formula into the lung and kidney.

The original name for the formula is *Ba Xian Chang Shou Wan,* "Eight Immortals Long Life Pills", indicating the use of eight ingredients. Later, it became known as *Mai Wei Di Huang Wan,* "Ophiopogon, Schisandra Rehmannia Pill".

BAI HE GU JIN TANG

Formula: *bǎi hé gù jīn tāng* (百合固金汤), "Lilium Secure Metal Decoction"
Author: Wāng Áng (汪昂)
Source: *Yī Fāng Jí Jiě* (医方集解), 1682
Literal: "Medical Formulas Collected, Explained"
Also attributed to:
Author: Zhōu Zhī-Gān (周之干) *aka* Zhōu Shèn-Zhāi (周慎斋)
Source: *Shèn Zhāi Yí Shū* (慎斋遗书), 1573
Literal: "Shen-Zhai's Dying Testament"

Availability:

Bai He Gu Jin Wan (PM, TL)
Bai He Gu Jin Tang (BP)
Lily Preserve Metal Formula (GF)
Lily Bulb Formula (HC)
Lily Combination (EG)
Lilium Teapills (MS, PF)

Ingredients: (from the standardized *"Lily Combination"*)

shú dì huáng (熟地黄), Radix Rehmanniae Praep.	23.0 %	AB
shēng dì huáng (生地黄), Radix Rehmanniae	15.3	DC
mài mén dōng (麦门冬), Radix Ophiopogonis	11.5	AD
bǎi hé (百合), Bulbus Lilii	7.6	AD
bái sháo (白芍), Radix Paeoniae Alba	7.6	AB
dāng guī (当归), Radix Angelicae Sinensis	7.6	AB
zhè bèi mǔ (浙贝母), Bulbus Fritillariae Thunbergii	7.6	CB
gān cǎo (甘草), Radix Glycyrrhizae	7.6	AA
xuán shēn (玄参), Radix Scrophulariae	6.1	DC
jié gěng (桔梗), Radix Platycodonis	6.1	CA

Nourishes lung yin, moistens the lung, nourishes kidney yin, clears heat, dissolves phlegm. Use for deficiency of lung *yin* with or without heat, causing dry unproductive cough. Other symptoms include dry sore throat or laryngitis, difficulty breathing, coughing small amounts of blood and low-grade tidal fever or night sweats. Recommended for dry cough that follows the lung fire stage, and in deficiency dry cough accompanying prolonged illness, including tuberculosis and AIDS. Helpful in pharyngitis and smoker's cough, and following radiation therapy to the face, neck and lungs.

Pulse: Thready, may be rapid
Tongue: Red with a dry, scanty yellow coat or no coat; possibly cracked or geographic

Comments: This is a successful formula for acute and chronic dry cough; and historically was used in the treatment of tuberculosis. Addressing lung dryness and heat with *shēng dì huáng, mài mén dōng* and *bǎi hé*, the addition of *zhè bèi mǔ* and *xuán shen* resolves sticky phlegm that may be due to residual heat further depleting *yin*. The formula can also be used following lung heat or phlegm-heat stages once the heat has cleared; it can help resolve any remaining of small amounts of sticky phlegm. Useful following radiation to the chest and throat. *Bai He Gu Jin Tang* is not intended for early dry cough due to pathogenic wind; instead, use *Sang Ju Yin* (see *Chapter 1B*). It is not intended for coughs with significant accumulation of phlegm.

Caution: *Dì huáng* can cause bloating, nausea, or loose stools in patients with a weak digestive system. Monitor and adjust accordingly.

Further Reading:

Bensky, p. 384
Chen & Chen, p. 1036
Ellis, p. 13

SHA SHEN MAI DONG TANG

Formula: *shā shēn mài dōng tāng* (沙参麦冬汤)
"Glehnia, Ophiopogon Decoction"
Author: Wú Táng (吴瑭) *aka* Wú Jū-Tōng (吴鞠通)
Source: *Wēn Bìng Tiáo Biàn* (温病条辨), 1798
Literal: "Warm Diseases Systematic Differentiation"

Availability:

Autumn Rain Teapills (PF)
Glehnia & Ophiopogon Combination (EG)
Glehnia and Ophiopogonis Formula (HS)
Sha Shen Mai Dong Wan (HT)
Sha Shen Mai Men Dong Tang (BP)
* Wise Judge (K)
* Jade Spring (TT)

Ingredients: (from the standardized *"Glehnia & Ophiopogon Combination"*)

běi shā shēn (北沙参), Radix Glehniae	22.2 %	AD
mài mén dōng (麦门冬), Radix Ophiopogonis	22.2	AD
yù zhú (玉竹), Rhizoma Polygonati Odorati	14.8	AD
sāng yè (桑叶), Folium Mori	11.1	BB
tiān huā fěn (天花粉), Radix Trichosanthis	11.1	CB
bǎi biǎn dòu (百扁豆), Semen Dolichos/Lablab Album	11.1	DF
gān cǎo (甘草), Radix Glycyrrhizae	7.5	AA

Ingredients: (from Herbal Times *"Sha Shen Mai Dong Wan"*)

bǎi biǎn dòu (百扁豆), Semen Dolichos/Lablab Album	21.7 %	DF
tiān huā fěn (天花粉), Radix Trichosanthis	17.4	CB
sāng yè (桑叶), Folium Mori	13.0	BB
yù zhú (玉竹), Rhizoma Polygonati Odorati	13.0	AD
mài mén dōng (麦门冬), Radix Ophiopogonis	13.0	AD
běi shā shēn (北沙参), Radix Glehniae	13.0	AD
gān cǎo (甘草), Radix Glycyrrhizae	8.9	AA

Nourishes lung yin, moistens the lung, clears heat, generates fluid, dispels wind, relieves cough, boosts lung qi. Use for deficiency of lung *yin* following fever, with symptoms of dry unproductive cough, sore throat, and dry nostrils and lips. Recommended for dry cough following the lung fire stage, and in deficiency dry cough following chronic illness, including tuberculosis and AIDS. Helpful in smoker's dry cough without excessive phlegm. Useful in asthmatic wheezing with deficiency of *yin* and *qi*, and signs of heat.

Pulses: Thin, weak, occasionally rapid
Tongue: Red with a dry, scanty yellow coat or no coat

Comments: This formula for dry cough addresses lung *yin* deficiency following lung fire or fever. *Běi shā shēn, mài mén dōng, yù zhú,* and *tiān huā fěn* boost *yin* and clear heat. *Běi shā shēn* also boosts lung *qi*. Patients with lung *yin* deficiency aggravate their dry cough when exposed to to wind pathogens; the addition of *sāng yè* addresses this concern. *Bǎi biǎn dòu* benefits stomach and spleen *qi* injured by heat. The author Wu Ju-Tong stated that the formula addresses autumn coughs due to dryness.

Different manufacturers will emphasize different ingredient percentages, affecting the formula. The standardized Taiwan extract granules, as well as Blue Poppy, have *běi shā shēn* and *mài mén dong,* the main herbs to moisten the lung, at 44% of the formula. Herbal Times, as an example, will have it at 26%, and Plum Flower, in their *Autumn Rain Teapills*, uses 33%.

Caution: *Tiān huā fěn* is contraindicated during pregnancy.

Further Reading:

Bensky et al, p. 669
Chen & Chen, p. 1047
Ellis, p. 255

SHENG MAI SAN

Author: Lǐ Gǎo (李杲) *aka* Lǐ Dōng-Yuán (李东垣)
Source: *Nèi Wài Shāng Biàn Huò Lùn* (内外伤辨惑论), 1247
Literal: "Internal External Injury, Clarify False-Notions Discussion"

Availability:

Ginseng & Ophiopogon Formula (EG)
Great Pulse Teapills (PF)
Sheng Mai Formula (GF)
Sheng Mai San (BP)

Ingredients: (from Golden Flower *"Sheng Mai Formula"*)

rén shēn (人参), Radix Ginseng	37.5 %	AA
mài mén dōng (麦门冬), Radix Ophiopogonis	37.5	AD
wǔ wèi zǐ (五味子), Fructus Schisandrae	25.0	L

Ingredients: (from Plum Flower *"Great Pulse Teapills"*)

dǎng shēn (党参), Radix Codonopsis	50.2 %	AA
mài mén dōng (麦门冬), Radix Ophiopogonis	33.3	AD
wǔ wèi zǐ (五味子), Fructus Schisandrae	16.5	L

Tonifies qi, tonifies and astringes yin, generates fluid, benefits lung and heart, stops sweating. Use for chronic cough or wheezing due to deficiency of *qi* and *yin,* with accompanying symptoms of fatigue, shortness of breath, dry throat and spontaneous sweating, or for dry cough following fever. Also be used for heart palpitation or arrhythmia due to deficiency of *qi* and *yin,* with accompanying symptoms of anxiety or anxiousness and fatigue. Useful as a geriatric tonic for lung and heart.

Pulse: Thin, weak, possibly rapid, possibly irregular
Tongue: Normal, or pale, or red with a dry coat

Comments: *Sheng Mai San* treats chronic cough and asthma due to a combined deficiency of *qi* and *yin*, or for the symptoms of dry throat and difficulty breathing. Originally, it was developed for patients who were overcome with summer-heat, where the *qi* and *yin* were consumed by excessive sweating. In the 19th century, it was commonly given to patients with tuberculosis, where exogenous and pathogenic factors damaged the *qi* and *yin*. The formula is currently popular in China for weakened heart conditions in the elderly, with symptoms of palpitation or irregularity. It can be given as a general geriatric tonic when deficiency of *qi* and *yin* predominates over deficiency of *yang*.

Rén shēn supports lung and heart *qi*. *Mài mén dōng* moistens lung and heart *yin*, and also clears heat in the heart causing irritability. *Wǔ wèi zǐ* astringes the formula into the lungs and also benefits kidney's ability to root the lungs to inhibit cough. Most manufacturers, including the extract granules from Taiwan, will use *rén shēn*. A few, such as Plum Flower, substitute *dǎng shēn*. For patients with significant deficiency of lung or heart *qi*, *rén shēn* is preferred.

Caution: Discontinue during colds and flu, as tonics tend to drive pathogenic factors into the interior. Not appropriate during fever or heat conditions.

Further Reading:

Bensky et al, p. 328
Chen & Chen, p. 557
Ellis, p. 275

Modern Formulas:

GU BEN WAN

Formula: *gù běn wán* (固本丸), "Secure the Root Pills"
Source: Modern patent medicine

Availability:

Gu Ben Wan (MS, TL)
Replenish The Root Teapills (PF)

Ingredients: (from Minshan's *"Gu Ben Wan"*)

shēng dì huáng (生地黄), Radix Rehmanniae	22.3 %	DC
tiān mén dōng (天门冬), Radix Asparagi	22.2	AD
mài mén dōng (麦门冬), Radix Ophiopogonis	22.2	AD
shú dì huáng (熟地黄), Radix Rehmanniae Praep.	22.2	AB
dǎng shēn (党参), Radix Codonopsis	11.1	AA

Nourishes lung yin, nourishes kidney yin, tonifies qi. Use for deficiency of lung and kidney *yin* causing dry cough, with dryness of the throat, lips and nose, and hoarseness. Useful for chronic deficiency dry cough in AIDS and tuberculosis, as well as chronic illness or with aging. Useful for dryness due to radiation to the throat or lungs, or to lung dryness following the use of steroids for the treatment of asthma. May be useful for autoimmune Sjögren's syndrome.

Pulse: Rapid, thin
Tongue: Red with scanty coat, or geographic or cracked

Comments: This formula addresses chronic dryness of the lungs and mucus membranes of the nose and mouth. Four of the five herbs are strong *yin* tonics (*shēng dì huáng, shú dì huáng, tiān mén dong* and *mài mén dong*), which comprise 89% of the formula. While *mài mén dong* and *tiān mén dong* direct the formula to the lungs, the combined use of *shēng dì huáng* and *shú dì huáng,* making up 44% of the formula, help "secure the root", that is, boost the kidney.

Gu Ben Wan is useful for very dry cough following chronic illness, and also for chronic *yin* deficiency of the mouth, throat and lungs. It may also be helpful in diabetes with symptoms of dryness and thirst.

Caution: The large amount of *dì huáng* (44.5%) can cause loose stools, bloating or nausea in patients with a weak digestive system. Monitor and adjust dosage accordingly.

OTHER FORMULAS APPROPRIATE FOR THIS CHAPTER:

Modern Formulas:

Astragalus 16 (SF)
Ginseng 6 (SF)
Jade Screen Tablets (SF)
Jade Spring (TT)
Lily 14 (SF)
Pseudostellaria 9 (SF)
Tremella 14 (SF)
Tremella and American Ginseng (HC)
Wise Judge (K)

3F. WHEEZING AND DIFFICULT BREATHING
(Asthma)

Classical Formulas:

Bu Fei Tang	*bŭ fèi tāng* (补肺汤)
Ding Chuan Wan	*dìng chuăn wán* (定喘丸)

Modern Formulas:

Ping Chuan Pian	*píng chuăn piàn* (平喘片)
Ping Chuan Wan	*píng chuăn wán* (平喘丸)

Asthma is characterized by wheezing respiration, or labored breathing aggravated by exertion; at times it can appear even during rest. The Chinese name for asthma, *xiào chuăn* (哮喘), translates as "wheezing panting". *Xiào* indicates short, rapid wheezing with a distinctive sound, while *chuăn* refers to panting, the more serious labored breathing where patients cannot lie flat, raising their shoulders and flaring their nostrils during inspiration. Clinically, we can offer two other differentiations in asthma and wheezing presentations. Basically, one type exhibits phlegm, and the other type does not.

All cases of asthma, a chronic condition, exhibit an underlying weakness of lung, spleen or kidney *qi*, and formulas typically contain herbs that tonify *qi*. Tonifying kidney *qi* supports the kidney function of "rooting the lungs" which facilitates a strong descent of the diaphragm, thereby maximizing air volume during inhalation.

These formulas can be used alone, or combined with other formulas. When there is phlegm, formulas from *Chapter 3B* or *3C* are appropriate. When there is a pronounced deficiency of lung *yin*, combine with formulas from *Chapter 3E*. With kidney *yang* or *jing* deficiency, combine with formulas from Chapter 17B.

Some cases of asthma are triggered by exposure to pathogenic wind-cold, and formulas from *Chapter 1A* that dispel wind and warm the lung are necessary.

In modern clinical practice, food allergies can contribute to asthma, and significant benefit may be gained by eliminating dairy and gluten grains (wheat, rye, barley and sometimes oats). Other allergen triggers include molds, fungus, animal hair, and dust mites. Supportive work with *qi* and *wei* formulas, or single herb tonics such as *huáng qí* (黄芪, Radix Astragali) and *dōng chóng xià căo* (冬虫夏草, Cordyceps), can be helpful in building resistance to exogenous irritants. These are found in *Chapters 16A, 18A* and *18B.*

The treatment of chronic asthma can be prolonged. The practitioner and patient should make effort to persevere through many months, or even years, but total cure is probable. The alternative – long term use of inhaled or ingested pharmaceutical steroids – can damage or inhibit the function of the adrenal glands, causing prolonged dependence on steroid medication.

Classical Formulas:

BU FEI TANG

Formula: *bǔ fèi tāng* (补肺汤), "Tonify Lung Decoction"
Author: Lǐ Zhòng-Nán (李仲南)
Source: *Yông Lèi Qián Fāng* (永类钤方), 1331
Literal: "Eternal Categories Inscribed Formulas"

Availability:

Bu Fei Teapills (PF)
Ginseng & Aster Combination (EG)
* Restore The Lung Formula (GF)

Ingredients: (from the standardized *"Ginseng & Aster Combination"*)

sāng bái pí (桑白皮), Cortex Mori	25.0 %	CC
shú dì huáng (熟地黄), Radix Rehmanniae Praep.	25.0	AB
huáng qí (黄芪), Radix Astragali	12.5	AA
rén shēn (人参), Radix Ginseng	12.5	AA
zǐ wǎn (紫菀), Radix/Rhizoma Asteris	12.5	CC
wǔ wèi zǐ (五味子), Fructus Schisandrae	12.5	L

Ingredients: (from Plum Flower "*Bu Fei Teapills*")

huáng qí (黄芪), Radix Astragali	28.5 %	AA
shú dì huáng (熟地黄), Radix Rehmanniae Praep.	28.5	AB
sāng bái pí (桑白皮), Cortex Mori	13.9	CC
zǐ wǎn (紫菀), Radix/Rhizoma Asteris	11.0	CC
míng dǎng shēn (明党参), Radix Changii	8.0	CB
wǔ wèi zǐ (五味子), Fructus Schisandrae	6.9	L
rén shēn (人参), Radix Ginseng	3.2	AA

Tonifies lung qi, nourishes lung yin, calms wheezing, relieves cough. Use for deficiency of lung *qi* causing shortness of breath or wheezing, habitual weak cough, frail constitution, tendency to common cold, difficult to expectorate phlegm, light sweating, pale complexion, low voice, and poor appetite. Symptoms can be aggravated by exertion. Useful in asthma, as well as lung deficiency with chronic illness.

Pulse: Weak, thin
Tongue: Normal, or pale with thin coat

Comments: *Bu Fei Tang* is a tonic for lung *qi* and *yin* in the absence of phlegm accumulation. It can act as a lung tonic for weakened patients in chronic illness, those with chronic asthma aggravated by exertion, or those with a frail constitution including the aged. *Huáng qí* and *rén shēn* are the chief herbs, tonifying *qi; sāng bái pí* and *zǐ wǎn* control cough and descend lung *qi; shú dì huáng* supports the *yin* and constitutional *jing;* and *wǔ wèi zǐ* astringes the formula into the lung and stabilizes lung *qi*.

Further Reading:

Bensky et al, p. 331
Chen & Chen, p. 560
Ellis, p. 31

DING CHUAN WAN

Formula: *dìng chuǎn wán* (定喘丸), "Relieve Panting Pill"
Author: Zhāng Shí-Chè (张时彻)
Source: *Shè Shēng Zhòng Miào Fāng* (摄生众妙方)
"Conserve Life Multitude (of) Marvelous Formulas", 1550

Availability:

Clear Mountain Air (PF)
Ding Chuan Wan (HT, TL)
Mahuang & Ginkgo Combination (EG)
* Clear Air (HC)

Ingredients: (from the standardized *"Mahuang & Ginkgo Combination"*)

bái guǒ (白果), Semen Ginkgo	20.0 %	L
má huáng (麻黄), Herba Ephedrae	13.3	BA
kuǎn dōng huā (款冬花), Flos Tussilaginis Farfarae	13.3	CC
sāng bái pí (桑白皮), Cortex Mori	13.3	CC
bàn xià (半夏), Rhizoma Pinelliae	13.3	CA
zǐ sū zǐ (紫苏子), Fructus Perillae	8.3	CC
xìng rén (杏仁), Semen Armeniacae Amarum	6.7	CC
huáng qín (黄芩), Radix Scutellariae	6.7	DB
gān cǎo (甘草), Radix Glycyrrhizae	5.1	AA

Ingredients: (from Herbal Times *"Ding Chuan Wan"*)

sāng bái pí (桑白皮), Cortex Mori	16.8 %	CC
bǎi bù (百部), Radix Stemonae	11.1	CC
huáng qín (黄芩), Radix Scutellariae	11.1	DB
xìng rén (杏仁), Semen Armeniacae Amarum	11.1	CC
zǐ wǎn (紫菀), Radix/Rhizoma Asteris	11.1	CC
bái guǒ (白果), Semen Ginkgo	8.3	L
bàn xià (半夏), Rhizoma Pinelliae	8.3	CA
jié gěng (桔梗), Radix Platycodonis	8.3	CA
zǐ sū zǐ (紫苏子), Fructus Perillae	8.3	CC
gān cǎo (甘草), Radix Glycyrrhizae	5.6	AA

Ingredients: (from Plum Flower *"Clear Mountain Air"*)

bái guǒ (白果), Semen Ginkgo	12.3 %	L
sāng bái pí (桑白皮), Cortex Mori	12.3	CC
jié gěng (桔梗), Radix Platycodonis	10.1	CA
zǐ sū zǐ (紫苏子), Fructus Perillae	10.1	CC
xìng rén (杏仁), Semen Armeniacae Amarum	10.1	CC
huáng qín (黄芩), Radix Scutellariae	10.1	DB
bàn xià (半夏), Rhizoma Pinelliae	10.1	CA
gān cǎo (甘草), Radix Glycyrrhizae	8.3	AA
bǎi bù (百部), Radix Stemonae	8.3	CC
zǐ wǎn (紫菀), Radix/Rhizoma Asteris	8.3	CC

Dispels wind, clears heat, dissolves phlegm, tonifies lung qi, diffuses and descends lung qi, calms panting, relieves cough. Use for asthmatic conditions marked by cough, wheezing or labored breathing, bronchial spasm and productive phlegm. Applicable for asthma, bronchitis, or emphysema with internal phlegm-heat aggravated by pathogenic wind.

Pulse: Slippery, may be rapid; may be tight in the superficial aspect
Tongue: White or yellow coat

Comments: This formula addresses asthma marked by cough with evidence of phlegm-damp, and is also applicable in cough with phlegm found in bronchitis and emphysema. The original formula was created for patients with accumulation of internal phlegm-heat who are then struck by exposure to wind-cold, leading to cough. It is useful for someone fighting a cough, who is then attacked by exogenous wind, aggravating the original cough.

Bu Fei Tang depended on *má huáng* as the chief herb to clear wind-cold and relax bronchial spasm, but this ingredient is now unavailable due to regulatory concerns. *Bái guǒ* dissolves phlegm and descends lung *qi* in order to control wheezing. It also roots the diaphragm by the kidney in order to open up breathing. Other herbs descend lung *qi*, eliminate phlegm, and stop cough.

The versions by Herbal Times and Plum Flower use the same formula, but with different ingredient percentages. Compared to the standardized prescription, they both remove *má huáng* and *kuǎn dōng huā*, and add *bǎi bù, zǐ wǎn* and *jié gěng*.

Further Reading:

Bensky et al, p. 540
Chen & Chen, 845
Ellis, p. 82

Modern Formulas:

PING CHUAN PIAN

Formula: *píng chuǎn piàn* (平喘片), "Calm Panting Tablet"
Source: Modern patent medicine

Availability:

Ping Chuan Pian (PF, PM, PIM)
Ping Chuan Wan (PM)

Ingredients: (from Plum Flower *"Ping Chuan Pian"*)

dǎng shēn (党参), Radix Codonopsis	15. %	AA
xìng rén (杏仁), Semen Armeniacae Amarum	15	CC
sāng bái pí (桑白皮), Cortex Mori	10	CC
wǔ zhǐ máo táo (五指毛桃), Radix Ficus Simplicissima	10	FA
mán hú tuí zǐ (蔓胡颓子), Fructus Elaeagni Glabrae	10	FA
gān cǎo (甘草), Radix Glycyrrhizae	10	AA
chén pí (陈皮), Pericarpium Citri Reticulatae	8	G
bái qián (白前), Radix/Rhizoma Cynanchi Stauntonii	8	CA
gé jiè (蛤蚧), Gecko	5	AC
dōng chóng xià cǎo (冬虫夏草), Cordyceps	5	AC
méng shí (礞石), Lapis	4	CB

Tonifies lung qi, tonifies kidney qi and yang, relieves cough. Use for asthma or labored breathing with cough due to underlying deficiencies of kidney and lung *qi,* without much accumulation of phlegm. Cough or shortness of breath is often worse following exertion.

Pulse: Weak, deep, thin
Tongue: Pale, white coat

Comments: The original *Ping Chuan Pian* appeared as the patent medicine *Ping Chuan Wan* from Sing-Kyn Drug House in Guangzhou; here, Plum Flower and Pine Mountain reproduce the formula as *Ping Chuan Pian*. It is essentially a lung-tonifying formula, using herbs such as *dǎng shēn*, *gé jiè*, and *dōng chóng xià cǎo* for 25% of the prescription. The formula contains two uncommon herbs, *wǔ zhǐ máo táo* and *mán hú tuí zǐ*, which help enhance lung function by descending lung *qi*. Combing with *xìng rén* and *sāng bái pí*, a total of 45% of the ingredients inhibits coughs and descends lung *qi.* The formula is used in asthma due to chronic deficiency without phlegm.

PING CHUAN WAN

Formula: *píng chuǎn wán* (平喘丸), "Calm Panting Pill"
Source: Modern patent medicine

Availability:

Ping Chuan Wan (HT)

Ingredients: (from Herbal Times *"Ping Chuan Wan"*)

dì lóng (地龙), Pheretima (Lumbricus)	11.9 %	O
wǔ wèi zǐ (五味子), Fructus Schisandrae	9.8	L
bái guǒ (白果), Semen Ginkgo	9.6	L
bàn xià (半夏), Rhizoma Pinelliae	7.2	CA
huáng qín (黄芩), Radix Scutellariae	7.2	DB
zhǐ shí (枳实), Fructus Aurantii Immaturus	7.2	G
shí gāo (石膏), Gypsum Fibrosum	5.6	DA
bái jiè zǐ (白芥子), Semen Sinapis	4.8	CA
lái fú zǐ (莱菔子), Semen Raphani	4.8	H
qián hú (前胡), Radix Peucedani	4.8	CA
qīng pí (青皮), Pericarpium Citri Reticulatae Viride	4.8	G
tíng lì zǐ (葶苈子), Semen Lepidii; Semen Descurainiae	4.8	CB
xìng rén (杏仁), Semen Armeniacae Amarum	4.8	CC
zǐ sū zǐ (紫苏子), Fructus Perillae	4.8	CC
gān cǎo (甘草), Radix Glycyrrhizae	2.4	AA
jié gěng (桔梗), Radix Platycodonis	2.4	CA
kuǎn dōng huā (款冬花), Flos Tussilaginis Farfarae	2.4	CC
shēng jiāng (生姜), Rhizoma Zingiberis Recens	0.7	BA

Clears heat, dispels wind-cold, dissolves phlegm, diffuses the lung and descends lung qi, calms wheezing. Use for asthma, difficult breathing, or wheezing aggravated by pathogenic wind-cold, or wind-cold transforming into heat, with accumulation of phlegm-heat or phlegm-fluid in the lung. Symptoms include wheezing, feelings of chest constriction, and cough with expectoration of frothy phlegm. Useful for emphysema and phlegm cough due to common cold.

Pulse: Weak, soft or slippery
Tongue: Pale, with wet white or yellow coat

Comments: Although having a similar same name to *Ping Chuan Pian*, above, this larger formula (17 herbs) addresses cough and wheezing aggravated by accumulation of phlegm-heat or phlegm-fluid. Use of cooling herbs (*huáng qín* and *shí gāo*) addresses heat in the lungs, while phlegm and phlegm-fluid resolving herbs account for 24% of the formula, including *bái jiè zǐ, lái fú zǐ*, and *tíng lì zǐ*. The synergistic effect of *dì long, bái guǒ* and *shí gāo* relaxes bronchial spasm, while other herbs directly relieve cough (*xìng rén, zǐ sū zǐ* and *kuǎn dōng huā*). The formula is preferred for asthma conditions showing damp or phlegm in the lung, and is particularly useful in frothy emphysema.

Caution: *Tíng lì zǐ* is contraindicated during pregnancy.

OTHER FORMULAS APPROPRIATE FOR THIS CHAPTER:

For asthma and wheezing due to phlegm-damp, see Chapter 3C:

Ban Xia Hou Po Tang
Su Zi Jiang Qi Tang
Xing Su San
Chuan Ke Wan

For asthma and wheezing due to deficiency of qi and yin, see Chapter 3E:

Sheng Mai San

For asthma and wheezing due to deficiency of *yang*, asthma formulas can be reinforced with products from Chapter 17B:

Ge Jie Bu Shen Wan / Ge Jie Da Bu Wan

Classical Formulas:

Ma Xing Shi Gan Tang

Great White Lung Clearing Formula (K)
Mahuang & Apricot Seed Combination (EG)
* Bai Xing Shi Gan Teapills (PF)

She Gan Ma Huang Tang

Belamcanda & Mahuang Combination (EG)

Xiao Qing Long Wan

Blue Green Lung Clearing Formula (K)
Minor Blue Dragon Formula (CC)
Minor Bluegreen Dragon Combination (EG)
* Blue Earth Dragon (SF)

Modern Formulas:

Cordyceps 9 (SF)
Ling Zhi Lung Formula (GF)
Minor Blue Perilla (HC)
Perilla Seed Tablets (SF)
Respitrol-Deficient (EV)
Strengthen Lung (CMS)
Wind Pearls (CP)

Also, Cordyceps Products

See Chapter 18B

4. BI SYNDROME
(Arthritis, Rheumatism, Back Pain)

BI SYNDROMES (*bì zhèng,* 痹证) are a group of disorders where joint or muscle pain is the main symptom. They include the medical diagnosis of rheumatism and arthritis, and are also applied to back pain and chronic joint pain following injury. *Bi* means painful-obstruction or blockage; in Chinese medicine it is due to stagnation of *qi* and blood, and may be complicated by damp, heat or cold. The cause often involves exogenous pathogenic factors intruding on an underlying deficiency of *qi*, blood or *yang*. Symptoms include pain, heaviness, numbness, tingling, difficulty of movement, or redness and swelling.

Bi Syndrome formulas are grouped into sub-chapters:

4A. WIND-COLD-DAMP BI
4B. BLOOD STAGNATION BI
4C. DEFICIENCY BI
4D. COLD BI
4E HEAT BI
4F. BACK PAIN AND SCIATICA

WIND-COLD DAMP BI, sometimes called "wandering *bi* syndrome", is characterized by pain that moves around various locations, and is aggravated by damp weather. The accumulation of damp impedes the flow of *qi* and blood, causing muscular and joint numbness, pain, swelling or feelings of heaviness. The pulse is full, and may be floating or slippery. The formulas use warm herbs to dispel wind-damp-cold and herbs to invigorate blood flow.

BLOOD STAGNATION BI is characterized by more severe pain in the joints and muscles, with numbness and poor circulation. Pain tends to be constant and fixed in the same location, and include pain following injury, surgery or degeneration. The tongue is sometimes dark and the pulse is choppy. The formulas rely on herbs that move *qi* and blood, and herbs that break blood stasis. They also use herbs to move wind-cold-dampness. They also use herbs to move wind-cold-dampness. The formulas are clinically useful following injury, and for the elderly who suffer poor blood circulation. Some of the herbal ingredients are contraindicated with Coumadin and other blood-thinners.

DEFICIENCY BI formulas use herbs that move *qi* and invigorate blood, but also address underlying deficiencies by using herbs that tonify *qi*, blood and/or *yang*. The pulse is weak, but may be floating or sunken. The formulas are beneficial in chronic and long-term *bi* syndrome presentations, and can also be used for numbness and tingling due to deficiency, as well as *wei* syndromes (*wěi zhèng,* 痿证), which involve weakness to the point of flaccid paralysis.

COLD BI formulas include herbs that are warming and invigorating, and are particularly useful for painful limbs that are worse in cold weather. In many patients, there may be underlying deficiency of kidney *yang,* and these patterns are often seen in the elderly. Sometimes very hot medicinals are used. The pulse is tight or choppy, and may be weak.

HEAT BI is characterized by red, warm and swollen joints. It includes attack of pathogenic heat or heat-toxins, and can include wind-cold-damp *bi* syndrome that has transformed into heat, or excessively warm constitutions that transform exogenous pathogens to heat. These formulas are also used for inflammatory joint illness such as rheumatoid arthritis or lupus. They are sometimes used for heat conditions resulting from trauma; other formulas can be found in *Chapter 5A.* The pulse is more rapid, and the tongue is red. Cold or cooling herbs are used in the formulas.

4. BI SYNDROME (Arthritis, Rheumatism, Back Pain)

4A. WIND-COLD-DAMP BI SYNDROME

Classical Formulas:

Juan Bi Tang – 1	*juān bì tāng* (蠲痹湯) (1)
Juan Bi Tang – 2	*juān bì tāng* (蠲痹湯) (2)
Shu Jing Huo Xue Tang	*shū jīng huó xuè tāng* (舒经活血汤)

Modern Formulas:

Guan Jie Yan Wan	*guān jié yán wán* (关节炎丸)

WIND-COLD DAMP BI, sometimes called "wandering *bi* syndrome", is characterized by pain that moves around various locations, and is aggravated by damp weather. The accumulation of damp impedes the flow of *qi* and blood, causing muscular and joint numbness, pain, swelling or feelings of heaviness. The pulse is full, and may be floating or slippery. The formulas use warm herbs to dispel wind-damp-cold and herbs to invigorate blood flow.

Classical Formulas:

JUAN BI TANG (1)

Formula: *juān bì tāng* (蠲痹汤), "Remove Blockage Decoction"
Author: Yáng Tán (杨倓)
Source: *Yáng Shì Jiā Cáng Fāng* (杨氏家藏方), 1178
Literal: "Yang Family Depository (of) Formulas"

Availability:

Chianghuo & Turmeric Combination (EG)
Graceful Branches (K)
Juan Bi Tang (BP, HT)
Notopterygium & Turmeric Combination (KP)

Ingredients: (from the standardized *"Notopterygium/Chianghuo & Turmeric Combination"*)

huáng qí (黄芪), Radix Astragali	11.2 %	AA
dāng guī (当归), Radix Angelicae Sinensis	11.1	AB
chì sháo (赤芍), Radix Paeoniae Rubra	11.1	K
qiāng huó (羌活), Radix Notopterygii	11.1	BA
fáng fēng (防风), Radix Saposhnikov./Ledebouriellae	11.1	BA
jiāng huáng (姜黄), Rhizoma Curcumae Longae	11.1	K
gān cǎo (甘草), Radix Glycyrrhizae	11.1	AA
shēng jiāng (生姜), Rhizoma Zingiberis Recens	11.1	BA
dà zǎo (大枣), Fructus Jujubae	11.1	AA

Ingredients: (from Blue Poppy *"Juan Bi Tang"*)

qiāng huó (羌活), Radix Notopterygii	15.8 %	BA
jiāng huáng (姜黄), Rhizoma Curcumae Longae	15.8	K
dāng guī (当归), Radix Angelicae Sinensis	15.8	AB
zhì huáng qí (炙黄芪), Radix Astragali Praep.	15.8	AA
bái sháo (白芍), Radix Paeoniae Alba	15.8	K
fáng fēng (防风), Radix Saposhnikov./Ledebouriellae	15.8	BA
gān cǎo (甘草), Radix Glycyrrhizae	5.2	AA

Disperses wind, removes damp, invigorates blood, boosts qi, nourishes blood, warms the channels and collaterals, relieves pain. Use for wind-damp *bi* syndrome characterized by painful joints, heaviness in the limbs and muscles or numbness. Use in rheumatism, osteoarthritis, bursitis and old injuries made worse in cold and damp conditions. The formula is particularly useful for neck and shoulder pain, or numbness in arms and hands. Helpful in older patients with deficiencies of *qi* and blood.

Pulse: Normal, weak, or slippery
Tongue: Normal, or pale with a white coat

Comments: This formula is effective for chronic joint pain or sore muscles aggravated by wind-cold-damp in patients with pre-existing deficiency of *qi* and blood, and in chronic conditions. Symptoms get worse with lack of movement or changes in the weather. This first version of *Juan Bi Tang* (from author Yang Tan, 1178) is both warming and invigorating, containing herbs for moving blood (*chì sháo* and *jiāng huáng*) and dispelling wind-damp (*qiāng huó* and *fáng fēng*), while boosting *qi* and blood (*huáng qí, dà zăo* and *dāng guī*).

Blue Poppy and Herbal Times follow the original formula. The Taiwan standardized versions add the "helpers" *shēng jiāng* and *dà zăo.*

Caution: *Jiāng huáng* is contraindicated during pregnancy, and for patients taking blood thinners such as Coumadin.

Further Reading:

Bensky et al, p. 756
Chen & Chen, p. 1158
Ellis, p. 177

JUAN BI TANG (2)

Formula: *juān bì tāng* (蠲痹汤), "Remove Blockage Decoction"
Author: Chéng Guó-Péng (程国彭)
Source: *Yī Xué Xīn Wù* (医学心悟), 1732
Literal: "Medical Studies Mind Awakening (eg, Insights)"

Availability:

Clear Channels Teapills (PF)
Juan Bi Formula (GF)
Juan Bi Tang (TZ)

Ingredients: (from Plum Flower *"Clear Channels Teapills"*)

sāng zhī (桑枝), Ramulus Mori	20.0 %	FA
hǎi fēng téng (海风藤), Caulis Piperis Kadsurae	20.0	FA
dāng guī (当归), Radix Angelicae Sinensis	13.0	AB
qiāng huó (羌活), Radix Notopterygii	6.5	BA
dú huó (独活), Radix Angelicae Pubescentis	6.5	FA
qín jiāo (秦艽), Radix Gentianae Macrophyllae	6.5	FA
chuān xiōng (川芎), Rhizoma Ligustici Chuanxiong	6.5	K
mù xiāng (木香), Radix Aucklandiae	6.5	G
guì zhī (桂枝), Ramulus Cinnamomi	6.5	BA
rǔ xiāng (乳香), Olibanum/Boswelliae	5.0	K
zhì gān cǎo (炙甘草), Radix Glycyrrhizae Praep	3.0	AA

Ingredients: (from Golden Flower *"Juan Bi Formula"*)

qiāng huó (羌活), Radix Notopterygii	14.8 %	BA
jiāng huáng (姜黄), Rhizoma Curcumae Longae	14.8	K
sāng zhī (桑枝), Ramulus Mori	14.8	FA
dāng guī (当归), Radix Angelicae Sinensis	14.8	AB
wēi líng xiān (威灵仙), Radix/Rhizoma Clematidis	14.8	FA
dú huó (独活), Radix Angelicae Pubescentis	4.9	FA
qín jiāo (秦艽), Radix Gentianae Macrophyllae	4.9	FA
rǔ xiāng (乳香), Olibanum	3.9	K
mù xiāng (木香), Radix Aucklandiae	3.9	G
chuān xiōng (川芎), Rhizoma Ligustici Chuanxiong	3.4	K
guì zhī (桂枝), Ramulus Cinnamomi	2.5	BA
zhì gān cǎo (炙甘草), Radix Glycyrrhizae Praep.	2.5	AA

Disperses wind, removes damp, invigorates blood and breaks stasis, nourishes blood, warms the channels and collaterals, relieves pain. Use for wind-cold-damp *bi* syndromes characterized by painful joints, heaviness in the limbs and muscles or numbness. Use in rheumatism, osteoarthritis, bursitis and old injuries marked by pain. Helpful for recent onset conditions or in acute aggravation due to cold and damp.

Pulse: Normal, excess, or slippery, may be slow
Tongue: Normal, or with a thick white coat

Comments: The version of *Juan Bi Tang* from Cheng Guo-Peng, 1732, is useful for joint pain or sore muscles due to wind-cold damp in patients with a recent onset, and more acute in nature. Lacking the *qi* tonics of the first *Juan Bi Tang* formula (above), this version more aggressively disperses wind and damp (*sāng zhī, qiāng huó, dú huó, qín jiāo*), while moving blood and breaking stasis (*chuān xiōng, rǔ xiāng*), dispersing cold and warming the channels (*hǎi fēng téng, guì zhī*).

The version from Golden Flower follows the same formula as Plum Flower, except that it removes *hǎi fēng téng* and adds *jiāng huáng* and *wēi líng xiān*.

Caution: *Rǔ xiāng* is contraindicated during pregnancy, and for patients on blood thinners including Coumadin.

Further Reading:

Bensky et al, p. 757
Chen & Chen, p. 1160

SHU JING HUO XUE TANG

Formula: *shū jīng huó xuè tāng* (舒经活血汤)
"Dredge Channels, Invigorate Blood Decoction"

Author: Gōng Tíng-Xián (龚廷贤)

Source: *Wàn Bìng Huí Chūn* (万病回春), 1587
Literal: "Thousand Diseases Returned to Spring (eg, Restored to Life)"

Availability:

Clematis & Stephania Combination (EG)
Course And Quicken Formula (GF)
Mobility 2 (HC)
Shu Jing Huo Xue Wan (HT)

Ingredients: (from the standardized *"Clematis & Stephania Combination"*)

shēng jiāng (生姜), Rhizoma Zingiberis Recens	11.0 %	BA
bái sháo (白芍), Radix Paeoniae Alba	9.1	AB
shēng dì huáng (生地黄), Radix Rehmanniae	7.3	DC
cāng zhú (苍术), Rhizoma Atractylodis	7.3	FB
chén pí (陈皮), Pericarpium Citri Reticulatae	7.3	G
táo rén (桃仁), Semen Persicae	7.3	K
dāng guī (当归), Radix Angelicae Sinensis	7.3	AB
fáng fēng (防风), Radix Saposhnikov./Ledebouriellae	5.7	BA
huái niú xī (怀牛膝), Radix Achyranthis Bidentatae	7.3	K
wēi líng xiān (威灵仙), Radix/Rhizoma Clematidis	7.3	FA
fú líng (茯苓), Poria	3.6	FC
lóng dǎn cǎo (龙胆草), Radix/Rhizoma Gentianae	3.6	DA
qiāng huó (羌活), Radix Notopterygii	3.6	BA
fáng fēng (防风), Radix Saposhnikoviae/Ledebouriella	3.6	BA
chuān xiōng (川芎), Rhizoma Ligustici Chuanxiong	3.6	K
hàn fáng jǐ (汉防己), Radix Stephaniae Tetrandrae	3.6	FC
bái zhǐ (白芷), Radix Angelicae Dahuricae	3.6	BA
gān cǎo (甘草), Radix Glycyrrhizae	3.6	AA

Ingredients: (from Herbal Times *"Shu Jing Huo Xue Wan"*)

bái zhú (白术), Rhizoma Atractylodis Macrocephalae	7.5 %	AA
chì sháo (赤芍), Radix Paeoniae Rubra	7.5	K
chuān xiōng (川芎), Rhizoma Ligustici Chuanxiong	7.5	K
dāng guī (当归), Radix Angelicae Sinensis	7.5	AB

shú dì huáng (熟地黄), Radix Rehmanniae Praep.	7.5	AB
fú líng (茯苓), Poria	7.5	FC
chén pí (陈皮), Pericarpium Citri Reticulatae	5.7	G
dú huó (独活), Radix Angelicae Pubescentis	5.7	FA
fáng fēng (防风), Radix Saposhnikoviae/Ledebouriella	5.7	BA
huái niú xī (怀牛膝), Radix Achyranthis Bidentatae	5.7	K
jī xuè téng (鸡血藤), Caulis Spatholobi/Millettiae	5.7	K
lóng dǎn cǎo (龙胆草), Radix/Rhizoma Gentianae	5.7	DA
qiāng huó (羌活), Radix Notopterygii	5.7	BA
shēng jiāng (生姜), Rhizoma Zingiberis Recens	5.7	BA
gān cǎo (甘草), Radix Glycyrrhizae	5.6	AA
bái zhǐ (白芷), Radix Angelicae Dahuricae	3.8	BA

Disperses wind-cold, removes damp, invigorates blood, strengthens tendon and bone, relieves pain. Use for excess patterns of wind-cold damp *bi* syndrome with blood stagnation causing painful joints on the upper or lower limbs, slow gait, stiff knees, and weak lower back. Use in arthritis, rheumatism, and also joint pain following injury.

Pulse: Excess, wiry or choppy
Tongue: Dark

Comments: This large prescription (18 herbs) addresses excess patterns of wind-damp *bi* syndrome complicated by blood stagnation. Symptoms include joint pain, as well as poor circulation or soreness in the muscles. *Huái niú xī* helps take the formula to the knees. The use of blood-invigorating herbs allows the formula to have a stronger effect.

The Herbal Times version changes the original formula by removing *táo rén, wēi líng xiān,* and *fáng jǐ*, and adding *dú huó* and *jī xuè téng*.

Caution: The herbs *táo rén* in the standardized version and *jī xuè téng* in the Herbal Times version are contraindicated during pregnancy, and for patients taking blood thinners such as Coumadin.

Further Reading:

Bensky et al, p. 571
Chen & Chen, p. 1169
Ellis, p. 288

Modern Formulas:

GUAN JIE YAN WAN

Formula: *guān jié yán wán* (关节炎丸), "Close-Down Joint Inflammation Pills"
Source: Modern patent medicine

Availability:

Guan Jie Yan Wan (HT, PM)
Joint Inflammation Teapills (PF)

Ingredients: (from Jianming Medical Works, Changzhou "Guan Jie Yan Wan")

hǎi tóng pí (海桐皮), Cortex Erythrinae	23.2 %	FA
cāng zhú (苍术), Rhizoma Atractylodis	18.8	FB
yì yǐ rén (薏苡仁), Semen Coicis	18.8	FB
hàn fáng jǐ (汉防己), Radix Stephaniae Tetrandrae	13.3	FC
qín jiāo (秦艽), Radix Gentianae Macrophyllae	6.5	FA
guì zhī (桂枝), Ramulus Cinnamomi	6.5	BA
huái niú xī (怀牛膝), Radix Achyranthis Bidentatae	6.5	K
dú huó (独活), Radix Angelicae Pubescentis	3.2	FA
gān jiāng (干姜), Rhizoma Zingiberis	3.2	E

Ingredients: (from Plum Flower *"Joint Inflammation Teapills"*)

yì yǐ rén (薏苡仁), Semen Coicis	20.9 %	FB
hàn fáng jǐ (汉防己), Radix Stephaniae Tetrandrae	13.9	FC
cāng zhú (苍术), Rhizoma Atractylodis	9.7	FB
hǎi tóng pí (海桐皮), Cortex Erythrinae	9.7	FA
guì zhī (桂枝), Ramulus Cinnamomi	7.7	BA
huái niú xī (怀牛膝), Radix Achyranthis Bidentatae	7.0	K
wú zhū yú (吴茱萸), Fructus Evodiae	7.0	E
qín jiāo (秦艽), Radix Gentianae Macrophyllae	7.0	FA
xiāng jiā pí (香加皮), Cortex Periplocae	6.9	FA
huáng qín (黄芩), Radix Scutellariae	3.5	DB
dú huó (独活), Radix Angelicae Pubescentis	3.5	FA
shēng jiāng (生姜), Rhizoma Zingiberis Recens	3.2	BA

Ingredients: (from Herbal Times, *"Guan Jie Yan Wan"*)

shēng jiāng (生姜), Rhizoma Zingiberis Recens	16.3 %	BA
cāng zhú (苍术), Rhizoma Atractylodis	15.3	FB

yì yǐ rén (薏苡仁), Semen Coicis	15.3	FC
sāng zhī (桑枝), Ramulus Mori	10.2	FA
hǎi tóng pí (海桐皮), Cortex Erythrinae	7.2	FA
guì zhī (桂枝), Ramulus Cinnamomi	5.1	BA
hǔ zhàng (虎杖), Rhizoma Polygoni Cuspidati	5.1	K
huái niú xī (怀牛膝), Radix Achyranthis Bidentatae	5.1	K
huáng qín (黄芩), Radix Scutellariae	5.1	DB
qín jiāo (秦艽), Radix Gentianae Macrophyllae	5.1	FA
dú huó (独活), Radix Angelicae Pubescentis	2.6	FA
jiāng huáng (姜黄), Rhizoma Curcumae Longae	2.6	K
xiāng rú (香薷), Herba Elsholtzia splendens	2.6	DF
hǎi fēng téng (海风藤), Caulis Piperis Kadsurae	1.2	FA
qiān nián jiàn (千年健), Rhizoma Homalomenae	1.2	FA

Disperses wind, removes damp, opens the channels and collaterals, warms the channels and collaterals, relieves pain. Use for wind-damp *bi* syndromes characterized by painful joints with swelling, especially in the knees or ankles. Also useful for a weak or sore lower back, sciatic pain, rheumatism and arthritis.

Pulse: Normal, wiry or slippery
Tongue: Normal, or slightly swollen

Comments: This formula is indicated for both hot and cold presentations of joint pain, particularly with puffiness or swelling, especially in the knees. The patent medicine is available in Chinatown pharmacies; GMP versions are available from Plum Flower and Herbal Times.

All three versions contain herbs that dispel wind-damp swelling and reduce inflammation. The original formula, from Jianming Medical Works patent medicine, contains 9 herbs. The Plum Flower formula (12 herbs) more closely resembles the original, using 8 of the original 9 herbs in the patent medicine. By combining *yì yǐ rén, fáng jǐ,* and *huái niú xī* for 42% of the formula, it particularly addresses swelling in the knees. It also adds in *xiāng jiā pí,* an infrequently used herb to dispel wind-damp.

The Herbal Times version (15 herbs) uses 7 of the original herbs, adding *hǔ zhàng* and *jiāng huáng* to move blood and reduce inflammation, and 3 uncommon herbs that enhance the dispelling of wind-damp: *xiāng rú, hǎi fēng téng* and *qiān nián jiàn.*

Caution: *Huái niú xī, jiāng huáng* and *yì yǐ rén* are contraindicated during pregnancy. *Jiāng huáng* is contraindicated for patients taking blood thinners such as Coumadin.

OTHER PRODUCTS APPROPRIATE FOR THIS CATEGORY:

Classical Formulas:

Fang Ji Huang Qi Tang

See Chapter 12

Gui Zhi Shao Yao Zhi Mu Tang

Cinnamon & Anemarrhena Combination (EG)
Clear Channels (K)

Modern Formulas:

AC-Q (HC)
Chase Wind, Penetrate Bone Formula (GF)
Chiang-Huo 13 (SF)
Drynaria 12 (SF)
Flex-CD (EV)
Meridian Comfort (K)
Mobility 3 (HC)

4B. BLOOD STAGNATION BI SYNDROME

Classical Formulas:

Shen Tong Zhu Yu Tang *shēn tòng zhú yū tāng* (身痛逐瘀丸)

Modern Formulas:

Zhong Guo Tong Xue Wan (China Tung Hsueh Pills)
zhōng guó tōng xuè wán (中国通血丸)

BLOOD STAGNATION BI is characterized by more severe pain in the joints and muscles, with numbness and poor circulation. Pain tends to be constant and fixed in the same location, and include pain following injury, surgery or degeneration. The tongue is dark and the pulse may be choppy. The formulas rely on herbs that move *qi* and blood, and herbs that break blood stasis. They also use herbs to move wind-cold-dampness. The formulas are clinically useful following injury, and for the elderly who suffer poor blood circulation. Some of the ingredients are contraindicated with Coumadin and other blood-thinners.

Classical Formulas:

SHEN TONG ZHU YU TANG

Formula: *shēn tòng zhú yū tāng* (身痛逐瘀丸)
"Body Pain Expel Stasis Decoction"
Author: Wáng Qīng-Rèn (王清任)
Source: *Yī Lín Gǎi Cuò* (医林改错), 1830
Literal: "Physicians' Circle, Correction (of) Errors"

Availability:

Cnidium & Notopterygium Combination (EG)
Great Invigorator Teapills (PF)
Ligusticum & Notopterygium Combination (KP)
Meridian Passage (K)
Shen Tong Zhu Yu Wan (HT)
* Sappan 12 (SF)

Ingredients: (from the standardized *"Ligusticum/Cnidium & Notopterygium Combination"*)

dāng guī (当归), Radix Angelicae Sinensis	12. %	AB
táo rén (桃仁), Semen Persicae	12	K
chuān niú xī (川牛膝), Radix Cyathulae	12	K
hóng huā (红花), Flos Carthami	12	K
gān cǎo (甘草), Radix Glycyrrhizae	8	AA
dì lóng (地龙), Pheretima/Lumbricus	8	O
mò yào (没药), Myrrha	8	K
chuān xiōng (川芎), Rhizoma Ligustici Chuanxiong	8	K
wǔ líng zhī (五灵脂), Faeces Trogopterori	8	K
qiāng huó (羌活), Radix Notopterygii	4	BA
qín jiāo (秦艽), Radix Gentianae Macrophyllae	4	FA
xiāng fù (香附), Rhizoma Cyperi	4	G

Ingredients: (from Herbal Times *"Shen Tong Zhu Yu Wan"* and Plum Flower "Great Invigorator Teapills")

dāng guī (当归), Radix Angelicae Sinensis	12. %	AB
táo rén (桃仁), Semen Persicae	12	K
chuān niú xī (川牛膝), Radix Cyathulae	12	K
hóng huā (红花), Flos Carthami	12	K

gān cǎo (甘草), Radix Glycyrrhizae	8	AA
dì lóng (地龙), Pheretima/Lumbricus	8	O
mò yào (没药), Myrrha	8	K
chuān xiōng (川芎), Rhizoma Ligustici Chuanxiong	8	K
wǔ líng zhī (五灵脂), Faeces Trogopterori	8	K
qiāng huó (羌活), Radix Notopterygii	4	BA
qín jiāo (秦艽), Radix Gentianae Macrophyllae	4	FA
xiāng fù (香附), Rhizoma Cyperi	4	G

Invigorates blood, expels blood stasis, opens the channels and collaterals, relieves pain. Use for stasis of *qi* and blood causing painful joints and limbs, or causing lower back pain, or general pain in the whole body. Use for *bi* syndromes due to blood stasis following invasion of wind-cold-dampness, or following injury. Effective for chronic deep pain in the limbs causing muscle aching, numbness and tingling. Use in arthritis, rheumatism and joint or muscle pain following trauma.

Pulse: Wiry or choppy; deep
Tongue: Dark, or dark spot

Comments: *Shen Tong Zhu Yu Tang* treats *bi* syndrome due to blood stasis; it is authored by Wang Qing-Ren, the 19th century master of blood stasis formulae. These cases exhibit stubborn or chronic fixed pain, and are often due to trauma or degeneration, including neck, spine, shoulder or hip pain.

The formula combines blood stasis breaking herbs (*táo rén, mò yào* and *wǔ líng zhī*) with blood moving herbs (*dāng guī, hóng huā, niú xī* and *chuān xiōng*), comprising 72% of the formula. *Qiāng huó* and *qín jiāo* dispel wind-dampness, allowing the formula to be used in *bi* syndrome.

In both the Herbal Times and Plum Flower versions, *wǔ líng zhī* has been removed.

Caution: Due to the inclusion of *táo rén, hóng huā, wǔ líng zhī, chuān niú* xī and *mò yào,* this formula is prohibited during pregnancy, and also when a patient is on blood thinners such as Coumadin.

Further Reading:

Bensky et al, p. 568
Chen & Chen, p. 893
Ellis, p. 268

Modern Formulas:

ZHONG GUO TONG XUE WAN
CHINA TUNG HSUEH PILLS

Formula: *zhōng guó tōng xuè wán* (中国通血丸), "China Unblock Blood Pills"
Source: Modern patent medicine

Availability:

China Tung Hsueh Pills (PM, PF)

Ingredients: (from Plum Flower *"China Tung Hsueh Pills"*)

dāng guī (当归), Radix Angelicae Sinensis	15. %	AB
rŭ xiāng (乳香), Olibanum/Boswelliae	10	K
mò yào (没药), Myrrha	10	K
tŭ mù xiāng (土木香), Radix Inulae	10	G
dān shen (丹参), Radix/Rhiz. Salviae Miltiorrhizae	10	K
ròu guì (肉桂), Cortex Cinnamomi	10	E
shú dì huáng (熟地黄), Radix Rehmanniae Praep.	10	AB
xù duàn (续断), Radix Dipsaci	10	K
xuè jié (血竭), Sanguis Draconis	5	K
yán hú suŏ (延胡索), Rhizoma Corydalis	5	K
ān xī xiāng (安息香), Benzoinum (Styrax)	5	R

Moves blood and dispels stasis, tonifies blood, benefits kidney and liver to strengthen tendon and bone. Use for poor circulation of *qi* and blood in the lumbar region, causing lumbar stiffness or weakness, joint pain, or cold or numb limbs. Useful in degenerative joints including spine, hip and knees. It can be used for acute trauma with swelling or post-traumatic swelling, and also other blood stasis conditions, such as arthrosclerosis and swelling due to thrombi.

Pulse: Wiry or choppy; deep
Tongue: Dark, or dark spots

Comments: This formula is effective for pain due to blood stasis and obstructed channels. It is used for lower back pain, painful rheumatism or arthritis, pain due to old injuries, or joint and spine degeneration. These formulas can be pricey.

Caution: Due to the inclusion of *ròu guì, rŭ xiāng, mò yào* and *xuè jié,* this formula is prohibited during pregnancy, and also when a patient is on blood thinners such as Coumadin.

OTHER FORMULAS APPROPRIATE FOR THIS CATEGORY:

Classical Formulas:

Bu Yang Huan Wu Wan

See Chapter 4C

Shu Jing Huo Xue Tang

See Chapter 4A

Modern Formulas:

Bone & Sinew Formula (GF)
Bonekinder (GC)
Channel Flow (HC)
Feng Shi Xiao Tong Wan (GC, TL)
Huo Xue Tong Mai Wan (GC, TL)
Invigorate The Collaterals (K)

4. BI SYNDROME (Arthritis, Rheumatism, Back Pain)

4C. DEFICIENCY BI SYNDROME

Classical Formulas:

Bu Yang Huan Wu Tang *bǔ yáng huán wǔ tāng* (补阳还五丸)
Huang Qi Gui Zhi Wu Wu Tang *huáng qí guì zhī wǔ wù tāng* (黄芪桂枝五物)
San Bi Tang *sān bì tāng* (三痹汤)

Modern Formulas:

Fu Fang Shou Wu Wan (Shou Wu Wan Compound) *fù fāng shǒu wū wán* (复方首乌丸)

DEFICIENCY BI formulas use herbs that move *qi* and invigorate blood, but also address underlying deficiencies by using herbs that tonify *qi*, blood and/or *yang*. The pulse is weak, but may be floating or sunken. The formulas are beneficial in chronic and long-term bi syndrome presentations, and can also be used for numbness and tingling due to deficiency, as well as *wei* syndromes (*wěi zhèng*, 痿证), which involve weakness to the point of flaccid paralysis.

Classical Formulas:

BU YANG HUAN WU TANG

Formula: *bǔ yáng huán wǔ tāng* (补阳还五湯)
"Tonify *Yang*, Return Five (50%) Decoction"
Author: Wáng Qīng-Rèn (王清任)
Source: *Yī Lín Gǎi Cuò* (医林改错), 1830
Literal: "Physicians Circle Correction (of) Errors"

Availability:

Astragalus & Peony Combination (EG)
Bu Yang Huan Wu Tang (BP)
Bu Yang Huan Wu Wan (HT, TL)
Great Yang Restoration Teapills (PF)

Ingredients: (from Plum Flower *"Great Yang Restoration Teapills"* and the standardized "*Astragalus & Peony Combination*")

huáng qí (黄芪), Radix Astragali	83.2 %	AA
chì sháo (赤芍), Radix Paeoniae Rubra	4.2	K
dāng guī (当归), Radix Angelicae Sinensis Wei	4.2	AB
chuān xiōng (川芎), Rhizoma Ligustici Chuanxiong	2.1	K
táo rén (桃仁), Semen Persicae	2.1	K
hóng huā (红花), Flos Carthami	2.1	K
dì lóng (地龙), Pheretima/Lumbricus	2.1	O

Ingredients: (from Herbal Times "*Bu Yang Huan Wu Wan*")

huáng qí (黄芪), Radix Astragali	23. %	AA
chì sháo (赤芍), Radix Paeoniae Rubra	14	K
dāng guī (当归), Radix Angelicae Sinensis	14	AB
chuān xiōng (川芎), Rhizoma Ligustici Chuanxiong	14	K
táo rén (桃仁), Semen Persicae	13	K
hóng huā (红花), Flos Carthami	13	K
dì lóng (地龙), Pheretima/Lumbricus	9	O

Tonifies qi, nourishes blood, invigorates blood, dredges and opens the channels and collaterals. Use for deficiency of *qi* and blood causing weakness or atrophy of the limbs or muscles, swelling, numbness or tingling. Use for atrophy conditions found in *wei* syndrome, including stroke, paralysis, facial paralysis, or urinary incontinence associated with stroke. Can be used for restless leg syndrome, as well as issues due to spinal stenosis.

Pulse: Weak, wiry or choppy; deep, slow
Tongue: Normal or pale or dark, with a white coat

Comments: This formula has been prescribed for hemiplegia as well as other problems due to stroke, and can also be used for weak and flaccid muscles following illness or with age. It can also be used for reactivated polio, and for muscle weakness due to spinal stenosis.

Using herbs to tonify *wei* and *ying qi*, additional blood movers circulate *qi* and blood through the channels and collaterals. The principal herb *huáng qí* comprises 83% of the classical formula, and is supported with 10% herbs to invigorate blood. For stroke and paralysis, giving large doses of *huáng qí* over a long period of time was perceived to be beneficial. In decoction form, dosages of 60-100 grams of *huáng qí* were given daily.

The Herbal Times version, containing 54% blood-moving herbs with only 23% *huáng qí*, is more appropriate for weakness and muscle flaccidity when accompanied by pain and swelling. It is useful for post-traumatic injury, progressive muscle weakening, and restless leg syndrome.

Lumbricus *dì long*, the common earthworm, follows the "law of signatures": giving movement within flaccidity; it activates *qi* in the channels and collaterals.

Combining either version with a strong blood mover (see formulas from *Chapter 4B*) can be used for weakness and flaccidity due to spinal degeneration and stenosis.

Caution: *Hóng huā* and *táo rén* are prohibited during pregnancy, and when a patient is taking pharmaceutical blood thinners, including Coumadin.

Further Reading:

Bensky et al, p. 568
Chen & Chen, p. 905
Ellis, p. 33

HUANG QI GUI ZHI WU WU TANG

Formula: *huáng qí guì zhī wǔ wù tāng* (黄芪桂枝五物汤)
"Astragalus, Cinnamon, Five Substance Decoction"
Author: Zhāng Zhòng-Jǐng (张仲景)
Source: *Jīn Guì Yào Lüè* (金匮要略), 220
Literal: "Golden Cabinet Essential Summary"

Availability:

Astragalus & Cinnamon Twig (EG)
Astragalus Five Combination (EG)
Huang Qi Gui Zhi Wu Wu Wan (HT)

Ingredients: (From Herbal Times *"Huang Qi Gui Zhi Wu Wu Wan"*)

dà zǎo (大枣), Fructus Jujubae	21.7 %	AA
gān jiāng (干姜), Rhizoma Zingiberis	21.7	BA
huáng qí (黄芪), Radix Astragali	21.7	AA
bái sháo (白芍), Radix Paeoniae Alba	17.4	AB
guì zhī (桂枝), Ramulus Cinnamomi	17.4	BA

Tonifies wei qi, dispels wind, warms the channels and collaterals, moves blood, unblocks painful obstruction. Use for deficiency *bi* syndrome causing numbness and tingling in the superficial flesh, without pain. Useful in mild conditions and as a *wei qi* tonic. Useful in diabetic neuropathy and restless leg syndrome.

Pulse: Faint, tight or choppy
Tongue: Normal, pale and quivering

Comments: *Huang Qi Gui Zhi Wu Wu Tang* addresses superficial numbness and tingling due to deficiency of *qi* and *wei qi* with wind-cold causing mild obstruction of the blood. It is useful in aged and weaker patients who are sensitive to wind and cold, and for cases of numbness or tingling due to deficiency. It can be used as a general tonic for *wei qi* for long periods. While *huáng qí* and *guì zhī* warm and tonify the *qi, bái sháo* moves the blood under the skin, resolving numbness and tingling. For stubborn cases of restless leg syndrome, combine with a formula from Chapter 4B.

Further Reading:

Bensky et al, p. 255
Chen & Chen, p. 500

SAN BI TANG

Formula: *sān bì tāng* (三痹汤), "Three Blockage Decoction"
Author: Chén Zì-Míng (陈自明)
Source: *Fù Rén Liáng Fāng* (妇人良方), 1237
Literal: "Women's Fine Formulas"

Also:
Author: Chén Zì-Míng (陈自明) 1237; edited by Xuē Jǐ (薛己)
Source: *Jiào Zhù Fù Rén Liáng Fāng* (校注妇人良方), mid-16th c.
Literal: "Corrections (and) Annotations (to) Women's Fine Formulas"

Availability:

San Bi Tang Teapills (PF)
Tuhuo & Astragalus Combination (EG)

Ingredients: (from Plum Flower *"San Bi Tang Teapills"*)

xù duàn (续断), Radix Dipsaci	7.5 %	AC
chǎo dù zhòng (炒杜仲), Cortex Eucommiae Praep.	7.5	AC
fáng fēng (防风), Radix Saposhnikov./Ledebouriellae	7.5	BA
ròu guì (肉桂), Cortex Cinnamomi	7.5	E
rén shēn (人参), Radix Ginseng	7.5	AA
fú líng (茯苓), Poria	7.5	FC
dāng guī (当归), Radix Angelicae Sinensis	7.4	AB
jiǔ chǎo bái sháo (酒炒白芍), Radix Paeoniae Alba Prep.	7.4	AB
huáng qí (黄芪), Radix Astragali	7.4	AA
huái niú xī (怀牛膝), Radix Achyranthis Bidentatae	7.4	K
zhì gān cǎo (炙甘草), Radix Glycyrrhizae Praep.	7.4	AA
qín jiāo (秦艽), Radix Gentianae Macrophyllae	4.5	FA
shēng dì huáng (生地黄), Radix Rehmanniae	4.5	DC
chuān xiōng (川芎), Rhizoma Ligustici Chuanxiong	4.5	K
dú huó (独活), Radix Angelicae Pubescentis	4.5	FA

Dispels wind, eliminates damp, tonifies kidney yang, boosts spleen qi, nourishes and invigorates blood, warms the channels and collaterals. Use for wind-damp *bi* syndromes accompanying deficiency of *qi* and blood and characterized by fatigue, painful joints, weakness, numbness or heaviness in the limbs and muscles, or tremors. Use in rheumatism and osteoarthritis, aching tendons, and deficiency tremors including Parkinson's.

Pulse: Thin or weak
Tongue: Normal, or pale with thin coat

Comments: This large prescription (15 herbs) was originally designed for women developing rheumatism after giving birth during cold and damp weather. Currently, it is used for rheumatism, joint soreness, and tendon or muscle pain in pronounced deficiency cases, and is particularly useful for the elderly. The formula treats three *bi* patterns: wind-*bi*, cold-*bi*, and deficiency-*bi* (of *qi*, blood and *yang*). About 50% of the formula includes tonifying herbs for *qi*, blood and *yang*, while 22% address wind-cold-damp.

The classical prescription included *xì xīn* (细辛, Radix/Rhizoma Asari), which has been deleted by Plum Flower due to regulatory concerns.

Caution: *Huái niú xī* and *ròu guì* are contraindicated during pregnancy.

Further Reading:

Bensky et al, p. 759
Chen & Chen, p. 1167
Ellis, p. 245

Modern Formulas:

FU FANG SHOU WU WAN
SHOU WU WAN COMPOUND

Formula: *fù fāng shǒu wū wán* (复方首乌丸)
"Medicinal Compound Polygonum Multiflorum Pills"
Source: Modern patent medicine
Availability:
Shou Wu Wan Compound (HT, TL)

Ingredients: (from Herbal Times *"Shou Wu Wan Compound"*)

hé shǒu wū (何首乌), Radix Polygoni Multiflori	35.1 %	AB
tù sī zǐ (菟丝子), Semen Cuscutae	9.2	AC
xī xiān cǎo (豨莶草), Herba Siegesbeckiae	9.2	FA
jīn yīng zǐ (金樱子), Fructus Rosae Laevigatae	8.1	L
sāng shèn (桑椹), Fructus Mori	8.1	AB
hàn lián cǎo (旱莲草), Herba Ecliptae	5.5	AD
bǔ gǔ zhī (补骨脂), Fructus Psoraleae	4.6	AC
huái niú xī (怀牛膝), Radix Achyranthis Bidentatae	4.6	K
nǚ zhēn zǐ (女贞子), Fructus Ligustri Lucidi	4.6	AD
sāng yè (桑叶), Folium Mori	4.6	BA
shú dì huáng (熟地黄), Radix Rehmanniae Praep.	2.3	AB
jīn yín huā (金银花), Flos Lonicerae Japonicae	2.3	DD
hēi zhī ma (黑芝麻), Semen Sesami Nigrum	1.8	AD

Tonifies blood, tonifies kidney yang and yin, dispels wind and dampness, strengthens tendon and bone, relieves pain. Use for *bi* syndrome due to deficiency of blood and deficiency of kidney *qi*, with symptoms of poor circulation, numbness or tingling into the limbs, dry or painful tendons, weak or painful lower back and knees. There may be also symptoms of fatigue, dry hair or skin, and lowered sexual drive.

Pulse: Weak, thin
Tongue: Pale

Comments: This modern formula addresses blood deficiency as an underlying cause of joint pain, back pain, weakness in the limbs, or stiff tendons. 35% of the formula consists of *hé shǒu wū*, a tonic for blood and *yin*, and is beneficial for moistening the tendons and aiding flexibility. 71% of the formula is a combination of tonic herbs (blood, *yin* and *yang*), while 18% of the formula uses herbs that target joints, especially the knees (*sāng yè, xī xiān cǎo, huái niú xī*). The small amount of *jīn yín huā* addresses joint inflammation.

The formula could be useful in neuropathy due to diabetes, where dryness of the tendons due to deficiency of *yin* and blood commonly occurs. The formula can also be used for general tonification of blood and kidney *qi*.

OTHER PRODUCTS APPROPRIATE FOR THIS CATEGORY:

Classical Formulas:

Da Fang Feng Tang

Major Siler Combination (EG)
* Acanthopanax 10 (SF)

Da Qin Jiao Tang

Major Chin-Chiu Combination (EG)

Modern Formulas:

AC-Q (HC)
Chui Feng Tou Gu Wan (PF)
Evergreen Pearls (CP)
Mobility 3 (HC)
Neuro Plus (EV)
Qiang Li Tian Ma Du Zhong Pian/Wan (GC)
Sea-Q (HC)

4D. COLD BI SYNDROME

Classical Formulas:

Dang Gui Si Ni Tang	*dāng guī sì nì tāng* (当归四逆汤)
Xiao Huo Luo Dan	*xiǎo huó luò dān* (小活络丹)

COLD BI formulas include herbs that are warming and invigorating, and are particularly useful for painful limbs that are worse in cold weather. In many patients, there may be underlying deficiency of kidney *yang,* and these patterns are often seen in the elderly. Sometimes very hot medicinals are used. The pulse is tight or choppy, and may be weak.

Classical Formulas:

DANG GUI SI NI TANG

Formula: *dāng guī sì nì tāng* (当归四逆汤)
"Angelica Dang Gui, Four (Limb) Counterflow Decoction"
Author: Zhāng Zhòng-Jǐng (张仲景)
Source: *Shāng Hán Lùn* (伤寒论), "Injury (by) Cold, Discussion", 220

Availability:

Dang Gui Si Ni Teapills (PF)
Dang Gui Si Ni Wan (HT)
Danggui/Tangkuei & Jujube Combination (EG)

Ingredients: (from Plum Flower *"Dang Gui Si Ni Teapills"*)

dāng guī (当归), Radix Angelicae Sinensis	19.5 %	AB
bái sháo (白芍), Radix Paeoniae Alba	19.5	AB
guì zhī (桂枝), Ramulus Cinnamomi	19.5	BA
gān cǎo (甘草), Radix Glycyrrhizae	14.0	AA
mù tōng (木通), Caulis Akebiae	14.0	FC
dà zǎo (大枣), Fructus Jujubae	13.5	AA

Ingredients: (from Herbal Times *"Dang Gui Si Ni Wan"*)

guì zhī (桂枝), Ramulus Cinnamomi	29.5 %	BA
bái sháo (白芍), Radix Paeoniae Alba	17.5	AB
dāng guī (当归), Radix Angelicae Sinensis	17.5	AB
gān cǎo (甘草), Radix Glycyrrhizae	12.0	AA
tōng cǎo (通草), Medulla Tetrapanacis	12.0	FC
dà zǎo (大枣), Fructus Jujubae	11.5	AA

Warms and opens the channels, dispels cold, tonifies qi and blood, relieves pain. Use for cold and blood deficiency affecting the channels and collaterals, causing cold hands and feet, numbness, tingling, cramping or joint pain. Can also be used for exogenous invasion of cold into the uterus, causing irregular periods. Applicable in arthritis, Raynaud's syndrome, neuropathy and frostbite.

Pulse: Weak or thin, deep
Tongue: Normal, or pale with thin coat

Comments: Zhang Zhong-Jing's formula originally addressed cold and stiff limbs due to an exogenous invasion of cold over a pre-existing blood deficiency. As a warm formula, it is currently used for any case of cold invasion affecting the channels, to treat cold limbs due to deficiency of kidney *yang,* and to treat cold limbs and poor circulation due to blood deficiency, especially during or following menses or postpartum. The formula elaborates Zhang's *Gui Zhi Tang* (*Chapter 1A*), adding *dāng guī* to enhance tonification of blood

"*Sì nì*", often translated as "four cold-limbs" or "four frigid extremities", is better translated as "four counterflow", indicating that the *qi* and blood in the four limbs are moving against their natural direction, resulting in cold limbs.

The original formula included a small amount of *xì xīn* (细辛, Radix/Rhizoma Asari), an important herb that opens and invigorates the channels; it is missing in most American versions due to regulatory concerns. Also, the original formula contains *tōng cǎo*, which is retained in the Herbal Times version. Most other manufacturers have substituted *mù tong*.

Further Reading:

Bensky et al, p. 252
Chen & Chen, p. 494
Ellis, p. 77

XIAO HUO LUO DAN

Formula: *xiǎo huó luò dān* (小活络丹), "Minor Invigorate Luo Channel Elixir"
Author: Imperial Medical Bureau (*tài yī jú*, 太医局);
revised by Chén Shī-Wén (陈师文)
Source: *Tài Píng Huì Mín Hé Jì Jú Fāng* (太平惠民和剂局方), 1078
Literal: "(Era of) Great Peace, Benefit People Harmonious Medicines, Office (of) Formulas"

Availability:

Myrrh & Aconite Formula (EG)
Xiao Huo Luo Dan Teapills (PF)
Xiao Huo Luo Wan (HT)

Ingredients: (from the standardized *"Myrrh & Aconite Formula"*)

tiān nán xīng (天南星), Rhizoma Arisaematis	21.1 %	CA
chuān wū (川乌), Radix Aconiti	21.1	E
cǎo wū (草乌), Radix Aconiti Kusnezoffii	21.1	E
dì lóng (地龙), Pheretima/Lumbricus	21.1	O
rǔ xiāng (乳香), Olibanum/Boswelliae	7.8	K
mò yào (没药), Myrrha	7.8	K

Dispels wind, warms and invigorates the channels and collaterals, moves qi and blood, resolving phlegm to clear the channels, relieves pain. Use for wind-cold-damp in the channels leading to blood stasis obstruction, resulting in sharp or dull pain, rheumatism, stiff joints, muscle spasm, or numbness. Can be used in sequelae of trauma or stroke, including spastic or flaccid hemiplegia, as well as *wei* syndromes marked by weakness or trembling. Useful in poor circulation in legs or arms with numbness, tingling, or pain, including Raynaud's syndrome and restless leg syndrome.

Pulse: Slow, deep, choppy
Tongue: Dark

Comments: This formula was originally intended, and still used for, sequelae of stroke leading to hemiplegia, spasticity or flaccidity, numbness, etc, in the limbs. It can also be used for poor circulation aggravated by cold and damp, employing herbs that invigorate blood while warming the channels. In this regard, it also used for arthralgia aggravated by deficiency of kidney *yang*. *Chuān wū* and *cǎo wū* are hot medicinals that dispel cold and dampness in the channels; *rǔ xiāng* and *mò yào* are strong herbs to break blood stasis. *Dì lóng*, earthworm, opens the channels and promotes movement within flaccidity or spasticity.

Note: Both Herbal Times and Plum Flower use *dǎn nán xīng* (胆南星, Rhizoma Arisaematis cum Bile) instead of *tiān nán xīng*. This herb is cold in nature, but stronger in transforming phlegm.

Caution 1: The formula uses strong invigorating herbs. Care should be taken with patients with weakened constitution.

Caution 2: *Cǎo wū, chuān wū, rǔ xiāng* and *mò yào* are prohibited during pregnancy. *Rǔ xiāng* and *mò yào* is contraindicated when the patient is on blood thinners, including Coumadin.

Further Reading:

Bensky et al, p. 631
Chen & Chen, p. 1177
Ellis, p. 349

OTHER FORMULAS APPROPRIATE FOR THIS CATEGORY:

Modern Formulas:

Cinnamon 14 (SF)

4. BI SYNDROME (Arthritis, Rheumatism, Back Pain)

4E. HEAT BI SYNDROME

Classical Formulas:

Dang Gui Nian Tong Tang	*dāng guī niān tòng tāng* (当归拈痛汤)
Si Miao Wan	*sì miào wán* (四妙丸)
Xuan Bi Tang	*xuān bì tang* (宣痹汤)

HEAT BI is characterized by red, warm and swollen joints. It includes attack of pathogenic heat or heat-toxins, and can include wind-cold-damp *bi* syndrome that has transformed into heat, or excessively warm constitutions that transform exogenous pathogens to heat. These formulas are also used for inflammatory joint illness such as rheumatoid arthritis or lupus. They are sometimes used for heat conditions resulting from trauma; other formulas can be found in *Chapter 5A.* The pulse is more rapid, and the tongue is red. Cold or cooling herbs are used in the formulas.

Classical Formulas:

DANG GUI NIAN TONG TANG

Formula: *dāng guī niān tòng tāng* (当归拈痛汤)
"Angelica *Dang Gui* Lift Pain Decoction"
Author: Zhāng Yuán-Sù (张元素) *aka* Zhāng Jié-Gǔ (张洁古)
Source: *Yī Xué Qǐ Yuán* (医学启源), 1186
Literal: "Medical Studies Informed Origins"
also referenced in:
Author: Lǐ Gǎo (李杲) *aka* Lǐ Dōng-Yuán (李东垣)
Source: *Lán Shì Mì Cáng* (兰室秘藏), date unknown, published 1276
Literal: "Orchid Chamber's Secrets Concealed"

Availability:

Dang Gui & Anemarrhena (BP)
Dong Quai & Anemarrhena (K)
Tangkuei & Anemarrhena Combination (EG)

Ingredients: (from the standardized *"Dang Gui & Anemarrhena Combination"*)

qiāng huó (羌活), Radix Notopterygii	10.6 %	BA
gān cǎo (甘草), Radix Glycyrrhizae	10.6	AA
huáng qín (黄芩), Radix Scutellariae	10.6	DB
yīn chén hāo (茵陈蒿), Herba Artemisiae Scopariae	10.6	FC
bái zhú (白术), Rhizoma Atractylodis Macrocephalae	6.4	AA
zé xiè (泽泻), Rhizoma Alismatis	6.4	FC
zhū líng (猪苓), Polyporus	6.4	FC
fáng fēng (防风), Radix Saposhnikov./Ledebouriellae	6.4	BA
zhī mǔ (知母), Rhizoma Anemarrhenae	6.4	DA
dāng guī (当归), Radix Angelicae Sinensis	4.3	AB
rén shēn (人参), Radix Ginseng	4.3	AA
kǔ shēn (苦参), Radix Sophorae Flavescentis	4.3	DB
shēng má (升麻), Rhizoma Cimicifugae	4.3	BB
gé gēn (葛根), Radix Puerariae Lobatae	4.2	BB
cāng zhú (苍术), Rhizoma Atractylodis	4.2	FB

Ingredients: (from Blue Poppy *"Dang Gui & Anemarrhena"*)

dāng guī (当归), Radix Angelicae Sinensis	7.2 %	AB
dang shēn (人参), Radix	7.2	AA
bái zhú (白术), Rhizoma Atractylodis Macrocephalae	7.2	AA
cāng zhú (苍术), Rhizoma Atractylodis	7.2	FB
zhū ling (猪苓), Polyporus	7.2	FC
zé xiè (泽泻), Rhizoma Alismatis	7.2	FC
zhī mŭ (知母), Rhizoma Anemarrhenae	7.2	DA
huáng qín (黄芩), Radix Scutellariae	7.2	DB
yīn chén hāo (茵陈蒿), Herba Artemisiae Scopariae	7.2	FC
kŭ shēn (苦参), Radix Sophorae Flavescentis	7.2	DB
gé gēn (葛根), Radix Puerariae Lobatae	7.2	BB
qiāng huó (羌活), Radix Notopterygii	7.2	BA
fáng fēng (防风), Radix Saposhnikov./Ledebouriellae	7.2	BA
shēng má (升麻), Rhizoma Cimicifugae	3.8	BB
gān căo (甘草), Radix Glycyrrhizae	2.6	AA

Dispels damp, clears heat, dispels wind, moves blood, relieves pain. Use for damp-heat *bi* syndromes marked by red, painful and swollen joints, especially affecting the knees and ankles. Also for heavy and achy shoulders and spine. Can also be used for damp-heat skin disorders involving eruptions, sores or raised wheals. Useful in rheumatoid arthritis, and in painful joints due to rheumatic fever, gout or lupus.

Pulse: Normal, or slippery, rapid
Tongue: Red with yellow greasy coat

Comments: *Dang Gui Nian Tong Tang* addresses painful warm joints with swelling. The disorder can be due to invasive heat-toxins, or transformation of chronic wind-cold-damp into heat. In damp-heat *bi* syndrome, the joints feel hot to the touch, appear red, and may be accompanied by swelling. It commonly affects the lower legs, and is very useful for acute gout. There may also be generalized body aching and irritability. The formula is also being used to treat eczema and skin ulcerations.

Within the formula, 25% of the herbs dispels wind, 21% clears heat, and 28% dispels dampness.

Further Reading:

Bensky et al, p. 707
Chen & Chen, p. 1191
Ellis, p. 73

SI MIAO WAN

Formula: *sì miào wán* (四妙丸), "Four Wonderful (Ingredients) Pill"
Author: Zhāng Bǐng-Chéng (张秉成)
Source: *Chéng Fāng Biàn Dú* (成方便读), 1904
Literal: "Established Formulas Convenient Reader"

Availability:

Four Marvel Formula (GF)
Four Marvel Teapills (PF)
Si Miao Wan (HT)

Ingredients: (from Herbal Times "Si Miao Wan")

huáng bǎi (黄柏), Cortex Phellodendri	33. %	DB
yì yǐ rén (薏苡仁), Semen Coicis	33	FC
cāng zhú (苍术), Rhizoma Atractylodis	17	FB
huái niú xī (怀牛膝), Radix Achyranthis Bidentatae	17	K

Historical Origins 1:

Formula: *èr miào sǎn* (二妙散), "Two Wonderful (Ingredients) Pill"
Author: *Zhū Zhèn-Hěng* (朱震亨) *aka* Zhū Dān-Xī (朱丹溪)
Source: *Dān Xī Xīn Fǎ* (丹溪心法), 1481
Literal: "Dan-Xi's Heart Method (eg, Personal Insights)"

Ingredients:

huáng bǎi (黄柏), Cortex Phellodendri	60. %	DB
cāng zhú (苍术), Rhizoma Atractylodis	40	FB

Historical Origins 2:

Formula: *sān miào sǎn* (三妙散), "Three Wonderful (Ingredients) Pill"
Author: Yú Tuán ***(虞抟)***
Source: *Yī Xué Zhèng Chuán* (医学正传), 1515
Literal: "Medical Studies Correct Transmission"
also attributed to:
Author: Fāng Zhào-Quán (方肇权)
Source: *Fāng Shì Mài Zhèng Zhèng Zōng* (方氏脉症正宗), 1749
Literal: "Fang's Pulse (and) Disease Orthodox Lineage"

Availability:

Atractylodes & Phellodendron Formula (EG)
San Miao San (BP)

Ingredients:

huáng bǎi (黄柏), Cortex Phellodendri	30. %	DB
cāng zhú (苍术), Rhizoma Atractylodis	20	FB
huái niú xī (怀牛膝), Radix Achyranthis Bidentatae	20	K

Dispels damp, clears heat, dredges and opens the channels and collaterals, relieves pain. Use for damp-heat *bi* syndrome marked by red swollen joints, especially affecting the knees. Also for *wei* syndrome due to accumulation of dampness and heat, with symptoms of heaviness, weakness, and flaccidity of the lower limbs, or numbness with slight swelling in the lower limbs. Useful in rheumatoid arthritis, and in painful joints due to rheumatic fever, gout or lupus. Can also be used in prostatitis and damp-heat leukorrhea.

Pulse: Normal, or slippery, rapid
Tongue: Normal, or yellow coat

Comments: *Si Miao Wan* addresses joint swelling marked by heat or redness, and is particularly directed towards the knees and ankles. It can be used for damp-heat *bi* patterns with pain, swelling and stiffness, and also *wei* patterns with numbness or weakness in the legs when due to damp-heat. Zhang Bing-Cheng's formula takes *sān miào sǎn* (above) and adds *yì yǐ rén* to increase the ability to drain dampness.

Caution: *Huái niú xī* and *yì yǐ rén* are contraindicated during pregnancy.

Further reading:

Bensky et al, p. 721; 720, 721
Chen & Chen, p. 1190; 1188

XUAN BI TANG

Formula: *xuān bì tāng* (宣痹汤), "Pacify Painful-Obstruction Decoction"
Author: Wú Táng (吴瑭) *aka* Wú Jū-Tōng (吴鞠通)
Source: *Wēn Bìng Tiáo Biàn* (温病条辨), 1798
Literal: "Warm Diseases Systematic Differentiation"

Availability:

Xuan Bi Teapills (PF, PM)

Ingredients: (from Plum Flower's *"Xuan Bi Teapills"*)

yì yĭ rén (薏苡仁), Semen Coicis	16.0 %	FB
hàn fáng jĭ (汉防己), Radix Stephaniae Tetrandrae	12.3	FC
kŭ xìng rén (苦杏仁), Semen Armeniacae Amarum	12.3	CC
lián qiào (连翘), Fructus Forsythiae	10.1	DD
huái niú xī (怀牛膝), Radix Achyranthis Bidentatae	10.1	K
huáng băi (黄柏), Cortex Phellodendri	10.1	DB
cāng zhú (苍术), Rhizoma Atractylodis	8.0	FB
zhī zĭ (栀子), Fructus Gardeniae	8.0	DA
jiāng bàn xià (姜半夏), Rhizoma Pinelliae Praep.	7.0	CA
mù tōng (木通), Caulis Akebiae	6.1	FC

Dispels damp, clears heat, dredges and opens the channels and collaterals, relieves pain. Use for damp-heat syndromes marked by red swollen joints, especially affecting the knees. Also for *wei* syndrome due to accumulation of damp and heat, with symptoms of heaviness, weakness, and flaccidity of the lower limbs, or numbness with slight swelling in the lower limbs. Useful in rheumatoid arthritis, and in painful joints due to rheumatic fever, gout or lupus.

Pulse: Normal, or slippery, rapid
Tongue: Normal, or red, swollen

Comments: This *wen bing* formula from 1798 is for inflammatory joints due to invasive heat-toxins, especially when accompanied by fever. In damp-heat *bi* syndrome, the joints feel hot to the touch, appear red, and may be accompanied by swelling. It is commonly seen following injury, or in pathogenic heat presentations found in rheumatoid arthritis or inflammatory fever such as rheumatic fever. It is particularly useful for swollen painful knees or ankles.

Xuan Bi Tang is an elaboration of *San Miao San* (1749, above), which uses *huáng bǎi, cāng zhú* and *niú xī*. Wu Ju-Tong reinforces the formula by adding *lián qiào* and *zhī zǐ* to clear heat; to reinforce the effects of moving dampness, *yì yǐ rén, hàn fáng jǐ, jiāng bàn xià* and *mù tōng* are added. The original formula included *huá shí* (滑石, Talcum), which is omitted here.

Caution: *Huái niú xī* is contraindicated during pregnancy.

Further Reading:

Bensky et al, p. 762

OTHER FORMULAS APPROPRIATE FOR THIS CATEGORY:

Modern Formulas:

Clerodendron 6 (SF)
Curcuma Longa Formula (GF)
Flex-Heat (EV)
Sea-Q (HC)

4F. BACK PAIN AND SCIATICA

Classical Formulas:

Du Huo Ji Sheng Tang	*dú huó jì shēng tāng* (独活寄生汤)

Modern Formulas:

Kang Gu Zeng Sheng Wan	*kàng gǔ zēng shēng wán* (抗骨增生丸)
Tian Qi Du Zhong Wan	*tián qī dù zhòng wán* (田七杜仲丸)
Yao Tong Pian	*yāo tòng piàn* (腰痛片)
Zuo Gu Shen Jing Tong Wan	*zuò gǔ shén jīng tòng wán* (坐骨神经痛丸)

BACK PAIN AND SCIATICA can be unilateral or bilateral; in some cases the hips and lower legs are affected and include sciatic pain. Triggers include traumatic injury, arthritic rheumatism, and structural disorders affecting the spine or hips. Underlying conditions include accumulation of dampness, or deficiency of kidney *yin, yang* or *jing*. Cases may also be complicated by blood deficiency or blood stagnation.

The formulas in this chapter strengthen the kidneys, support the fascia of the lower back, and relieve pain. They generally combine tonifying herbs with herbs that move stagnation of *qi*, blood and dampness. Most chronic cases of lower back pain (lumbago) involve a deficiency of kidney *yang*, especially as patients age beyond 40. Deficiency of kidney combined with blood deficiency can lead to spinal degeneration and stenosis.

Most of these formulas provide support for *yang*, *qi* and blood, thereby strengthening the lumbar region. Because the kidney channel nourishes the knees, deficiency of kidney *yang* or *qi* can lead to weak or degenerative knees, and these formulas are helpful.

For practitioners using spinal manipulation or *tui na* on lower back problems, these formulas can help hold spinal adjustments. Products in this chapter may also be useful for general *bi* syndromes causing rheumatism and arthralgia. Conversely, products found in the chapters for *bi* syndrome (Chapters 4A-4E) may be used for lower back pain, particularly *Chapter 4C. Deficiency Bi Syndrome*. Also, formulas from *Chapter 17B. Kidney Yang and Jing Tonics* will be useful. Precautions should be taken during pregnancy when formulas include herbs that break blood stasis.

Classical Formulas:

DU HUO JI SHENG WAN

Formula: *dú huó jì shēng tāng* (独活寄生汤)
"Angelica Du Huo, Loranthus Decoction"
Author: Sūn Sī-Miǎo (孙思邈)
Source: *Qiān Jīn Yào Fāng* (千金要方), 652
Literal: "Thousand Gold (Pieces) Important Formulas"
aka:
Bèi Jí Qiān Jīn Yào Fāng (备急千金要方), 652
Literal: "Prepare (for) Emergency Thousand Gold (Pieces) Important Formulas"

Availability:

Angelica Pubescens and Sangjisheng Formula (HS)
Du Huo & Loranthus Formula (GF)
Du Huo Ji Sheng Wan (BP, HT, TL)
Solitary Hermit Teapills (PF)
Tuhuo & Loranthus Combination (EG)
Invigorate the Root (TT)
Meridian Circulation (K)

Ingredients: (from the standardized *"Duhuo/Tuhuo & Loranthus Combination"*)

dú huó (独活), Radix Angelicae Pubescentis	9.0 %	FA
sāng jì shēng (桑寄生), Herba Taxilli	6.5	AD
dù zhòng (杜仲), Cortex Eucommiae	6.5	AC
huái niú xī (怀牛膝), Radix Achyranthis Bidentatae	6.5	K
xì xīn (细辛), Radix/Rhizoma Asari	6.5	BA
qín jiāo (秦艽), Radix Gentianae Macrophyllae	6.5	FA
fú líng (茯苓), Poria	6.5	FC
guì zhī (桂枝), Ramulus Cinnamomi	6.5	BA
fáng fēng (防风), Radix Saposhnikov./Ledebouriellae	6.5	BA
chuān xiōng (川芎), Rhizoma Ligustici Chuanxiong	6.5	K
rén shēn (人参), Radix Ginseng	6.5	AA
gān cǎo (甘草), Radix Glycyrrhizae	6.5	AA
dāng guī (当归), Radix Angelicae Sinensis	6.5	AA
bái sháo (白芍), Radix Paeoniae Alba	6.5	AB
shú dì huáng (熟地黄), Radix Rehmanniae Praep.	6.5	AB

Dispels wind-cold, eliminates damp, tonifies qi and blood, invigorates blood, tonifies kidney, nourishes liver, strengthens tendon and bone, relieves pain. Use for wind-cold-damp *bi* syndrome with deficiency of *qi* and blood, affecting the lower back and legs. Symptoms include aversion to cold, fatigue, slow gait, stiff knees, weak lower back, numbness into the limbs, and painful joints and tendons. Applicable for chronic lumbago, sciatica, numbness in the limbs, arthritis and rheumatism.

Pulse: Normal, or pale
Tongue: Normal, or thin, weak, deep

Comments: Sun Si-Miao's large formula for lower-back pain (15 herbs) addresses underlying deficiency of *qi* and blood complicated by exogenous wind and damp. It is applicable for arthritic conditions when weak lower back or weak aching knees are predominant. It is often taken by older patients for arthritis and rheumatism, and can be used for long periods.

Outide of the *Shang Han Lun* formulas, this is one of the oldest formulas in our modern clinical repertoire, from the 7th century. It is formulated for prolonged exposure to cold and dampness causing chronic back or joint pain. The two lead herbs, *dú huó* and *qín jiāo*, address wind-cold-damp, while *sāng jì shēng* and *dù zhòng* herbs support weak kidney *qi.* Other herbs tonify *qi* and blood, and include the *qi*-tonifying herbs found in *Si Jun Zi Tang* (Chapter 6A).

The original formula includes Asarum *xì xīn,* which is removed by American companies due to regulatory concerns. Herbal Times has substituted *mù guā* (木瓜, Fructus Chaenomelis).

Caution: *Huái niú xī* is contraindicated during pregnancy.

Further Reading:

Bensky et al, p. 758
Chen & Chen, p. 1161
Ellis, p. 85

Modern Formulas:

KANG GU ZENG SHENG WAN

Formula: *kàng gǔ zēng shēng wán* (抗骨增生丸), "Fight Bone Hyperplasia Pill"
Source: Modern patent medicine

Availability:

Kang Gu Zeng Sheng Pian (PF, PM)
Kang Gu Zeng Sheng Wan (GC, HT, TL)

Ingredients: (from Plum Flower *"Kang Gu Zeng Sheng Pian"*)

shú dì huáng (熟地黄), Radix Rehmanniae Praep.	15.0 %	AB
ròu cōng róng (肉苁蓉), Herba Cistanches	12.5	AC
lù xián cǎo (鹿衔草), Herba Pyrolae	10.0	FA
lù lù tōng (路路通), Fructus Liquidambaris	10.0	K
cháng chūn téng (长春滕), Caulis/Folium Hederae	10.0	AC
chuān shān lóng (穿山龙,) Rhizoma Dioscoreae Nippon.	8.2	FA
lǎo hè cǎo (老鹤草), Herba Geranii	8.0	FA
yín yáng huò (淫羊藿), Herba Epimedii	3.5	AC

Ingredients: (from Herbal Times *"Kang Gu Zeng Sheng Wan"*)

shú dì huáng (熟地黄), Radix Rehmanniae Praep.	28.6 %	AB
gǔ suì bǔ (骨碎补), Rhizoma Drynariae	17.5	AC
jī xuè téng (鸡血藤), Caulis Spatholobi/Millettiae	17.5	K
yín yáng huò (淫羊藿), Herba Epimedii	17.5	AC
huái niú xī (怀牛膝), Radix Achyranthis Bidentatae	6.3	K
lái fú zǐ (莱菔子), Semen Raphani	6.3	H
nǚ zhēn zǐ (女贞子), Fructus Ligustri Lucidi	6.3	AD

Tonifies qi and yang, benefits the kidney, nourishes the liver, benefits tendon and bone, invigorates blood, relieves pain. Use for vertebral calcification and degeneration following injury or with aging. It is useful in chronic vertebral subluxations and spinal inflammations causing dull aching pain or numbness. Applicable for spontaneous multiplicative spondylitis and deformities resulting from rheumatoid arthritis.

Pulse: Normal, or weak, deep, thin
Tongue: Normal, or pale

Comments: This formula is based on a special patent medicine from China intended for spinal calcification and degeneration, including spondylitis, and can also be used for cervical, thoracic, or lumbar pain. The Plum Flower version follows the original formula (with the exclusion of 8% *māo gǔ*, 猫骨, Os Felis). It contains unusual plant medicinals*: lù xián cǎo, chuān shān lóng* and *lǎo hè cǎo* to dispel wind-damp, and *cháng chūn téng,* which boosts kidney *yang*.

Although the intention is the same, the Herbal Times version has a more conventional formula, using herbs to boost kidney *qi* (*gǔ suì bǔ, yín yáng huò, nǚ zhēn zǐ*), and nourish and invigorate blood (*shú dì huáng, jī xuè téng*). To slow damage due to autoimmune spondylitis, I would recommend the Plum Flower version, combined with a heat-toxin formula such as *Huang Lian Jie Du Tang* (*Chapter 2A*). For progressive stenosis or vertebral degeneration, either formula is helpful when taken over a prolonged course.

Caution: *Jī xuè téng, huái niú xī* and *lù lù tōng* are contraindicated during pregnancy, and for patients taking blood thinners such as Coumadin.

TIAN QI DU ZHONG WAN

Formula: *tián qī dù zhòng wán* (田七杜仲丸)
Source: Modern patent medicine

Availability:

Tian Qi Du Zhong Wan (GC, PF, PM, TL)

Ingredients: (from Plum Flower *"Tian Qi Du Zhong Wan"*)

wǔ wèi zǐ (五味子), Fructus Schisandrae	20. %	L
tián qī (田七), Radix/Rhizoma Notoginseng	18	J
dù zhòng (杜仲), Cortex Eucommiae	16	AC
ròu guì (肉桂), Cortex Cinnamomi	10	E
rǔ xiāng (乳香), Olibanum/Boswelliae	10	K
sāng jì shēng (桑寄生), Herba Taxilli/Loranthi	10	AD
rén shēn (人参), Radix Ginseng	8	AA
dú huó (独活), Radix Angelicae Pubescentis	8	FA

Ingredients: (from Tanglong *"Tian Qi Du Zhong Wan"*:

tián qī (田七), Radix/Rhizoma Notoginseng	16. %	J
dù zhòng (杜仲), Cortex Eucommiae	15	AC
xù duàn (续断), Radix Dipsaci	10	AC
rǔ xiāng (乳香), Olibanum/Boswelliae	10	K
sāng jì shēng (桑寄生), Herba Taxilli/Loranthi	10	AD
rén shēn (人参), Radix Ginseng	8	AA
dú huó (独活), Radix Angelicae Pubescentis	8	FA
huái niú xī (怀牛膝), Radix Achyranthis Bidentatae	7	K
gǒu jǐ (狗脊), Rhizoma Cibotii	6	AC
ròu guì (肉桂), Cortex Cinnamomi	5	E
wǔ wèi zǐ (五味子), Fructus Schisandrae	5	L

Tonifies kidney yang, dispels wind and eliminates damp, tonifies qi and blood, nourishes kidney yin, invigorates blood, relieves pain. Use for weak lower back due to underlying deficiency of *qi* and kidney *yang*. Symptoms include chronic weak lower back, weakness and pain of the waist and knees, and muscle stiffness.

Pulse: Normal, or weak, deep. May be choppy or wiry.
Tongue: Normal, or dark, or pale.

Comments: This formula treats lower back pain and rheumatism due to kidney deficiency and aggravated by wind-damp. *Dù zhòng, sāng jì shēng* and *ròu guì*, in combination, support kidney *qi* and *yang*. *Rǔ xiāng* and *tián qī* move blood, and *dú huó* dispels wind and dampness. *Rén shēn* reinforces *qi,* and *wǔ wèi zǐ* astringes the formula into the kidney and lower back.

The Tanglong product includes all of the herbs in the Plum Flower version, adding the kidney *yang* tonics *xù duàn* and *gǒu jǐ*, and *huái niú xī*, further supporting the back and knees.

Caution: Prohibited during pregnancy due to the inclusion of *ròu guì* and *rǔ xiāng*, and in the Tanglong version, *huái niú xī*. *Rǔ xiāng* is contraindicated when patients are on blood thinners, including Coumadin.

YAO TONG PIAN

Formula: *yāo tòng piàn* (腰痛片), "Lower-Back Pain Tablets"
Source: Modern patent medicine

Availability:

Angelica and Eucommia Support (K)
Anti-Lumbago Tablets (PM)
Specific Lumbaglin (PM)
Yao Tong Pian (PF)
Yao Tong Wan (HT)

Ingredients: (from Plum Flower *"Yao Tong Pian"*)

dāng guī (当归), Radix Angelicae Sinensis	17.6 %	AB
dù zhòng (杜仲), Cortex Eucommiae	17.5	AC
xù duàn (续断), Radix Dipsaci	13.1	AC
bái zhú (白术), Rhizoma Atractylodis Macrocephalae	13.1	AA
bǔ gǔ zhī (补骨脂), Fructus Psoraleae	13.1	AC
huái niú xī (怀牛膝), Radix Achyranthis Bidentatae	13.1	K
gǒu jǐ (狗脊), Rhizoma Cibotii	12.5	AC

Ingredients: (from Herbal Times *"Yao Tong Wan"*)

xù duàn (续断), Radix Dipsaci	19.9 %	AC
dāng guī (当归), Radix Angelicae Sinensis	13.3	AB
dù zhòng (杜仲), Cortex Eucommiae	13.3	AC
bái zhú (白术), Rhizoma Atractylodis Macrocephalae	9.9	AA
bǔ gǔ zhī (补骨脂), Fructus Psoraleae	9.9	AC
huái niú xī (怀牛膝), Radix Achyranthis Bidentatae	9.9	K
zé xiè (泽泻), Rhizoma Alismatis	6.6	FC
chì sháo (赤芍), Radix Paeoniae Rubra	5.3	K
tǔ biē chóng (土鳖虫), Eupolyphaga seu Steleophaga	5.3	K
ròu guì (肉桂), Cortex Cinnamomi	3.3	E
rǔ xiāng (乳香), Olibanum/Boswelliae	3.3	K

Ingredients: (from Guangzhou Zhongyi Pharmaceutical "*Specific Lumbaglin*")

dù zhòng (杜仲), Cortex Eucommiae	15.3 %	AC
dāng guī (当归), Radix Angelicae Sinensis	15.3	AB
bā jǐ tiān (巴戟天), Radix Morindae Officinalis	15.3	AC
huái niú xī (怀牛膝), Radix Achyranthis Bidentatae	10.3	K

bái zhǐ (白芷), Radix Angelicae Dahuricae	10.3	BA
sāng jì shēng (桑寄生), Herba Taxilli/Loranthi	8.3	AD
bái fù zǐ (白附子), Rhizoma Typhonii	6.3	CA
hóng huā (红花), Flos Carthami	5.2	K
qín jiāo (秦艽), Radix Gentianae Macrophyllae	5.2	FA
gǔ suì bǔ (骨碎补), Rhizoma Drynariae	5.2	AC
dú huó (独活), Radix Angelicae Pubescentis	3.3	FA

Tonifies and warms kidney yang, tonifies blood, moves blood and breaks stasis, strengthens tendon and bone, strengthens the back and knees. Use for deficient kidney *yang* causing lower back pain, weak lower back, slow gait, and stiff knees. Useful in chronic lumbar disorders, sciatica, arthritis and rheumatism and back disorders due to overstrain. Can be used for other kidney *yang* deficiency disorders including frequent urination and urinary dribbling.

Pulse: Normal, or weak, deep or thin, or choppy
Tongue: Normal, or pale or dark

Comments: These formulas are intended for chronic or acute lumbar pain or weak lower back, and are useful as people age. There are numerous *Yao Tong Pian* formulas from China, including *Anti-Lumbago Tablets* and *Specific Lumbaglin*. Three versions are described here.

The Plum Flower version uses the same formula and ingredient percentages as the original *Anti-Lumbago Tablets* from Hu Qing Yu Tang Medicine Factory, Hangzhou, and contains seven herbs. This version is appropriate for chronically weak lower back due to weakened kidney *yang*.

The Herbal Times version includes all of the herbs of the Plum Flower version with the exception of *gǒu jǐ*. It adds 3 herbs to move blood and break stasis (*chì sháo, tǔ biē chóng* and *rǔ xiāng*), and 2 herbs to support the kidney: *ròu guì* and *zé xiè*. This version may be more appropriate for back pain due to trauma, and for sciatica.

Specific Lumbaglin (*té xiào yāo tòng líng*, 特效腰痛) has a similar application, but only shares 3 herbs from the original formula (*dù zhòng, dāng guī,* and *huái niú xī*). The insert paper reminds us, "the waist is the home of the kidneys".

All three versions are equally effective for lower back pain.

Caution: *Huái niú xī, ròu guì, rǔ xiāng* and *hóng huā* are contraindicated during pregnancy. *Rǔ xiāng* is contraindicated when patients are on blood thinners, including Coumadin.

ZUO GU SHEN JING TONG WAN
SCIATICA PILLS

Formula: *zuò gǔ shén jīng tòng wán* (坐骨神经痛丸), "Sciatic Nerve Pain Pill"
Source: Modern patent medicine

Availability:

Sciatica Pills (PM)
Zuo Gu Shen Jing Tong San (PF)
Zuo Gu Shen Jing Tong Wan (GC, HT, TL)

Ingredients: (from Herbal Times *"Zuo Gu Shen Jing Tong Wan"*)

xī xiān cǎo (豨莶草), Herba Siegesbeckiae	15. %	FA
jī xuè téng (鸡血藤), Caulis Spatholobi/Millettiae	10	K
jīn yīng zǐ (金樱子), Fructus Rosae Laevigatae	10	L
qiān jīn bá (千斤拔), Radix Moghaniae	10	FA
tòu gǔ cǎo (透骨草), Herba Speranskiae	10	FA
wēi líng xiān (威灵仙), Radix/Rhizoma Clematidis	10	FA
zǒu mǎ tāi (走马胎), Rhizoma Ardisiae Gigantifoliae	10	FA
shú dì huáng (熟地黄), Radix Rehmanniae Praep.	5	AB
dú huó (独活), Radix Angelicae Pubescentis	5	FA
qiān nián jiàn (千年健), Rhizoma Homalomenae	5	FA
shēn jīn cǎo (伸筋草), Herba Lycopodium clavatum	5	FA
tù sī zǐ (菟丝子), Semen Cuscutae	5	AC

Ingredients: (from Tanglong *"Zuo Gu Shen Jing Tong Wan"*)

shú dì huáng (熟地黄), Radix Rehmanniae Praep.	13.0 %	AB
lù jiǎo shuāng (鹿角霜), Cornu Cervi Degelatinatum	11.0	AC
jī xuè téng (鸡血藤), Caulis Spatholobi/Millettiae	9.9	K
gǒu jǐ (狗脊), Rhizoma Cibotii	9.9	AC
wēi líng xiān (威灵仙), Radix/Rhizoma Clematidis	9.9	FA
jiāng huáng (姜黄), Rhizoma Curcumae Longae	9.9	K
xī xiān cǎo (豨莶草), Herba Siegesbeckiae	6.6	FA
rǔ xiāng (乳香), Olibanum/Boswelliae	6.6	K
mò yào (没药), Myrrha	6.6	K
yán hú suǒ (延胡索), Rhizoma Corydalis	6.6	K
jīn yīng zǐ (金樱子), Fructus Rosae Laevigatae	6.6	L
chuān xiōng (川芎), Rhizoma Ligustici Chuanxiong	3.3	K

Dispels wind, eliminates damp, frees the channels and collaterals, invigorates blood, strengthens sinew and bone, relieves pain. Use for lumbar or sciatic pain with symptoms of numbness, tingling or pain radiating down the legs. Can be used for lumbar or knee pain due to wind-damp and blood stasis.

Pulse: Normal, or deep with weak or wiry.
Tongue: Normal, or dark.

Comments: This formula is specifically formulated for sciatic pain, but also can be applied in acute or chronic lower-back pain. Two versions are discussed here, each containing five herbs as a common foundation: *shú dì huáng, jī xuè téng, wēi líng xiān, xī xiān cǎo* and *jīn yīng zǐ.* Both formulas are equally effective, although one emphasizes dispelling wind-damp while the other emphasizes moving blood and breaking stasis.

The Herbal Times version, listed first, prioritizes dispelling wind and dampness, comprising 65% of the formula (versus 16.5% of our second formula). It includes uncommon herbs that are also found in the original patent medicine *Sciatica Pills*: *qiān jīn bá, tòu gǔ cǎo, zǒu mǎ tāi, qiān nián jiàn* and *shēn jīn cǎo.* All of these dispel wind and move dampness, and are known to benefit sciatic pain.

Our second version, manufactured by both Tanglong and Plum Flower, is stronger in blood-moving and stasis-breaking herbs, comprising 43% of the formula (versus 10% in the Herbal Times formula). Additional blood-moving herbs include *jiāng huáng, rǔ xiāng, mò yào, yán hú suǒ* and *chuān xiōng.* In addition, they further support kidney *yang* with *lù jiǎo shuāng* and *gǒu jǐ.*

Caution: Due to the inclusion of *jī xuè téng, mò yào, rǔ xiāng* and *jiāng huáng*, the Tanglong and Plum Flower versions are prohibited during pregnancy and for patients on blood thinners, including Coumadin.

OTHER PRODUCTS FOR LUMBAR PAIN OR WEAKNESS:

Classical Formulas:

Jin Gui Shen Qi Wan

See Chapter 17B

You Gui Wan

See Chapter 17B

Modern Formulas:

Cong Rong Bu Shen Wan

See Chapter 17B

Ge Jie Bu Shen Wan / Ge Jie Da Bu Wan

See Chapter 17B

Zhong Guo Tong Xue Wan

See Chapter 17B

Others:

Ba Ji Yin Yang Teapills (PF, PM)
Back Support-Acute (EV)
Back Support-Chronic (EV)
Backbone (HC)
Qixing Zhuangyao Tablets (PM)
Zhuang Yao Tonic (PM)

PRODUCTS FOR NECK STIFFNESS AND PAIN

Modern Formulas:

Jing Zhui Tong Wan (TI)
Neck & Shoulder-Acute (EV)
Neck & Shoulder-Chronic (EV)
Neck Formula (PF)
Pueraria 10 (SF)

5. TRAUMA AND PAIN

5A. TRAUMATIC INJURY

Classical Formulas:

Huo Luo Xiao Ling Dan	*huó luò xiào líng dān* (活络效灵丹)
Qi Li San	*qī lí sǎn* (七厘散)

Modern Formulas:

Jin Gu Die Shang Wan	*jīn gǔ diē shāng wán* (筋骨跌伤丸)

Chinese herbal formulas for traumatic injuries have their origins in a subspecialty of Chinese medicine called *diē dǎ yào* (跌打葯), literally "fall-hit medicine" or "hit medicine". This trauma subspecialty developed in the martial arts schools and the military, both as medicines for injuries in training, or injuries sustained in actual combat. They have an impressive clinical history dating back at least 2500 years. The formulas use herbs that invigorate blood and break stasis, move *qi* and warm the channels. Some may also clear heat associated with acute inflammation. If the *qi* and blood can flow unimpeded, the site of the injury will heal more quickly while overall pain is reduced. We have divided the medicines into two groups. This chapter addresses medicines to be taken internally. Chapter 5B addresses products for topical application.

The formulas and products offer a valuable repertoire for management of the bruising, swelling and pain associated with acute trauma. They also promote healing in fractures and sprains. The use of internal medicines allows healing when the site of the injury is isolated within a cast or splint.

Because the formulas use strong blood invigorating herbs, they are prohibited during pregnancy and for patients taking blood thinners such as Coumadin. These formulas can be reinforced with products from *Chapter 5C. Pain Medicines*.

Classical Formulas:

HUO LUO XIAO LING DAN

Formula: *huó luò xiào líng dān* (活络效灵丹)
"Invigorate Collaterals Effective Efficacious Elixir"
Author: Zhāng Xī-Chún (张锡纯)
Source: *Yī Xué Zhōng Zhōng Cān Xī Lù* (医学衷中参西录), 1918-1934
Literal: "Medical Studies Heartfelt (towards) Chinese, Respecting Western, Records"

Availability:

Huo Luo Xiao Ling Dan (PM)
Invigorate The Collaterals (K)
Red Vessel Teapills (PF)

Ingredients: (from Plum Flower *"Red Vessel Teapills"*)

dāng guī (当归), Radix Angelicae Sinensis	25. %	AB
dān shen (丹参), Radix/Rhizoma Salviae Miltiorrhizae	25	K
rŭ xiāng (乳香), Olibanum/Boswelliae	25	K
mò yào (没药), Myrrha	25	K

Invigorates blood, breaks blood stasis, tonifies blood, stops bleeding, dredges and opens the channels and collaterals, relieves pain. Use internally for blood stasis causing swelling, in both soft tissue and internal organs. Applicable for acute bruising or swelling accompanying traumatic sprain, fracture or dislocation, injury to internal organs, and internal or external ulcerations. Besides traumatic injury, the formula is used for ectopic pregnancy, embolism and thrombosis, hepatomegaly, splenomegaly, angina and headaches following injury. It can also be combined with formulas for *bi* syndromes (arthritis, rheumatism, sciatica) and pelvic inflammatory disease (PID).

Pulse: Normal, or wiry or choppy
Tongue: Normal, or dark

Comments: This small formula is used for blood stasis with swelling, most often for acute trauma. It can also be used for hepatomegaly (liver swelling) and splenomegaly (spleen swelling), regardless of the cause; it is also used in heart blood stasis causing angina and chest pain. Zhang Xu-Chun, the formulator, recommended taking the product with wine, allowing the herbal medicine to enter the blood and reach affected areas more quickly. The name *huó luò*, "invigorate the collaterals" applies to microcirculation throughout the body, including organs and connective tissue.

The version from Kan, *Invigorate the Collaterals*, adds *yán hú suŏ* (延胡索, Rhizoma Corydalis) and *huái niú xī* (怀牛膝, Radix Achyranthis Bidentatae).

Caution: *Rŭ xiāng* and *mò yào* are prohibited during pregnancy, and contraindicated for patients on blood thinners such as warfarin or Coumadin.

QI LI SAN

Formula: *qī lí sǎn* (七厘散), "Seven Li Powder"
Author: Xiè Yuán-Qìng (谢元庆)
Source: *Liáng Fāng Jí Yè* (良方集腋), 1842
Literal: "Fine Formulas Collection Small"

Availability:

Qi Li San (PM)
Resinall K (HC)

Ingredients: (From the classical formula *Qi Li San*)

xuè jié (血竭), Sanguis Draconis	54.2 %	K
ér chá (儿茶), Catechu	13.6	R
hóng huā (红花), Flos Carthami	8.1	K
rŭ xiāng (乳香), Olibanum/Boswelliae	8.1	K
mò yào (没药), Myrrha	8.1	K
zhū shā (朱砂), Cinnabaris	6.5	N
shè xiāng (麝香), Moschus	.65	M
bīng piàn (冰片), Borneolum	.65	R

Ingredients: (From Health Concerns *"Resinall K"*. Ingredient percentages are not given.)

xuè jié (血竭), Sanguis Draconis	K
yán hú suŏ (延胡索), Rhizoma Corydalis	K
hóng huā (红花), Flos Carthami	K
mò yào (没药), Myrrha	K
rŭ xiāng (乳香), Olibanum/Boswelliae	K
ér chá (儿茶), Catechu	R
Kava, Radix Piper Metystici	N
bīng piàn (冰片), Borneolum	R
Alcohol, Glycerin	

Invigorates blood, breaks blood stasis, opens the channels and collaterals, relieves pain. Use internally or externally for acute bruising or swelling with pain accompanying traumatic sprain, fracture or dislocation. Can also be used for torn or inflamed ligaments, with or without swelling.

Pulse: Normal, or wiry or choppy
Tongue: Normal, or dark

Comments: *Qi Li San* was recorded in 1842 by author Xie Yuan-Qing. It was originally created for both topical application (surviving as *Tieh Ta Yao Gin*, Chapter 5B) as well as internal use, and has become a foundation formula for many modern products used in acute trauma. The name "seven *li*" is an indication regarding dosage. It can mean 7%, or it could be a unit of measurement for a prepared powder (about .22 gram).

In the original formula, *xuè jié* comprised 54% of the formula. This is an important herb for moving blood, breaking stasis, and stopping pain. It is used for both bruising and fractures, and here it is supported by the blood movers *hóng huā, rŭ xiāng* and *mò yào. Ér chá* clears heat, astringes bleeding, and helps repair tissue. *Shè xiāng* and *bīng piàn* are strong aromatics to open channels blocked by swelling, and are useful in topical application to drive the formula deeper into the skin. Cinnabar *zhū shā* may have been added to calm fright and shock.

The formula is hard to find in its original form. Health Concerns, in its tincture *Resinall K,* uses six of the original herbs, adding in *yán hú suŏ* to reduce pain, and the Hawaiian herb Kava as a substitute for *zhū shā*.

The combining of *rŭ xiāng* and *mò yào* is common to most formulas addressing acute trauma. These two herbs originated in the Arabian Peninsula as frankincense and myrrh, and were traded as a fuel for lighting indoor lamps over two thousand years ago. The Chinese recognized their importance in treating traumatic swelling and fracture during military campaigns, as well as discharging retained lochia following childbirth. For the Chinese, it was considered a traditional gift following the birth of wealthy or important people.

Caution: *Rŭ xiāng, mò yào, hóng huā* and *xuè jié* are prohibited during pregnancy, and contraindicated for patients on blood thinners, including Coumadin.

Further Reading:

Bensky et al, p. 573
Chen & Chen, p. 903

Modern Formulas:

JIN GU DIE SHANG WAN

Formula: *jīn gǔ diē shāng wán* (筋骨跌骨丸)
"Muscle, Bone Traumatic Injury Pill"
Source: Modern patent medicine
based on:
Formula: *qī lí sǎn* (七厘散), "Seven Li Powder"
Author: Xiè Yuán-Qìng (谢元庆)
Source: *Liáng Fāng Jí Yè* (良方集腋), 1842
Literal: "Fine Formulas Collection Small"

Availability:

Great Mender Teapills (PF)
Jin Gu Die Shang Wan (HT, TL)
Joint Invigorator (JD)
Tieh Ta Formula (GF)

Ingredients: (From Golden Flower *"Tieh Ta Formula"*)

tián qī (田七), Radix/Rhizoma Notoginseng	14.3 %	J
dāng guī (当归), Radix Angelicae Sinensis	14.3	AB
yù jīn (郁金), Radix Curcumae	9.5	K
bái dòu kòu (白豆蔻), Fructus Amomi Kravanh	9.5	FB
huáng qín (黄芩), Radix Scutellariae	9.5	P
hóng huā (红花), Flos Carthami	7.1	K
niú xī (牛膝), Radix Achyranthis Bidentatae	7.1	K
xù duàn (续断), Radix Dipsaci	7.1	AC
gǔ suì bǔ (骨碎补), Rhizoma Drynariae	7.1	AC
xiāng fù (香附), Rhizoma Cyperi	4.8	G
rǔ xiāng (乳香), Olibanum	4.8	K
mò yào (没药), Myrrha	4.8	K

I

Ingredients: (From Herbal Times *"Jin Gu Die Shang Wan"*)

tián qī (田七), Radix/Rhizoma Notoginseng	20. %	J
dāng guī (当归), Radix Angelicae Sinensis	15	AB
rŭ xiāng (乳香), Olibanum/Boswelliae	15	K
xù duàn (续断), Radix Dipsaci	15	AC
xuè jié (血竭), Sanguis Draconis	15	K
hóng huā (红花), Flos Carthami	10	K
mò yào (没药), Myrrha	10	K

Ingredients: (from Plum Flower *"Great Mender Teapills"*. The current formula is proprietary; the following is based on a previous published version, and may be the same.)

xù duàn (续断), Radix Dipsaci	25.8 %	AC
tián qī (田七), Radix/Rhizoma Notoginseng	5.2	J
chì sháo (赤芍), Radix Paeoniae Rubra	5.2	K
rŭ xiāng (乳香), Olibanum/Boswelliae	3.9	K
mò yào (没药), Myrrha	3.9	K
hóng huā (红花), Flos Carthami	3.9	K
xuè jié (血竭), Sanguis Draconis	3.9	K
sān léng (三棱), Rhizoma Sparganii	3.9	K
bái sháo (白芍), Radix Paeoniae Alba	3.9	AB
sū mù (苏木), Lignum Sappan	3.9	K
gān căo (甘草), Radix Glycyrrhizae	3.9	AA
yán hú suŏ (延胡索), Rhizoma Corydalis	2.6	K
dāng guī (当归), Radix Angelicae Sinensis	2.6	AB
tŭ biē chóng (土鳖虫), Eupolyphaga seu Steleophaga	2.6	K
mŭ dān pí (牡丹皮), Cortex Moutan	2.6	DC
tián guā zĭ (甜瓜子), Semen Curcumis	2.6	CC
táo rén (桃仁), Semen Persicae	2.6	K
fáng fēng (防风), Radix Saposhnikov./Ledebouriellae	2.6	BA
mù tōng (木通), Caulis Akebiae	2.6	FC
gŭ suì bŭ (骨碎补), Rhizoma Drynariae	2.6	AC
zhĭ shí (枳实), Fructus Aurantii Immaturus	2.6	G
liú jì nú (刘寄奴), Herba Artemisiae Anomalae	2.6	K
jié gĕng (桔梗), Radix Platycodonis	2.6	CA
jiāng huáng (姜黄), Rhizoma Curcumae Longae	1.9	K

Invigorates blood, breaks blood stasis, tonifies blood, stops bleeding, strengthens sinew and bone, opens the channels and collaterals, relieves pain. Use internally for acute bruising or swelling with pain accompanying traumatic sprain, fracture or dislocation. Also for torn or inflamed ligaments, with or without swelling.

Pulse: Normal, or wiry or choppy
Tongue: Normal, or dark

Comments: There are several versions of *Jin Gu Die Shang Wan*, all of which are used for acute trauma with swelling. They can also be used for chronic injury, especially if swelling involved. Each features Notoginseng *tián qī,* an important trauma herb that stops bleeding while also breaking stasis.

As an internal medicine, *Jin Gu Die Shang Wan* is useful for treating bone fractures with swelling when a limb is in a cast. It is less effective for injuries without swelling, such as inflamed tendon, but can still be helpful.

We can look at the six herbs of the Herbal Times version as the basic formula. It takes four herbs from *Qi Li San* (described above) to break stasis and stop pain: *xuè jié, hóng huā, rǔ xiāng* and *mò yào*. To this, a large amount of *tián qī* is added (20%), making the formula more effective for bleeding wounds or wounds with swelling. Finally, it adds *xù duàn*, which helps mend fractured bone.

Golden Flower's *Tieh Ta Formula* adds six herbs to the basic formula, using 14% *tián qī*. Plum Flower's *Great Mender Teapills*, a large formula of 24 herbs, gives priority to *xù duàn* (26%), which addresses bone fracture. In both formulas, the additional herbs reinforce the treatment of trauma with swelling.

Caution: These formulas are prohibited during pregnancy, and are contraindicated for patients on blood thinners such as Coumadin.

OTHER FORMULAS APPROPRIATE FOR THIS CATEGORY:

Modern Formulas:

Yan Hu Suo Zhi Tong Wan
See Chapter 5C

Zhong Guo Tong Xue Wan
See Chapter 4B

Other:

Bone And Sinew Formula (GF)
Ox Bone Pearls (CP)
Recovery Pills (SF)
Resinall E (HC)
Resinall K (HC)
San Qi 17 (SF)
Trauma 1 Formula (GF)
Trauma 2 Formula (GF)
Traumanex (EV)
Yunnan Bai Yao Capsule (*See Chapter 5D*)

5B. TOPICAL APPLICATIONS FOR TRAUMATIC INJURY & BI SYNDROME

Modern Formulas:

Die Da Yao Jing (Tieh Ta Yao Gin)	*diē dǎ yào jīng* (跌打药精)
Die Da Zhi Tong Gao (Plaster for Bruise)	*diē dǎ zhǐ tòng gāo* (跌打止痛散膏)
Jing Wan Hong (Ching Wan Hung)	*jīng wàn hóng* (京万红)
Shang Shi Bao Zhen Gao	*shāng shī bǎo zhēn gāo* (伤湿宝珍膏)
/ Shang Shi Zhi Tong Gao	*shāng shī zhǐ tòng gāo* (伤湿止痛膏)
Yun Nan Bai Yao (Yunnan Paiyao)	*yún nán bái yào* (云南白药)
Zheng Gu Shui	*zhēng gǔ shuǐ* (正骨水)

Self-sticking plasters and liniments for topical application are an established part of traditional Chinese medicine, developing as *diē dǎ yào* (跌打药), the medicine associated with the martial arts. In both ancient and modern clinical medicine, water-extracted decoctions are used for topical application, using cloth as a topical poultice. Today in China, topical applications are still used for fractures by TCM doctors who specialize in bone setting, applying treatments 2-3 times weekly.

Over the centuries, products emerged that were ready for immediate application. Plasters started as *gǒu pí gāo* (狗皮膏). These used powdered or cooked herbs mixed with sticky carriers and applied to dried leather; later they could be steamed and applied to the skin. In modern times, plasters are made on disposable pre-cut cloth and do not require steaming or heating. These plasters have cellophane protection, which is removed prior to application. They are typically left on for 8-24 hours, and need to be replaced following bathing.

There are various liquid liniments that are available from domestic as well as Chinese sources; some are for acute injury, others are for chronic pain in the joints and muscles. They can be applied to cloth to cover the affected areas, or can also be rubbed directly to the skin using gentle but rapid *tui na* massage. Liniments can cause stinging to the eyes, and may stain clothes. Precautions should be taken.

Topical applications can be cooling, warming or neutral. Cooling plasters and liniments are used for acute injury with heat and inflammation, while warming formulas are used for chronic pain due to arthritism or old injury. Both cooling and warming formulas include herbs that move *qi*, invigorate blood, and dispel wind and dampness.

For patients with acute traumatic swelling or chronically painful joints and sore muscles, these products are both effective and convenient, allowing an opportunity to treat a problem on a daily basis. Patients report significant relief of pain with topical applications.

Several of the products listed here are for special application. *Ching Wan Hung* is specific for acute burns; *Zheng Gu Shui* is intended as a soak for fracture.

Caution is required for patients with sensitive skin. Remove any plaster with the development of itch, redness or burning, and never cover with a plastic wrap. Also, topical plasters and liniments should not be applied to the lower back or abdomen during pregnancy.

Modern Formulas:

DIE DA YAO JING
TIEH TA YAO GIN

Formula: *diē dǎ yào jīng* (跌打药精), "Traumatic Injury Medicinal Essence"
Source: Modern patent medicine
based on:
Formula: *qī lí sǎn* (七厘散), "Seven Mile Powder"
Author: Xiè Yuán-Qìng (谢元庆)
Source: *Liáng Fāng Jí Yè* (良方集腋), 1842
Literal: "Fine Formulas Collection Small"

Availability:

Tieh Ta Yao Gin (PM)

Ingredients: (From Guangzhou Heping Pharmaceutical *"Tieh Ta Yao Gin"*)

xuè jié (血竭), Sanguis Draconis	18. %	K
rǔ xiāng (乳香), Olibanum/Boswelliae	15	K
mò yào (没药), Myrrha	15	K
hóng huā (红花), Flos Carthami	15	K
tián qī (田七), Radix/Rhizoma Notoginseng	15	J
lú huì (芦荟), Aloe	10	PA
dāng guī (当归), Radix Angelicae Sinensis	8	AB
ér chá (儿茶), Catechu	4	R

Invigorates blood, breaks blood stasis, tonifies blood, stops bleeding, strengthens tendon and bone, dredges and opens the channels and collaterals, relieves pain. Apply topically for pain, bruising and swelling associated with acute injury, including fracture. Can be applied in torn or inflamed ligaments, with or without swelling. Can also be used for pain associated with chronic arthritis or rheumatism.

Comments: Based on the formula *Qi Li San* (see Chapter 5A), this liniment is excellent for acute or chronic injury with pain, swelling or bruising, and for mending fractured bone. Most of the formula (83%) consists of herbs that move blood and break blood-stasis, which causes swelling and bruising. Additional herbs include *lú huì,* which pulls heat out of inflamed tissue, and *ér chá*, which stops internal bleeding. Use until swelling or bruising is gone, changing the application every day or after bathing.

External Application:
Bottles of liquid: 10 ml, 30 ml or 100 ml.
Injuries should be clean and dry before applying the lotion. Apply 3 to 4 times day to gauze, and place over wound. May be covered if desired. Or can be applied to skin with light tui na massage.

Caution: Do not apply to lower abdomen or lumbar spine during pregnancy. Do not apply to open wounds or close to the eyes. Not recommended for internal use.

DIE DA ZHI TONG GAO
PLASTER FOR BRUISE

Formula: *diē dǎ zhǐ tòng gāo* (跌打止痛散膏)
"Traumatic Injury Stop Pain Plaster"
Source: Modern patent medicine

Availability:

Plaster For Bruise And Analgesic (PM)
Wu Yang Brand Pain Relieving Medicated Plaster (PM)
Yang Cheng Brand Medicated Herbal Plaster (PM)

Packing and Dosage:

Boxes of 10 sheets (10 x 28 cm). Also available in a can with a single extended length of 10 x 200 cm. Cut to size, remove plastic, and apply to affected area. Change the application every day, or after bathing.

Ingredients: (From *"Wu Yang Brand Pain Relieving Medicated Plaster"*, Guangzhou Medicines & Health Products. Ingredient percentages are not given.)

ér chá (儿茶), catechu	R
dà huáng (大黄), Radix/Rhizoma Rhei	PA
pú gōng yīng (蒲公英), Herba Taraxaci	DD
xuè jié (血竭), Sanguis Draconis	K
gǔ suì bǔ (骨碎补), Rhizoma Drynariae	AC
lóng gǔ (龙骨), Os Draconis	N
zhī zǐ (栀子), Fructus Gardeniae	DA
jīn yín huā (金银花), Flos Lonicerae Japonicae	DD
hóng huā (红花), Flos Carthami	K
xù duàn (续断), Radix Dipsaci	AC
mò yào (没药), Myrrha	K

Ingredients: (From *"Plaster For Bruise and Analgesic"*, Guangzhou Hygienic Material Factory)

jīn yín huā (金银花), Flos Lonicerae Japonicae	20.0 %	DD
tǔ biē chóng (土鳖虫), Eupolyphaga seu Steleophaga	10.4	K
lóng gǔ (龙骨), Os Draconis	10.4	N
hóng huā (红花), Flos Carthami	9.2	K
dà huáng (大黄), Radix/Rhizoma Rhei	8.3	PA
pú gōng yīng (蒲公英), Herba Taraxaci	8.3	DD
zhī zǐ (栀子), Fructus Gardeniae	8.3	DA
mò yào (没药), Myrrha	6.3	K
ér chá (儿茶), Catechu	6.2	R
xuè jié (血竭), Sanguis Draconis	4.2	K
gǔ suì bǔ (骨碎补), Rhizoma Drynariae	4.2	AC
xù duàn (续断), Radix Dipsaci	4.2	AC

Invigorates blood, breaks blood stasis, clears heat, strengthens tendon and bone, dredges and opens the channels and collaterals, relieves pain. Reduces bruising, swelling and inflammation in acute injury. Apply topically, change daily.

Comments: There are several versions of *Die Da Zhi Tong Gao*, with the original called *Plaster for Bruise*. It is an effective topical plaster from China that can reduce a bruise by 75% in the first fifteen hours. It is also indicated for swelling and pain associated with recent injury. For application, cut the plaster to cover the bruise, and, if necessary, tape down the corners.

Ingredients are the same in the various versions, although may be in different percentages. Certain herbs clear heat (*jīn yín huā, dà huáng, pú gōng ying, zhī zǐ*), while others move blood and break stasis. The version from Yang Cheng Brand *Medicated Herbal Plaster* also contains *tǔ biē chóng* (土鳖虫, Eupolyphaga seu Steleophaga).

Caution: Do not apply to lower abdomen or lumbar spine during pregnancy. Do not apply to open wounds.

JING WAN HONG
CHING WAN HUNG

Formula: *jīng wàn hóng* (京万红), "Capital Ten-Thousand Red"
eg, "Capital (City) Myriad (number of) Red (Ingredients)"
Source: Modern patent medicine

Availability:

Ching Wan Hung, (Tientsin Drug Manufactory; Tianjin)

Packing and Dosage:

In small tubes of 10 g. or larger plastic cups of 50 g.
Apply topically, cover with bandage. Wipe clean and change daily.

Ingredients: (from Tientsin Drug Manufactory, *"Ching Wan Hung"*

bàn biān lián (半边莲), Herba Lobeliae Chinensis	27.5 %	FC
mò yào (没药), Myrrha	17.5	K
dāng guī (当归), Radix Angelicae Sinensis	12.0	AB
bīng piàn (冰片), Borneolum Syntheticum	12.0	R
dì yú (地榆), Radix Sanguisorbae	8.5	J
mù guā (木瓜), Fructus Chaenomelis	8.5	FA
rŭ xiāng (乳香), Olibanum/Boswelliae	8.5	K
hóng huā (红花), Flos Carthami	5.5	K
Plus base of oil and wax		

Ingredients: (from Great Wall Brand, Tianjin Darentang Da'Er Pharmaceutical *"Ching Wan Hung"*). Ingredient percentages not listed.

dāng guī (当归), Radix Angelicae Sinensis	AB
rŭ xiāng (乳香), Olibanum/Boswelliae	K
mò yào (没药), Myrrha	K
mù guā (木瓜), Fructus Chaenomelis	FA
hóng huā (红花), Flos Carthami	K
dì yú (地榆), Radix Sanguisorbae	J
Plus base of sesame oil and yellow wax	

Clears heat, disperses swelling, invigorates blood, relieves pain, generates tissue. Use topically for first, second, and third degree burns with blistering, redness and pain. Also for sunburn, eczema, psoriasis, external hemorrhoids, and festering sores including bedsores and boils. Useful in pediatric eczema.

Comments: This is China's major herbal medicine for burns, so much so that it is used for serious third degree burns in hospitals. The product is recommended as a topical first-aid for first and second degree burns, and patients should be encouraged to keep a tube in their first-aid kit. It reduces the blistering and pain of a burn, promotes tissue regeneration, and prevents scarring. It is also excellent for bed-sores, and as an antiseptic for open wounds showing heat and blood stasis. Clinically, it can also be used for eczema and psoriasis.

The lead herb (in the first version) is *bàn biān lián*, an unusual herb with the properties of clearing heat and resolving toxins, and very good for repairing burned tissue. Other herbs move and tonify blood (*mò yào, dāng guī, rǔ xiāng* and *hóng huā*). Other versions may contain *dà huáng* (大黄, Radix/Rhizoma Rhei) and *zhī zǐ* (栀子, Fructus Gardeniae). Burns should be covered to protect the ointment from being wiped off. For serious burns, the ointment is put on, covered with gauze, and then wiped off with dead skin every 24 hours, until healing is complete.

The name refers to the number of red ingredients, including the flowers of sanguisorba, boswellia and safflower (carthamus). The product is reddish, and can stain clothes.

Caution: Caution applying to lower abdomen or lumbar spine during pregnancy.

SHANG SHI BAO ZHEN GAO / SHANG SHI ZHI TONG GAO

Formula: *shāng shī bǎo zhēn gāo* (伤湿宝珍膏)
"Injury (from) Damp, Precious Treasure Plaster"
Source: Modern patent medicine

Availability:

Shang Shi Bao Zhen Gao (PM)
Shang Shi Bao Zhen Medicated Plaster (PM)

Ingredients: (from Shanghai Lei Yun Shang Pharmaceutical *"Shang Shi Bao Zhen Gao"*. Ingredient percentages are not given.)

hú jiao (胡椒), Fructus Piperis	E
gān song (甘松), Radix/Rhizoma Nardostachyos	FB
dà huáng (大黄), Radix/Rhizoma Rhei	PA
guì zhī (桂枝), Ramulus Cinnamomi	BA
dīng xiāng (丁香), Flos Caryophylli	E
mù xiāng (木香), Radix Aucklandiae	G
bái zhǐ (白芷), Radix Angelicae Dahuricae	BA
rǔ xiāng (乳香), Olibanum/Boswelliae	K
gāo liáng jiāng (高良姜), Rhizoma Alpiniae Offic.	E
qīng pí (青皮), Pericarpium Citri Reticulatae Viride	G
cǎo dòu kòu (草豆蔻), Semen Alpiniae Katsumadai	FB
xīn yí huā (辛夷花), Flos Magnoliae	BA
fēng xiāng zhī (枫香脂), Resina Liquidambaris	K
xiāng jiā pí (香加皮), Cortex Periplocae	FA
gān jiāng (干姜), Rhizoma Zingiberis	E
dú huó (独活), Radix Angelicae Pubescentis	FA
tán xiāng (檀香), Lignum Santali Albi	G
jīng jiè (荆芥), Herba Schizonepetae	BA
chuān xiōng (川芎), Rhizoma Ligustici Chuanxiong	K
mò yào (没药), Myrrha	K
mǔ dān pí (牡丹皮), Cortex Moutan	DC
zhāng nǎo (樟脑), Camphora	R
bò hé nǎo (薄荷脑), Mentholum	BB

in a base of wintergreen oil (methyl salicylate), ester gum, lanolin, mineral oil, petroleum jelly and zinc oxide

Formula: *shāng shī zhǐ tòng gāo* (伤湿止痛膏)
"Injury (from) Damp Stop Pain Plaster"
Source: Modern patent medicine

Availability:

Shang Shi Zhi Tong Gao (PM)
Shang Shi Zhi Tong Medicated Plaster (PM)

Ingredients: (from Shanghai Chinese Medicine Works *"Shang Shi Zhi Tong Pain Relief Patches"*)

fēng xiāng zhī (枫香脂), Resina Liquidambaris	17.7 %	K
dīng xiāng yóu (丁香油), Flos Caryophylli	14.2	DD
zhāng nǎo (樟脑), Camphora	7.1	R
bò hé nǎo (薄荷脑), Mentholum	7.1	BB
Proprietary blend	53.2	

plus wintergreen oil (methyl salicylate), ester gum, lanolin, mineral oil, petroleum jelly and zinc oxide.

Ingredients: (from Shanghai Chinese Medicine Works *"Shang Shi Zhi Tong Gao"*. Previously published, this may be a discontinued version.)

dīng xiāng yóu (丁香油), Flos Caryophylli	42.5 %	E
zhāng nǎo (樟脑), Camphora	17.0	R
máo dōng qīng (毛冬青), Radix Ilex Pubescens	12.8	DD
fēng xiāng zhī (枫香脂), Resina Liquidambaris	10.6	K
bò hé nǎo (薄荷脑), Mentholum	8.6	BB
bīng piàn (冰片), Borneolum	8.5	R

plus carrier base

continued

Dredges, opens and warms the channels and collaterals, invigorates blood, moves qi, relieves pain. Use as a topical plaster for wind-cold-damp *bi* syndrome causing stiffness, poor circulation or sore muscles. Can be applied to joints and lower back, and can also be used for pain due to traumatic injury.

Comments: The *Shang Shi* plasters are well known topicals for localized aches and pains. They are warming and invigorating, and suited to chronic arthritic conditions aggravated by cold and damp. They can also be used for chronic pain following injury. Two versions are available.

Shang Shi Bao Zhen Gao uses numerous herbs that dispel wind-dampness combined with herbs that move *qi* and blood. Most versions don't list the ingredients, but the version from Shanghai Lei Yun Shang Pharmaceutical (above) is probably typical.

A similar but more warming formula is available as *Shang Shi Zhi Tong Gao*. Ingredients are proprietary, although they list percentages for *fēng xiāng zhī*, a blood mover, and *dīng xiāng yóu,* the very warming clove oil. The proprietary mixture probably consists of herbs similar to those listed in *Shang Shi Bao Zhen Gao*.

The small plasters are convenient for patients, and can be applied daily, providing effective though temporary relief.

Packing and Dosage: Boxes of 5 packets, 10 sheets. Apply one medicated adhesive to the area for 8 to 24 hours (typically 12 hours). Change after bath or shower.

Caution 1: Certain skin-sensitive patients may react to this product: remove in the event of heat or itching so as to avoid a skin reaction. Do not cover with plastic. Do not apply to open wounds. Avoid contact with eyes.

Caution 2: Do not apply to lower abdomen or lumbar spine during pregnancy.

YUN NAN BAI YAO
YUNNAN PAI YAO POWDER

Formula: *yún nán bái yào* (云南白药), "Yunnan (Province) White Medicine"
Source: Modern patent medicine

Availability:

Yunnan Baiyao Plaster (PM)
Yunnan Baiyao Powder (PM)
Yunnan Pai Yao Powder (PM)

Ingredients: (from Yunnan Baiyao Group, China)

tián qī (田七), Radix Notoginseng	40.0 %	J
sǎn yū cǎo (散瘀草), Herba Ajuga Forrestii	17.0	
huái shān yào (淮山药), Rhizoma Dioscoreae	13.3	AA
chuān shān lóng (穿山龙,) Rhizoma Dioscoreae Nip.	11.5	FA
lǎo hè cǎo (老鹤草), Herba Geranii	7.2	
kǔ liáng jiāng (苦良姜), Dioscoreae Parviflora	6.0	
bái niú dǎn (白牛胆), Herba Inulae Cappae	5.0	

Stops bleeding, clears heat, resolves toxins. Apply topically to stop bleeding in acute wounds, and to control infection.

Comments: *Yunnan Bai Yao* comes as capsule, powder, or topical plaster. The powder form is appropriate for topical application in traumatic bleeding, while the capsules are taken internally (see Chapter 5D). The complete formula has only been revealed recently; besides *shān yào* and *tián qī* (the main ingredient and a strong hemostatic agent), all the other ingredients are little known plants from Yunnan province.

Topically, it is an extraordinary formula for stopping bleeding wounds. Sprinkle the powder on bleeding wounds, and the bleeding stops within a minute or so. The red pill is a hypotensive agent meant to lower blood pressure in severe bleeding due to arterial or venous puncture. We recommend against using it except for that reason.

For internal applications, see *Chapter 5D.*

ZHENG GU SHUI

Formula: *zhēng gǔ shuǐ* (正骨水), "Rectify Bone Liquid"
Source: Modern patent medicine

Availability:

Zheng Gu Shui (PM)

Packing and Dosage: Bottles of 30 cc or 100 cc. Also available in 60 cc (2 fl. oz.) spray bottles and in 88 cc rub-on bottles. Soak cotton balls, gauze or cloth, and apply directly to injury. Cover with gauze, and leave in place for 1 to 2 hours. Repeat 2 x day.

Ingredients: (from Yulin Pharmaceutical Co, Guangxi. Percentages not given.)

hǔ zhàng (虎杖), Rhizoma Polygoni Cuspidati	K
jī gǔ xiāng (鸡骨香), Radix Croton Crassifoli	FA
bái zhǐ (白芷), Radix Angelicae Dahuricae	BA
qiān jīn bá (千斤拔), Radix Moghaniae	FA
é zhú (莪术), Rhizoma Curcumae	K
tián qī (田七), Radix/Rhizoma Notoginseng	J
Alcohol and water	

Invigorates blood, breaks blood stasis, moves qi, stops bleeding, disperses swelling, strengthens tendon and bone, dredges and opens the channels and collaterals, relieves pain. Use to heal bone fracture, and for inflammation, bruising and swelling due to acute trauma. May be helpful in torn or inflamed ligaments, with or without swelling. Analgesic for pains of muscles, joints, bruises, and strains.

Comments: This liniment is designed to address bone fracture, but is also very good for bruising and swelling due to trauma. Gauze, cotton balls or cloth is soaked in the liquid, and applied directly to the fracture or wound for thirty minutes up to two hours. In China, TCM doctors reset the bones every three days, following with wraps soaked in *Zheng Gu Shui* (or a formula like it) before applying splints. As a trauma liniment, it is applicable for other acute injuries including torn tendon, sprain with swelling, bruises, and localized pain.

The lead herb, *hǔ zhàng*, clears heat and inflammation while also moving blood; it is supported by *é zhú* and *tián qī.* The herbs *jī gǔ xiāng* and *qiān jīn bá* are unusual and unique to this product; they promote bone healing.

Caution: Do not apply to lower abdomen or lumbar spine during pregnancy.

OTHER PRODUCTS FOR TOPICAL APPLICATION:

Amber Massage Salve (SW)
Burn Cream (SW)
Burn Ointment (BP)
Chinese Herbal Sports Massage Oil (BP)
Clear Heat Ointment (BP)
Cut & Sore Ointment (BP)
Dr. Bob's Medicated Oil (BP)
Dr. Shir's Liniment (SW)
Dragon's Blood Liniment (BP)
Green Willow Liniment (BP)
Resinall K (HC)
Shang Shi Zhi Tong Gao (PM)
Shaolin Dee Dat Jow (BP)
Sprain Ointment (BP)
Spring Wind Muscle And Joint Rub (SW)
Stop Pain Tincture (BP)
Three Angels Liniment (BP)
Wan Hua Oil (PM)
White Flower Analgesic Ointment (PM)
Yun Xiang Jing (PM)

5. TRAUMA AND PAIN

5C. PAIN

Classical Formulas:

Shao Yao Gan Cao Tang — *sháo yào gān cǎo tāng* (芍药甘草汤)

Modern Formulas:

Yan Hu Suo Zhi Tong Wan — *yán hú suǒ zhǐ tòng wán* (延胡索止痛丸)

Two formulas are discussed in this chapter. The first is for pain due to muscle contraction and spasm. The second refers to a group of products that rely on *yán hú suǒ* (延胡索, Rhizoma Corydalis), an herb with strong analgesic effect. The *yán hú suǒ* variations contain between two to five herbs, and can be taken alone or to reinforce other products. They are useful for pain due to trauma as well as headache, toothache, joint pain, epigastric pain and so on.

These formulas can be taken alone, or to reinforce other formulas when specific differentiations are being treated, such as heat or cold, excesses of phlegm or damp, or deficiencies of *qi,* blood, *yin* or *yang*, or events involving toxins.

Herbs that have an analgesic effect in Chinese medicine invigorate blood and break stasis. They tend to be bitter, and excessive consumption can lead to nausea. Blood invigorating herbs should not be used while patients are taking Coumadin or other blood thinning medicines.

Products specific for menstrual cramps can be found in *8C. Uterine Blood Stasis*.

SHAO YAO GAN CAO TANG

Formula: *sháo yào gān cǎo tāng* (芍药甘草汤),"Paeonia, Glycyrrhiza Decoction"
Author: Zhāng Zhòng-Jǐng (张仲景)
Source: *Shāng Hán Lùn* (伤寒论), 220
Literal: "Injury (by) Cold, Discussion"

Availability:

Peony & Licorice Combination (EG)
Peony & Licorice Formula (K)
Peony & Licorice Teapills (PF)
Peony And Licorice Formula (HS)
Shao Yao Gan Cao Wan (HT)
* Flex-Sc (EV)
* SPZM (HC)

Ingredients: (from the standardized *"Peony & Licorice Combination"*)

bái sháo (白芍), Radix Paeoniae Alba	50.0 %	AB
zhì gān cǎo (炙甘草), Radix Glycyrrhizae Praep.	50.0	AA

Invigorates blood, tonifies qi and blood, dredges the liver, harmonizes liver and spleen, relieves pain. Use for blood stagnation causing spasm, cramps and pain, especially in the calf muscles or abdomen. Useful for pain accompanying diarrhea in irritable bowel syndrome, as well as muscle pain found in back pain, sciatica and dysmenorrhea. Also useful in relaxing spasm around kidney stone. The formula can be used for pain accompanying hepatomegaly and splenomegaly.

Pulse: Normal, or slightly pale
Tongue: Normal, or slightly wiry or choppy

Comments: This *Shang Han Lun* formula from the 3rd century is a two-herb combination for relieving pain associated with muscle spasm. It was originally used for muscle spasms following over-use of diaphoretic formulas and dehydration, and has also been the formula of choice for chronic spasms in the calf muscles or abdominal cramping. It is currently used for a variety of pain presentations. The synergistic combination of the two herbs moves *qi* and blood in the liver and along the liver and gallbladder channels.

YAN HU SUO ZHI TONG WAN

Formula: *yán hú suǒ zhǐ tòng wán* (延胡索止痛丸), "Corydalis Relieve Pain Pills"
Source: Modern patent medicine

Availability:

Corydalis 5 (SF)
Corydalis Formula (GF)
Great Corydalis Teapills (PF)
Herbal Analgesic (EV)
Yan Hu Suo Zhi Tong Wan (HT)

Ingredients: (from Plum Flower *"Great Corydalis Teapills"*)

yán hú suǒ (延胡索), Rhizoma Corydalis	66.6 %	K
bái zhǐ (白芷), Radix Angelicae Dahuricae	33.3	BA

Ingredients: (from Golden Flower "*Corydalis Formula*")

yán hú suǒ (延胡索), Rhizoma Corydalis	33.3 %	K
bái sháo (白芍), Radix Paeoniae Alba	33.3	AB
gān cǎo (甘草), Radix Glycyrrhizae	33.3	AA

Ingredients: (from Seven Forest *"Corydalis 5"*)

yán hú suǒ (延胡索), Rhizoma Corydalis	40. %	K
bái sháo (白芍), Radix Paeoniae Alba	15	AB
gān cǎo (甘草), Radix Glycyrrhizae	15	AA
pú huáng (蒲黄), Pollen Typhae	15	J
wǔ líng zhī (五灵脂), Faeces Trogopterori	15	K

Ingredients: (from Herbal Times *"Yan Hu Suo Zhi Tong Wan"*)

yán hú suǒ (延胡索), Rhizoma Corydalis	25. %	K
chì sháo (赤芍), Radix Paeoniae Rubra	25	K
mù xiāng (木香), Radix Aucklandiae	25	G
sān léng (三棱), Rhizoma Sparganii	25	K

Ingredients: (from Evergreen *"Herbal Analgesic"*. Percentages are not given.)

yán hú suǒ (延胡索), Rhizoma Corydalis	K
rǔ xiāng (乳香), Olibanum/Boswelliae	K
mò yào (没药), Myrrha	K
guì zhī (桂枝), Ramulus Cinnamomi	BA
dāng guī (当归), Radix Angelicae Sinensis	AB

Invigorates blood, moves qi, relieves pain. Use for pain due to blood stasis, including trauma, epigastric pain, headache, sinus pain, dysmenorrhea, postpartum pain and tooth pain. Also used for pain found in hemorrhoids, arthritis, angina, and sciatica. Used in hemiplegia following stroke to move *qi* and blood.

Comments: *Yán hú suǒ* is considered a principal Chinese herb for relieving pain, especially the dull lingering type. Here we have five different formulas represented, containing between two and five herbs. The first, *Great Corydalis Teapills* (Plum Flower), combines *yán hú suǒ* with *bái zhǐ* on a 2:1 ratio. In this formula, *bái zhǐ* helps to invigorate *qi* in aiding the blood-moving qualities of *yán hú suǒ*. In the second, *Corydalis Formula* (Golden Flower), we find *yán hú suǒ* combined with the two herbs of the formula *Shao Yao Gan Cao Tang* (above), namely *bái sháo* and *gān cǎo*. The third formula, *Corydalis 5* (Seven Forest), takes this 3-herb combination, and adds *pú huáng* and *wǔ líng zhī*, making this formula appropriate for menstrual pain with cramping.

The Herbal Times formula, *Yan Hu Suo Zhi Tong Wan*, combines *yán hú suǒ* with *chì sháo* and *sān léng* to move blood and break stasis; *mù xiāng* helps move qi. Finally, *Herbal Analgesic* (Evergreen) reinforces *yán hú suǒ* with *rǔ xiāng, mò yào, guì zhī* and *dāng guī*, making it appropriate in chronic or acute pain due to trauma or menstrual cramping.

Caution: *Sān léng, pú huáng, wǔ líng zhī, rǔ xiāng* and *mò yào* are prohibited during pregnancy, and for patients taking blood thinners, including Coumadin. These are found in the last three of the included products.

OTHER FORMULAS APPROPRIATE FOR THIS CATEGORY:

Classical Formulas:

Fu Yuan Huo Xue Tang

Tangkuei & Persica Combination (EG)

Modern Formulas:

Eupolyphaga Tablets (SF)
Flex-NP (EV)
Herbal Analgesic (EV)
Lindera 15 (SF)
Qi Ye Lian (PF)

6. DIGESTIVE DISORDERS

6A. SPLEEN QI DEFICIENCY

Classical Formulas:

Bu Zhong Yi Qi Tang	*bǔ zhōng yì qì tāng* (补中益气汤)
Si Jun Zi Tang	*sì jūn zǐ tāng* (四君子汤)
Liu Jun Zi Tang	*liù jūn zǐ tāng* (六君子汤)
Xiang Sha Liu Jun Zi Tang	*xiāng shā liù jūn zǐ tāng* (香砂六君子汤)
Ping Wei San	*píng wèi sǎn* (平胃散)
Shen Ling Bai Zhu San	*shēn líng bái zhú sǎn* (参苓白术散)

Deficiency of spleen *qi* manifests as poor digestion, with symptoms of abdominal bloating, discomfort after eating, and irregular bowel movements. When the digestive function is weak, there is poor absorption and conversion of food into *qi* (energy), affecting both the acupuncture channels and the *zang-fu* organs. This also affects blood production, and it is common for people with chronic spleen *qi* deficiency to have deficiency of *qi* and blood, leading to fatigue, poor sleep and poor mental concentration. In terms of modern physiology, deficiency of spleen *qi* can be measured as lowered hydrochloric acid and/or pancreatic enzyme production.

Spleen energetics relate to the whole digestive tract. For example, the spleen's function of taking nutrients and fluid to create *qi* and blood starts in the small intestine, in both modern physiology and TCM energetic physiology. Also, spleen and stomach meridian applications apply to the length of the digestive tract, from the mouth and pharynx to the anus. Spleen *qi* affects all the organs of digestion, and can underlie problems of the mouth, esophagus, stomach and the small and large intestines, contributing to gum disease, esophageal reflux, esophageal constriction, stomach ulcer, irritable bowel syndrome, food allergies and Inflammatory Bowel Disease. Deficiencies of spleen *qi* can affect absorption of essential nutrients, leading to both underweight and overweight conditions.

Cases of deficiency of spleen *qi* need to be distinguished from deficiency of spleen *yang* (see *Chapter 6B*), and cases involving stagnation of food, *qi*, and damp (*Chapter 6C*). All of these cases may show signs of poor digestion, bloating, and erratic stools. In deficiency of spleen *qi* cases (this chapter and *Chapter 6B*), the pulses are weak, deep or soft and there are accompanying symptoms of fatigue, lethargy and low vitality. It also leads to a weakened immune response, affecting the production of both *ying* and *wei qi.*

Deficiency of spleen *yang* (*Chapter 6B*) will also show weak or deep pulses, but there are also symptoms of a cold lower abdomen, loose stools or diarrhea, and aggravation of pain or bloating when eating cold or raw foods.

Food stagnation (*Chapter 6C*) – a combined stagnation of *qi*, phlegm and damp - is a pattern of excess , and will show a full pulse with a greasy tongue coat. In cases of chronic accumulation of food, phlegm, or damp - even with accompanying deficiency of spleen *qi* - it is best to start therapy with a formula that clears the excess first before tonifying, using formulas from *Chapter 6C*. Once the phlegm and mucus has cleared, true deficiency will begin to show on the pulse. At this point, one can move to the formulas listed in this chapter. Liver *qi* stagnation can also lead to digestive problems by inhibiting the flow of spleen or stomach *qi*. In these cases, refer to formulas in *Chapter 7A*.

Clinically, for any digestive problem, the spleen, stomach and liver all have to be evaluated. The acupuncture channels for the spleen and stomach act in a vertical direction, with spleen *qi* moving upwards and stomach *qi* moving downwards. Deficiency of spleen *qi* can stop stomach *qi* from descending, while stagnation of stomach *qi* can keep spleen *qi* from rising. On the horizontal plane, liver and spleen and stomach also have a relationship. The *qi* of spleen provides movement for liver *qi* and blood. Weak spleen will lead to stagnation of liver, and conversely, stagnant liver *qi* will inhibit the rising or movement of spleen *qi*. Also, stagnation of liver, for any reason, can stop the stomach from descending, and contribute to stomach stagnation.

The pulse can help determine the amount each *zang* organ plays in digestive issues. Stagnation of stomach *qi* shows as excess in the stomach position; deficiency of spleen *qi* shows as deficiency in the spleen position. Excess in the stomach can be due to stagnation of *qi*, or accompanied by excess of food or phlegm stasis. Liver stagnation will show as either as excess in the liver position, or excess in the gallbladder position (with weakness in the liver position). Once the scenario is determined, then one can more readily choose the appropriate formula. Cases of combined excess and deficiency should prioritize clearing the excess first; tonifying formulas will aggravate stagnation.

Caution. *Qi* tonics are by nature warming and can be slightly stagnating to the *qi*. Caution is advised if the following symptoms develop: heat or dryness, oppressive feelings in the chest, or abdominal congestion and bloating. Overuse of spleen *qi* tonics by the mother may cause colic in breast-fed infants.

Tonics not be used alone during the early stages of pathogenic wind (common cold), as they tend to drive pathogens deeper into the body.

Classical Formulas:

BU ZHONG YI QI TANG

Formula: *bǔ zhōng yì qì tāng* (补中益气汤)
"Tonify Center, Increase *Qi* Decoction"
Author: Lǐ Gǎo (李杲) *aka* Lǐ Dōng-Yuán (李东垣)
Source: *Pí Wèi Lùn* (脾胃论), 1249
Literal: "Spleen, Stomach Discussion"
also attributed to:
Author: *Lǐ Gǎo* (李杲) *aka* Lǐ Dōng-Yuán (李东垣)
Source: *Nèi Wài Shāng Biàn Huò Lùn* (内外伤辨惑论), 1247
Literal: "Internal External Injury, Clarify False-Notions Discussion"

Availability:

Arouse Vigor (K)
Breaking Clouds (TT)
Bu Zhong Yi Qi Tang (BP)
Bu Zhong Yi Qi Wan (HT, MS, PIM, PM, TL)
Central Chi Teapills (PF)
Ginseng & Astragalus Combination (EG)
Ginseng & Astragalus Formula (CC, GF)
Raise Qi (HC)
Tonify The Middle And Augment The Qi Formula (HS)

Ingredients: (from the standardized *"Ginseng & Astragalus Combination"*)

huáng qí (黄芪), Radix Astragali	22.3 %	AA
zhì gān cǎo (炙甘草), Radix Glycyrrhizae Praep.	14.8	AA
rén shēn (人参), Radix Ginseng	14.8	AA
shēng jiāng (生姜), Rhizoma Zingiberis Recens	11.1	BA
dāng guī (当归), Radix Angelicae Sinensis	7.4	AB
chén pí (陈皮), Pericarpium Citri Reticulatae	7.4	G
dà zǎo (大枣), Fructus Jujubae	7.4	AA
bái zhú (白术), Rhizoma Atractylodis Macrocephalae	7.4	AA
shēng má (升麻), Rhizoma Cimicifugae	3.7	BB
chái hú (柴胡), Radix Bupleuri	3.7	BB

Tonifies spleen qi, warms the middle jiao, supports spleen yang, harmonizes liver and stomach, raises prolapse. Use for deficiency in the spleen channel causing deficiency fever, headache, or the prolapse of major organs, including stomach, intestines, and uterus. Can be used for a variety of complaints due to spleen *qi* deficiency, including poor digestion, distension, fatigue and lethargy, loose stools, chronic diarrhea, and flatulence. Applicable for uterine bleeding due to spleen deficiency, poor digestion due to chronic hepatitis or cirrhosis, and certain *wei* patterns, including myasthenia gravis and multiple sclerosis. Can be used as a *qi* tonic during deficiency fever.

Pulse: Weak, sunken or thin
Tongue: Normal, or pale with teeth marks

Comments: Li Dong-Yuan, the author, perceived a situation where deficiency of *qi* in the exterior fails to control the upward movement of *yang*, allowing *yang* stasis to develop into fever, headache, dizziness and palpitations. Historically, the formula has also been applied to a variety of situations where clear *yang* cannot rise or reinforce *wei qi* on the surface. It does these using herbs that boost spleen *qi* and *yang* (*huáng qí, zhì gān cǎo, rén shen, dà zǎo,* and *bái zhú*), and reinforced with *chái hú* and *shēng má,* herbs with an upward direction that raise spleen *qi*.

Applications have included organ prolapse due to depletion of spleen *qi*, particularly following childbirth; deficiency of *wei qi* leading to frequent common cold; leakage of fluids in the lower burner (chronic diarrhea, urinary incontinence, spermatorrhea, bleeding disorders); and accumulation of turbid *yin* in the upper burner (dizziness, tinnitus, etc.)

In modern times, the formula has become a popular prescription for a variety of digestive disorders based in spleen *qi* deficiency, and is finding new applications in treating liver-spleen disorders causing blood sugar dysregulation, epigastric distension, esophageal reflux (GERDS) and irritable bowel syndrome.

Note: Many manufacturers will substitute *dǎng shēn* (党参, Radix Codonopsis) for *rén shēn* (人参, Radix Ginseng), due to cost concerns.

Caution: For fever, only use in cases due to *qi* deficiency.

Further Reading:

Bensky et al, p. 317
Chen & Chen, p. 542
Ellis, p. 33

THE JUN ZI TANG FORMULAS

sì jūn zǐ tāng (四君子汤) - 1078 CE
liù jūn zǐ tāng (六君子汤) - 1237 CE
xiāng shā liù jūn zǐ tāng (香砂六君子汤) - 1675 CE

SI JUN ZI TANG

Formula: *sì jūn zǐ tāng* (四君子汤), "Four Gentlemen Decoction"
Author: Imperial Medical Bureau (*tài yī jú*, 太医局);
revised by Chén Shī-Wén (陈师文)
Source: *Tài Píng Huì Mín Hé Jì Jú Fāng* (太平惠民和剂局方), 1078
Literal: "(Era of) Great Peace, Benefit People Harmonious Medicines, Office (of) Formulas"

Availability:

Four Gentlemen Formula (HS)
Four Gentlemen Teapills (PF)
Major Four Herb Combination (EG)
Si Jun Zi Tang (BP)
Si Jun Zi Wan (HT, PM, TL)

Ingredients: (from Herbal Times *"Si Jun Zi Wan"*)

rén shēn (人参), Radix Ginseng	27. %	AA
bái zhú (白术), Rhizoma Atractylodis Macrocephalae	27	AA
fú líng (茯苓), Poria	27	FC
gān cǎo (甘草), Radix Glycyrrhizae.	19	AA

Ingredients: (from the standardized *"Major Four Herb Combination"*)

rén shēn (人参), Radix Ginseng	23.1 %	AA
bái zhú (白术), Rhizoma Atractylodis Macrocephalae	23.1	AA
fú líng (茯苓), Poria	23.1	FC
zhì gān cǎo (炙甘草), Radix Glycyrrhizae Praep.	11.5	AA
shēng jiāng (生姜), Rhizoma Zingiberis Recens	11.5	BA
dà zǎo (大枣), Fructus Jujubae	7.7	AA

Tonifies spleen and lung qi, dispels damp. Use for deficiency of *qi* causing fatigue, weak voice, pale complexion, weak limbs, poor appetite and loose stools. Use for chronic digestive disorders including ulcer, acid reflux, belching, and digestive tract epithelial repair. Can be used adjunctively as a *qi* tonic for chronic weak cough, lowered immune response, difficulty breathing, recovery from childbirth or following chronic illness.

Pulse: Weak, sunken or thin
Tongue: Normal, or pale with teeth marks

Comments: This four-herb formula from the 11th century is considered the foundation for boosting the spleen's ability to convert food into *qi*-energy. It is the basis for *Liu Jun Zi Tang* and *Xiang Sha Liu Jun Zi Tang*, below, and *Xiang Sha Yang Wei Tang* (*Chapter 6C*). *Rén shēn* and *zhì gān cǎo* tonify and build *qi*, while *bái zhú* and *fú líng* dispel spleen dampness, allowing spleen *qi* to clarify and rise.

Many manufacturers substitute *dǎng shēn* (党参, Radix Codonopsis) for the more expensive *rén shēn*, but *rén shēn* is superior for building *qi*. Also, the original formula calls for *zhì gān cǎo* (honey-stirred fried Glycyrrhiza), a stronger *qi* tonic. Numerous versions, such as Herbal Times and Plum Flower, use the normal *gān cǎo.*

The modern English convention is to translate *jūn zǐ* (君子) as "gentlemen". The classical meaning refers to a Confucian scholar who cultivates higher consciousness, moderation and harmony. (In Wilhelm and Baynes' translation of the *yì jīng,* 易经 - *aka* I Ching - *jūn zǐ* is translated as "the superior man".) The four ingredients are considered *jūn zǐ* because they act harmoniously with each other, are moderate, and raise the *qi* to the purest level.

Caution: Tonifying formulas are generally not employed when fighting an exogenous event such as common cold. They can drive the pathogen deeper into the interior.

Further Reading:

Bensky et al, p. 309
Chen & Chen, p. 522
Ellis, p. 291

LIU JUN ZI TANG

Formula: *liù jūn zǐ tāng* (六君子汤), "Six Gentlemen Decoction"
Author: Chén Zì-Míng (陈自明)
Source: *Fù Rén Liáng Fāng* (妇人良方), 1237
Literal: "Women's Fine Formulas"

also:

Author: Chén Zì-Míng (陈自明) 1237; edited by Xuē Jǐ (薛己)
Source: *Jiào Zhù Fù Rén Liáng Fāng* (校注妇人良方), mid-16th c.
Literal: "Corrections (and) Annotations (to) Women's Fine Formulas"

also attributed to:

Author: Imperial Medical Bureau (*tài yī jú*, 太医局);
revised by Chén Shī-Wén (陈师文)
Source: *Tài Píng Huì Mín Hé Jì Jú Fāng* (太平惠民和剂局方), 1078
Literal: "(Era of) Great Peace, Benefit People Harmonious Medicines, Office (of) Formulas"

Availability:

Liu Jun Zi Tang (BP)
Liu Jun Zi Wan (HT, PM, TL)
Major Six Herb Combination (EG)
Six Gentlemen (HC, K)
Six Gentlemen Formula (GF, HS)
Six Gentlemen Teapills (PF)

Ingredients: (from the standardized *"Major Six Herb Combination"*)

rén shēn (人参), Radix Ginseng	16.7 %	AA
bái zhú (白术), Rhizoma Atractylodis Macrocephalae	16.7	AA
fú líng (茯苓), Poria	16.7	FC
bàn xià (半夏), Rhizoma Pinelliae	16.7	CA
zhì gān cǎo (炙甘草), Radix Glycyrrhizae Praep.	8.3	AA
chén pí (陈皮), Pericarpium Citri Reticulatae	8.3	G
shēng jiāng (生姜), Rhizoma Zingiberis Recens	8.3	BA
dà zǎo (大枣), Fructus Jujubae	8.3	AA

Ingredients: (from Herbal Times *"Liu Jun Zi Wan"*)

dǎng shēn (党参), Radix Codonopsis	20. %	AA
bái zhú (白术), Rhizoma Atractylodis Macrocephalae	20	AA
jiāng bàn xià (姜半夏), Rhizoma Pinelliae Praep.	20	CA
fú líng (茯苓), Poria	20	FC
chén pí (陈皮), Pericarpium Citri Reticulatae	10	G
gān cǎo (甘草), Radix Glycyrrhizae	10	AA

Tonifies spleen qi, transforms phlegm, harmonizes the stomach, directs counterflow ascent of stomach qi downwards, moves damp, stops vomiting. Use for deficiency of spleen *qi* with some stagnation of food, phlegm and *qi*. Symptoms include poor digestion, poor appetite, nausea or vomiting, epigastric or abdominal bloating, and loose, pasty, or poorly formed stools. Useful for deficiency morning sickness; and also as a general tonic for chronic deficiency cough with phlegm.

Pulse: Thin, weak, sunken. May be soft or slippery
Tongue: Normal, or pale, swollen, teeth marks, and coated

Comments: Chen Zi-Ming's variation of *Si Jun Zi Tang* (above) adds *bàn xià* and *chén pí*. *Bàn xià* and *chén pí* clears phlegm and food stasis, and helps to descend stomach *qi*. The additions are useful when additional symptoms include belching, distension, and acid reflux. Some versions use *dǎng shēn*, although the original formula uses *rén shēn*.

The formula, minus *rén shēn/dǎng shēn* and *bái zhú,* may be based on Chen Shi-Wen's *Er Chen Tang* (see *Chapter 3C*), a foundation formula for clearing phlegm.

Caution: Tonifying formulas are generally not employed when fighting an exogenous event such as common cold. They can drive the pathogen deeper into the interior.

Further Reading:

Bensky et al, p. 311
Chen & Chen, p. 527
Ellis, p. 187

XIANG SHA LIU JUN ZI TANG

Formula: *xiāng shā liù jūn zǐ tāng* (香砂六君子汤)
"Aucklandia, Amomum Six Gentlemen Decoction"
Author: Luō Měi (罗美)
Source: *Míng Yī Fāng Lùn* (名医方论), 1675
Literal: "Famous Doctors' Formulas Discussion"
aka:
Gǔ Jīn Míng Fāng (古今名方), 1675
Literal: "Ancient, Modern Famous Formulas"

Availability:

Aplotaxis-Amomum Pills - Xiang Sha Liu Jun Wan (MS)
Saussurea & Cardamon Combination (EG)
Saussurea & Cardamon Formula (CC)
Six Gentlemen Plus Teapills (PF)
Six-Gentlemen Formula with Aucklandia and Amomum (HS)
Soothe The Center (TT)
Vladimiria & Cardamon Combination (KP)
Xiang Sha Liu Jun Wan (HT, PM, TL)
Xiang Sha Liu Jun Zi Tang (BP)
* Prosperous Farmer (K)

Ingredients: (from the standardized *"Saussurea & Cardamon Combination"*)

bái zhú (白术), Rhizoma Atractylodis Macrocephalae	18.0 %	AA
fú ling (茯苓), Poria	17.9	FC
shēng jiāng (生姜), Rhizoma Zingiberis Recens	17.9	BA
rén shēn (人参), Radix Ginseng	8.9	AA
bàn xià (半夏), Rhizoma Pinelliae	8.9	CA
shā rén (砂仁), Fructus Amomi	7.1	FB
chén pí (陈皮), Pericarpium Citri Reticulatae	7.1	G
mù xiāng (木香), Radix Aucklandiae	7.1	G
gān cǎo (甘草), Radix Glycyrrhizae	7.1	AA

Tonifies spleen qi, warms the middle jiao, harmonizes the stomach, descends stomach qi, moves damp, transforms phlegm. Use for deficiency of spleen *qi* with some stagnation of food and *qi*, causing poor digestion, appetite, epigastric or abdominal bloating, hiccough and loose, pasty, or poorly formed stools. Useful for nausea, vomiting, belching, acid reflux, distension and deficiency morning sickness. Use for deficiency ulcer, intestinal inflammation, Crohn's disease, chronic diarrhea, and chronic gastritis due to deficiency.

Pulse: Weak and deep, or slippery or wiry
Tongue: Normal, or pale with greasy coat

Comments: This formula is based on Chen Zi-Ming's *Liu Jun Zi Tang*, and was recorded 600 years later by Luo Mei. (See comments to *Si Jun Si Tang* and *Liu Jun Zi Tang*, above.) It adds *mù xiāng* and *shā rén* to aid in the downward movement of stomach *qi* and damp. Of the three *Jun Zi Tang* formulas, it is the best for balancing tonification of spleen *qi* with descent of stomach *qi* and removal of phlegm and food stasis. The formula is useful for abdominal distension due to deficiency, belching, acid reflux and GERDS, and is a good formula for deficiency morning sickness. It is preferred in cases of deficiency with food stasis. Once food stasis is cleared, one can move back to *Liu Jun ZI Tang* in order to enhance tonification of spleen *qi*.

For cases with less deficiency and more stagnation, consider *Xiang Sha Yang Wei Tang* (Chapter 6C), a formula from Gong Ting-Xian in 1587 that may have served as the origin for this formula.

Note: *Dǎng shēn* (党参, Radix Codonopsis) is often substituted for the more expensive *rén shen*.

Caution: Tonifying formulas are generally not employed when fighting an exogenous event such as common cold. They can drive the pathogen deeper into the interior.

Further Reading:

Bensky et al, p. 312
Chen & Chen, p. 531
Ellis, p. 335

PING WEI SAN

Formula: *píng wèi sǎn* (平胃散), "Calm the Stomach Powder"
Author: Imperial Medical Bureau (*tài yī jú,* 太医局);
revised by Chén Shī-Wén (陈师文)
Source: *Tài Píng Huì Mín Hé Jì Jú Fāng* (太平惠民和剂局方), 1078
Literal: "(Era of) Great Peace, Benefit People Harmonious Medicines, Office (of) Formulas"

also attributed to:
Author: Zhōu Yìng (周应)
Source: *jiǎn yaò jǐ zhòng fāng* (简要济众方), 1051
Literal: "Simple Important Aid (the) Multitude Formulas"

Availability:

Calm Stomach Teapills (PF)
Calm The Stomach Formula (HS)
Magnolia & Ginger Formula (EG)
Ping Wei San (BP, HT, PM)
Ping Wei San Wan (TL)

Ingredients: (from Minshan *"Ping Wei San"*)

cāng zhú (苍术), Rhizoma Atractylodis	33.3 %	FB
hòu pò (厚朴), Cortex Magnoliae Officinalis	25.0	FB
chén pí (陈皮), Pericarpium Citri Reticulatae	25.0	G
gān cǎo (甘草), Radix Glycyrrhizae	16.7	AA

Ingredients: (from the standardized *"Magnolia & Ginger Formula"*)

cāng zhú (苍术), Rhizoma Atractylodis	28.5 %	FB
hòu pò (厚朴), Cortex Magnoliae Officinalis	14.3	FB
chén pí (陈皮), Pericarpium Citri Reticulatae	14.3	G
gān cǎo (甘草), Radix Glycyrrhizae	14.3	AA
dà zǎo (大枣), Fructus Jujubae	14.3	AA
shēng jiāng (生姜), Rhizoma Zingiberis Recens	14.3	BA

Tonifies spleen qi, descends stomach qi, harmonizes spleen and stomach, dries dampness, dispels turbid dampness. Use for deficiency of spleen *qi* with accumulation of damp. Symptoms include poor appetite, dyspepsia, epigastric pain or distension, acid regurgitation, hiccoughs, nausea, watery stools, and borborygmus (intestinal gurgling). Also used for fatigue with heavy limbs. Useful in gastric reflux, chronic gastritis, pediatric diarrhea and colic. May be used for morning sickness.

Pulse: Slippery, wide, full
Tongue: Swollen, with greasy, wet or sticky coat

Comments: This formula is used for stagnant dampness in the middle *jiao* due to either deficiency of spleen *qi* or stagnation of stomach *qi*. Clinically, it is used for chronic digestive complaints marked by poor digestion or appetite, abdominal gurgling, and heaviness in the body. *Cāng zhú, hòu pò* and *chén pí* descend *qi* and dampness; *cāng zhú* and *gān cǎo* nourish *qi*. Both the Plum Flower and Nuherb versions follow the Taiwan extract granule example, adding *dà zǎo* and *shēng jiāng*, digestion's "little helpers". For spleen damp causing loose stools, consider *Shen Ling Bai Zhu Tang*, below.

Caution: Do not use for extended periods during pregnancy. Also, do not use in cases with deficiency heat.

Further Reading:

Bensky et al, p. 687
Chen & Chen, p. 1068
Ellis, p. 206

SHEN LING BAI ZHU TANG

Formula: *shēn líng bái zhú sǎn* (参苓白术散)
"Ginseng, Poria, Atractylodes Powder"

Author: Imperial Medical Bureau (*tài yī jú*, 太医局);
revised by Chén Shī-Wén (陈师文)

Source: *Tài Píng Huì Mín Hé Jì Jú Fāng* (太平惠民和剂局方), 1078
Literal: "(Era of) Great Peace, Benefit People Harmonious Medicines, Office (of) Formulas"

Availability:

Ginseng & Atractylodes Formula (EG)
Ginseng, Poria And Atractylodes Formula (HS)
Shen Ling Bai Zhu Pian (PF)
Shen Ling Bai Zhu San (BP, TL)
Shen Ling Bai Zhu Wan (HT, PM)
Shen Ling Spleen Support (K)
* Central Mansion (TT)
* GI Tonic (EV)
* Shen Ling (HC)

Ingredients: (from the standardized *"Ginseng & Atractylodes Formula"*)

bái zhú (白术), Rhizoma Atractylodis Macrocephalae	12.1 %	AA
rén shēn (人参), Radix Ginseng	12.1	AA
shān yào (山药), Rhizoma Dioscoreae	12.1	AA
fú ling (茯苓), Poria	12.1	FC
gān cǎo (甘草), Radix Glycyrrhizae	12.1	AA
biǎn dòu (扁豆), Semen Dolichos/Lablab Album	9.5	FC
lián zǐ (莲子), Semen Nelumbinis	6.0	L
yì yǐ rén (薏苡仁), Semen Coicis	6.0	FC
shā rén (砂仁), Fructus Amomi	6.0	FB
jié gěng (桔梗), Radix Platycodonis	6.0	CA
dà zǎo (大枣), Fructus Jujubae	6.0	AA

Tonifies spleen qi, harmonizes stomach and spleen, descends stomach qi, dispels damp, transforms phlegm, relieves diarrhea. Use for deficiency of spleen *qi* with accumulation of damp. Symptoms include loose or pasty stools or diarrhea, borborygmus (intestinal gurgling), poor appetite, fatigue, weight loss, lassitude, indigestion, nausea and vomiting. Useful in pediatric diarrhea, loose stools during pregnancy, and as a tonic in chronic disease, including chronic cough and chronic illness. Can be used in watery-phlegm cough aggravated by accumulation of stomach phlegm-dampness, as found in emphysema. Also used in leukorrhea due to accumulation of dampness; myasthenia and weakness of the limbs and as a general *qi* tonic to boost immunity.

Pulse: Weak, wide or submerged
Tongue: Swollen with a wet, white or greasy coat; may be pale

Comments: This formula treats deficiency of spleen *qi* with accumulation of damp in the intestines, particularly with chronic loose stools or diarrhea not related to parasites, food poisoning or inflammation. It has been used for pediatric accumulation of water in the inner ear, and for leukorrhea in women. As a spleen *qi* tonic, it can be beneficial even in the absence of accumulation of damp. It is also commonly used for chronic wet cough.

Using *Si Jun Zi Tang* as a foundation (see above), it adds several herbs. *Biǎn dòu* and *yì yǐ rén* add diuretic properties to help drain dampness. The addition of *jié gěng* helps bring the formula to the lung to resolve chronic lung phlegm due to stomach phlegm-dampness. *Jié gěng* also allows clear *yang* to rise so that turbid dampness can descend. *Lián zǐ*, an astringent, helps check diarrhea and leukorrhea.

Note: *Dǎng shēn* (党参, Radix Codonopsis) is often substituted for the more expensive *rén shen*.

Caution 1: Tonifying formulas are generally not employed when fighting an exogenous event such as common cold. They can drive the pathogen deeper into the interior.

Caution 2: *Yì yǐ rén* is contraindicated during pregnancy.

Further Reading:

Bensky et al, p. 314
Chen & Chen, p. 535
Ellis, p. 264

OTHER PRODUCTS APPROPRIATE FOR THIS CATEGORY:

Single Herb and Two-Herb Combinations

See Chapter 16A

Feng Wang Jiang (Royal Jelly)
Huang Qi (Astragalus)
Ren Shen (Ginseng)
Xi Yang Shen (American Ginseng)
Ren Shen Feng Wang Jiang (Ginseng Royal Jelly)

Classical Formulas:

Li Zhong Wan

Ginseng & Ginger Combination (EG)
Rectify The Center Pill (BP)
Regulate The Middle Formula (HS)

Ling Gui Zhu Gan Wan

Hoelen, Cinnamon, Atractylodes, Licorice Formula (HS)
Ling Gui Zhu Gan Wan (TL)
Poria/Hoelen & Atractylodes Combination (EG)
* Cinnamon Pearls (CP)

Yu Ping Feng San

See Chapter 16A

Modern Formulas:

Astra 8 (HC)
Bupleurum-S (SF)
Consolidate Qi (CMS)
Earth Pearls (CP)
Ginseng 18 (SF)
Grow and Thrive (GW)
Harmonize Spleen And Kidney (CMS)
Prosperous Earth (TT)
Prosperous Farmer (K)
Rejuvenate and Regulate Decoction (AL)
Resolve The Middle Formula (GF)
Source Qi (HC)
Soothe The Center (TT)
Stomach Tabs (HC)
Strengthen Spleen (CMS)

6B. SPLEEN YANG DEFICIENCY
(Poor Digestion - Cold Type)

Classical Formulas:

Fu Zi Li Zhong Wan	*fù zǐ lǐ zhōng wán* (附子理中丸)
Xiao Jian Zhong Tang	*xiǎo jiàn zhōng tāng* (小建中汤)

Modern Formulas:

Mu Xiang Shun Qi Wan	*mù xiāng shùn qì wán* (木香顺气丸)

Deficiency of spleen *yang* can be considered a subcategory of deficiency of spleen *qi*. (For a further description, see the introduction to *Chapter 6A*.) It is a deficiency presentation showing a weak and sometimes slow pulse with symptoms of poor digestion, acid reflux, fatigue, lethargy and low vitality. There is often loose stools and occasional diarrhea. Daybreak diarrhea, between the hours of 4 am and 8 am, is a sign of this pattern. Deficiency of spleen *yang* is often characterized by a cold lower abdomen and aggravation of pain or bloating when eating raw or cold foods, especially iced drinks or foods from the refrigerator.

Spleen *yang* and stomach fire are responsible for the production of hydrochloric acid (HCl). Hypochloridia – a deficiency of hydrochloric acid – is often the real cause behind acid reflux. Strong HCl secretion keeps the gastroesophageal junction closed during digestion. When HCl is weak, this junction weakens, allowing normal acid secretion to spray into the esophagus and pharynx. The key to curing conditions like GERDS (gastroesophageal reflux disease) and acid reflux, therefore, is boosting natural HCl production, by boosting spleen *qi* and stomach *yang* and fire.

When spleen *yang* is reduced, other *yang* deficiency signs may be present, including cold limbs, weak lower back and lowered sex drive. In these cases, kidney *yang* and *mingmen* fire may also be deficient, and require supportive tonification. (One can combine with products from *Chapter 17B*.) *Mingmen* fire diminishes with age, and can affect hydrochloric acid production in the elderly. Conversely, prolonged dampening down of stomach fire by a diet of cold or raw foods, or reduced intake of animal protein, can weaken *mingmen* fire, even in young adults.

Qi and *yang* tonics are by nature warming and slightly stagnating to the *qi*. Caution is advised if the following symptoms develop: heat or dryness, oppressive feelings in the chest, or abdominal congestion and bloating. It is recommended that spleen *yang* tonics be discontinued during the early stages of pathogenic wind (common cold), as they tend to drive wind deeper into the body.

Classical Formulas:

FU ZI LI ZHONG WAN

Formula: *fù zǐ lǐ zhōng wán* (附子理中丸),"Aconite Regulate the Center Pill"
Author: Imperial Medical Bureau (*tài yī jú,* 太医局);
revised by Chén Shī-Wén (陈师文)
Source: *Tài Píng Huì Mín Hé Jì Jú Fāng* (太平惠民和剂局方), 1078
Literal: "(Era of) Great Peace, Benefit People Harmonious Medicines, Office (of) Formulas"

Availability:

Aconite, Ginseng & Ginger Combination (EG)
Fu Zi Li Zhong Wan (PF, MS)

Ingredients: (from the standardized *"Aconite, Ginseng & Ginger Combination"*)

rén shēn (人参), Radix Ginseng	20. %	AA
bái zhú (白术), Rhizoma Atractylodis Macrocephalae	20	AA
gān jiāng (干姜), Rhizoma Zingiberis	20	BA
zhì gān cǎo (炙甘草), Radix Glycyrrhizae Praep.	20	AA
fù zǐ (附子), Radix Aconiti Lateralis Praeparata	20	E

Ingredients: (from Minshan and Plum Flower *"Fu Zi Li Zhong Wan"*)

dǎng shēn (党参), Radix Codonopsis	30.7 %	AA
bái zhú (白术), Rhizoma Atractylodis Macrocephalae	23.1	AA
gān jiāng (干姜), Rhizoma Zingiberis	15.4	BA
gān cǎo (甘草), Radix Glycyrrhizae	15.4	AA
fù zǐ (附子), Radix Aconiti Lateralis Praeparata	15.4	E

Tonifies spleen qi, dispels cold, warms the middle burner, supports stomach fire. Use for deficiency of spleen *qi* and *yang* with symptoms of poor digestion, acid reflux, nausea, loose stools, weight loss or overweight, poor appetite, fatigue, and cold cramping in the epigastrium or abdomen. Can be used for acute cases of exogenous cold attack into the middle *jiao*, with symptoms of epigastric or abdominal pain, nausea, vomiting, or diarrhea.

Pulse: Slow, deep, weak
Tongue: Normal, or pale possibly swollen with wet coat

Comments: This formula is probably the best for digestive problems due to accumulation of internal cold and spleen *yang* deficiency, using both *fù zǐ* and *gān jiāng*, very warming herbs for the middle burner. It is applicable in a wide variety of chronic digestive disorders, including bloating, indigestion, poor appetite and acid reflux (GERDS). Symptoms often are due to, and aggravated by, cold or raw foods, which should be avoided. The large amount of *fù zǐ* makes this an effective formula for chronic deficiency of stomach fire.

The original formula calls for *rén shēn*, which is used by the Taiwan extract granule manufacturers. The Minshan and Plum Flower versions substitute *dǎng shēn*.

The version by Lanzhou Foguang Pharmaceutical Co, lists *bái fù zǐ* (白附子, Rhizoma Typhonii) instead of *fù zǐ* (附子, Radix Aconiti Lateralis). This can be an error of labeling, or an error of manufacturing. Although similar in appearance and Chinese name, *bái fù zǐ* is used for wind-phlegm-cold, while *fù zǐ* is used for internal cold in the stomach and spleen. It is not a suitable substitute.

Caution: *Zhì fù zǐ* is used with caution during pregnancy. Also, tonifying formulas are generally not employed when fighting an exogenous event such as common cold. They can drive the pathogen deeper into the interior.

Further Reading:

Bensky et al, p. 261
Chen & Chen, p. 463
Ellis, p. 101

XIAO JIAN ZHONG TANG

Formula: *xiǎo jiàn zhōng tāng* (小建中汤), "Small Fortify Center Decoction"
Author: Zhāng Zhòng-Jǐng (张仲景)
Source: *Shāng Hán Lùn* (伤寒论), 220
Literal: "Injury (by) Cold, Discussion"

Availability:

Astragalus Formula (GF)
Minor Cinnamon & Peony Combination (EG)
Minor Restore The Middle Teapills (PF)
Xiao Jian Zhong Tang (BP)
* Xiao Jian Zhong Wan (HT)

Ingredients: (from the standardized *"Minor Cinnamon & Peony Combination"*)

bái sháo (白芍), Radix Paeoniae Alba	30. %	AB
guì zhī (桂枝), Ramulus Cinnamomi	15	BA
shēng jiāng (生姜), Rhizoma Zingiberis Recens	15	BA
dà zǎo (大枣), Fructus Jujubae	15	AA
yí táng (饴糖), Saccharum Granorum	15	
gān cǎo (甘草), Radix Glycyrrhizae	10	AA

Ingredients: (from Plum Flower *"Minor Restore the Middle Teapills"*)

yí táng (饴糖), Saccharum Granorum	35.7 %	AA
bái sháo (白芍), Radix Paeoniae Alba	21.3	AB
dà zǎo (大枣), Fructus Jujubae	14.2	AA
guì zhī (桂枝), Ramulus Cinnamomi	10.7	BA
shēng jiāng (生姜), Rhizoma Zingiberis Recens	10.7	E
gān cǎo (甘草), Radix Glycyrrhizae	7.5	AA

Ingredients: (from Herbal Times *"Xiao Jian Zhong Wan"*)

bái sháo (白芍), Radix Paeoniae Alba	44. %	AB
guì zhī (桂枝), Ramulus Cinnamomi	22	BA
gān cǎo (甘草), Radix Glycyrrhizae	12	AA
shēng jiāng (生姜), Rhizoma Zingiberis Recens	12	BA
dà zǎo (大枣), Fructus Jujubae	10	AA

Tonifies spleen qi, warms the middle jiao, harmonizes the stomach, relieves pain. Use for deficiency of spleen *qi* and *yang* with symptoms of epigastric or abdominal pain or spasm, acid reflux and poor appetite. Other symptoms can include pale complexion, palpitation, or fever with abdominal pain. Used as a *qi* tonic following birth or after a long sickness, especially when *qi* and *yang* have been depleted. Also useful for pediatric colic, fussiness, and loose stool.

Pulse: Deep, thin; can be weak or soft
Tongue: Normal, or pale with white coat

***Comments*:** This formula addresses depletion of spleen *qi* with cold in the mididle *jiao*. The ingredient *yí táng* is basically sugar made from barley malt. In classical times, malt sugar was used for a rapid infusion of energy – both *qi* and calories – for malnourished patients. It was especially suitable following childbirth, where spleen *qi* had become exhausted. In addition, *dà zăo* and *gān căo* support spleen *qi*, while *guì zhī* and *shēng jiāng* warm the middle *jiao*. Also, the combination of *bái sháo* and *gān căo* helps relieve abdominal cramping and spasm. Currently, it is a popular pediatric formula in Japan for digestive complaints including colic and loose stool.

In the original prescription, 18 to 30 grams of *yí táng* were added to the herbal decoction for a daily dose. Given the excesses of sugar in the modern diet, even though *yí táng* is considered less cooling or damaging to the spleen than cane sugar, one should be cautious when using the available products. The Taiwan extract-granule formulas contain 15% *yí táng*, while Plum Flower contains 36%, Golden Flower's *Astragalus Formula* contains 32%, and Blue Poppy's contains 25%.

Herbal Times (Nuherbs) avoids the issue by omitting *yí tang* from the formula.

Further Reading:

Bensky et al, p. 264
Chen & Chen, p. 471
Ellis, p. 350

Modern Formulas:

MU XIANG SHUN QI WAN

Formula: *mù xiāng shùn qì wán* (木香顺气丸), "Aucklandia Normalize *Qi* Pills"
Source: Modern patent medicine

Availability:

Mu Xiang Shun Qi Wan (MS, PM, TL)

Ingredients: (from Minshan *"Mu Xiang Shun Qi Wan"*)

dāng guī (当归), Radix Angelicae Sinensis	13.6 %	AB
hòu pò (厚朴), Cortex Magnoliae Officinalis	10.8	FB
mù xiāng (木香), Radix Aucklandiae	8.1	G
bái dòu kòu (白豆蔻), Fructus Amomi Kravanh	8.1	FB
cāng zhú (苍术), Rhizoma Atractylodis	8.1	FB
yì zhì rén (益智仁), Fructus Alpiniae Oxyphyllae	8.1	E
zé xiè (泽泻), Rhizoma Alismatis	5.4	FC
qīng pí (青皮), Pericarpium Citri Reticulatae Viride	5.4	G
wú zhū yú (吴茱萸), Fructus Evodiae	5.4	E
gān jiāng (干姜), Rhizoma Zingiberis	5.4	E
chén pí (陈皮), Pericarpium Citri Reticulatae	5.4	G
fú líng (茯苓), Poria	5.4	FC
bàn xià (半夏), Rhizoma Pinelliae	5.4	CA
shēng má (升麻), Rhizoma Cimicifugae	2.7	BB
chái hú (柴胡), Radix Bupleuri	2.7	BB

Tonifies spleen qi, dispels damp, harmonizes liver and stomach, descends stomach qi, removes food stagnation, frees the stool, warms spleen and stomach. Use for digestive complaints due to spleen *yang* deficiency with accumulation of food and dampness. Symptoms include indigestion, epigastric or abdominal distension, poor appetite, borborygmus (abdominal gurgling), loose or erratic stools, and sensitivity to cold foods.

Pulse: Weak and soft; or wiry or slippery
Tongue: Swollen, pale, greasy coat

Comments: There are several versions of *Mu Xiang Shun Qi* Wan available as Chinese patent medicines. They each have unique formulas, but the intent is the same: to warm the stomach, boost *qi* and *yang*, harmonize liver and stomach, and dispel food stasis and phlegm-dampness. The Minshan version contains 19% herbs that warm spleen *yang*: *yì zhì rén*, *wú zhū yú* and *gān jiāng*. However, most of the formula (62%) concerns itself with dispelling phlegm and dampness and descending stomach *qi*, making it useful for chronic digestive complaints exhibiting both excess and deficiency.

This formula should not be confused with *Mu Xiang Bing Lang Wan* (Chapter 6E), which is used for damp-turbidity and parasites.

OTHER PRODUCTS APPROPRIATE TO THIS CATEGORY:

Classical Formulas:

An Zhong San

An Zhong San (TZ)
Calm The Middle Formula (HS)
Fennel & Galanga Formula (EG)

Da Jian Zhong Tang

Major Zanthoxylum Combination (EG)

Huang Qi Jian Zhong Tang

Astragalus Combination (EG)
Astragalus Formula (GF)
Huang Qi Jian Zhong Tang (BP)

Li Zhong Wan

Ginseng & Ginger Combination (EG)
Li Zhong Wan (TZ)
Rectify The Center Pill (BP)

Si Ni Tang

Aconite, Ginger & Licorice Combination (EG)

Si Shen Tang

Si Shen Wan (BP)

Wu Zhu Yu Tang

Evodia Combination (EG)
Evodia Formula (HS)
* Ginkgo Pearls (CP)

6C. FOOD STAGNATION AND INDIGESTION

Classical Formulas:

Bao He Wan	*bǎo hé wán* (保和丸)
Jian Pi Wan	*jiàn pí wán* (健脾丸)
Xiang Sha Yang Wei Tang	*xiāng shā yǎng wèi tāng* (香砂养胃汤)
Zi Sheng Wan	*zī shēng wán* (资生丸)

Modern Formulas:

Kang Ning Wan (Curing/Culing Pills) *kāng níng wán* (康宁丸)

Food stagnation results when food matter accumulates in the stomach, and can be considered a combined stasis of *qi*, phlegm and dampness. Generally, symptoms include epigastric or abdominal discomfort, bloating, poor appetite, irregular stools, belching and hiccoughs, and weight gain. Formulas for food stagnation are useful for morning sickness, hangover, and discomfort brought about by overeating, as well pediatric cases of colic and bloating.

Chronic cases occur when the stomach fails to descend *qi* properly, due to either liver *qi* stasis over-controlling the descent of stomach *qi*, or deficiency of spleen *qi* failing to ascend, thereby inhibiting the descent of stomach *qi.* It can also be caused by a combination of these factors. In addition, acute episodes can develop by over-eating, or consuming cold food and drink. Acute episodes of food stasis due to microbial pathogenic factors are treated with formulas found in *Chapter 6D. Damp Turbidity.*

In the main, food stagnation is treated as an excess condition. The pulses are full or slippery, and the tongue tends to be coated or even greasy. With stomach stagnation, the superficial aspect of the right middle pulse (*guān* 關) is wiry. With spleen deficiency, the right middle *guan* pulse is soft or wide. For liver stagnation contributing to stomach stagnation, the left medial *guan* pulse is wiry, especially in the superficial aspect.

Chronic food stagnation often involves an underlying deficiency of spleen *qi*. In these cases, the pulses may be weak or soft, but also show as wide or slippery, or wiry in isolated positions. In acute episodes it is more effective to clear food stagnation first before tonifying spleen *qi;* chronic cases can be treated with formulas in this chapter that clear excess while also tonifying deficiency. Once signs of food stagnation are gone, formulas may be chosen from chapter *6A. Spleen Qi Deficiency* or *6B. Spleen Yang Deficiency.*

When epigastric distension and fullness is due to liver *qi* stagnation overacting on the stomach and spleen, refer to products in chapter *7A. Liver Stagnation,* particularly *Shu Gan Wan.* Food stagnation due to food poisoning with vomiting or diarrhea can be treated with products found in chapter *6D. Damp Turbidity.*

In general, food stagnation formulas are considered safe and can be taken as needed or on a long-term basis.

Classical Formulas:

BAO HE WAN

Formula: *bǎo hé wán* (保和丸), "Preserve Harmony Pill"
Author: Zhū Zhèn-Hěng (朱震亨) *aka* Zhū Dān-Xī (朱丹溪)
Source: *Dān Xī Xīn Fǎ* (丹溪心法), 1481
Literal: "Dan-Xi's Essential Teachings"

Availability:

Bao He Wan (BP, HT, MS, PIM, TL)
Citrus & Crataegus Formula (EG)
Preserve Harmony Formula (HS)

Ingredients: (from the standardized *"Citrus & Crataegus Formula"*)

shān zhā (山楂), Fructus Crataegi	35.1 %	H
bàn xià (半夏), Rhizoma Pinelliae	11.8	CA
shén qū (神曲), Massa Medicata Fermentata	11.8	H
fú líng (茯苓), Poria	11.8	FC
mài yá (麦芽), Fructus Hordei Germinatus	11.8	H
lái fú zǐ (莱菔子), Semen Raphani	5.9	H
jú hóng (橘红), Exocarpium Citri Rubrum	5.9	G
lián qiào (连翘), Fructus Forsythiae	5.9	DD

Ingredients: (from the Herbal Times *"Bao He Wan"*)

shān zhā (山楂), Fructus Crataegi	37.5 %	H
bàn xià (半夏), Rhizoma Pinelliae	12.5	CA
shén qū (神曲), Massa Medicata Fermentata	12.5	H
fú líng (茯苓), Poria	12.5	FC
chén pí (陈皮), Pericarpium Citri Reticulatae	6.25	G
lái fú zǐ (莱菔子), Semen Raphani	6.25	H
lián qiào (连翘), Fructus Forsythiae	6.25	DD
mài yá (麦芽), Fructus Hordei Germinatus	6.25	H

Resolves food stasis, harmonizes the stomach, descends stomach qi, clears heat, dispels damp, promotes digestion. Use for acute or chronic food stagnation, with symptoms of indigestion, epigastric or abdominal bloating or distension, belching, hiccoughs, nausea, poor appetite, or poorly formed stools. Useful in morning sickness due to excess, motion sickness, overeating, and to alleviate hangover. Also for infantile disorders due to food stagnation, including colic, poor appetite, abdominal distension and nocturnal cough with abundant expectoration.

Pulse: Excess or slippery
Tongue: Greasy yellow or white coat

Comments: *Bao He Wan* is the standard-bearing formula for resolving excess food stagnation. In food stagnation, the stomach fails to descend *qi* properly, causing an accumulation of food and mucus in the digestive tract. This formula addresses accumulation of food and mucus in the middle burner, without addressing the causative factor.

Bao He Wan can be considered an elaboration of *Er Chen Tang* (*Chapter 3D*), using *bàn xià* and *fú líng* as the basis to dissolve and discharge phlegm and dampness. *Shān zhā* is the main herb to clear phlegm, turbid dampness and food stasis, and is supported by *shén qū, mài yá,* and *lái fú zǐ*. Also, *lái fú zǐ* with *jú hóng* (or *chén pí*) descends stomach *qi*. *Lián qiào* clears heat generating from stasis.

Caution: *Shén qū* contains a wheat binder and is contraindicated for people with celiac disease or gluten sensitivity.

Further Reading:

Bensky et al, p. 828
Chen & Chen, p. 1266
Ellis, p. 28

JIAN PI WAN

Formula: *jiàn pí wán* (健脾丸), "Strengthen Spleen Pill"
Author: Wāng Áng (汪昂)
Source: *Yī Fāng Jí Jiě* (医方集解), 1682
Literal: "Medical Formulas Collected, Explained"

Availability:

Healthy Digestion Teapills (PF)
Jian Pi Wan (MS, TL)
Ren Shen Jian Pi Wan (PM)

Ingredients: (from Minshan *"Jian Pi Wan"*)

bái zhú (白术), Rhizoma Atractylodis Macrocephalae	24. %	AA
zhǐ shí (枳实), Fructus Aurantii Immaturus	16	G
dǎng shēn (党参), Radix Codonopsis	16	AA
chén pí (陈皮), Pericarpium Citri Reticulatae	16	G
mài yá (麦芽), Fructus Hordei Germinatus	16	H
shān zhā (山楂), Fructus Crataegi	12	H

Resolves food stasis, harmonizes stomach and spleen, descends stomach qi, tonifies spleen qi, promotes digestion. Use for chronic deficiency of spleen *qi* with accumulation of food matter. Symptoms include poor digestion or appetite, distension in the epigastrium or abdomen, borborygmus (abdominal gurgling), nausea, fatigue, and poorly formed stools. Useful in morning sickness due to deficiency, and as a foundation formula for weight loss.

Pulse: Weak and slippery or wide
Tongue: Normal or greasy coat

Comments: *Jian Pi Wan* is an efficient formula for chronic cases of accumulated food stasis with underlying deficiency of spleen *qi*. *Mài yá* and *shān zhā* dispel food stasis; *bái zhú* and *dǎng shēn* tonify *qi,* while *zhǐ shí* and *chén pí* descend *qi* through the intestinal tract. Combined with caloric restriction, this is a good formula for weight loss.

Note: A larger formula of the same name but different composition was authored by Wáng Kěn-Tāng (王肯堂) in the *Zhèng Zhì Zhǔn Shéng* (证治准绳, "Pattern Treatment Standards", 1602). See Bensky p. 835 or Chen, p. 1277. It is not available in product form.

Further Reading: Bensky et al, p. 837

XIANG SHA YANG WEI TANG

Formula: *xiāng shā yǎng wèi tāng* (香砂养胃汤)
"Aucklandia, Amomum Nourish Stomach Decoction"
Author: Gōng Tíng-Xián (龚廷贤)
Source: *Wàn Bìng Huí Chūn* (万病回春), 1587
Literal: "Thousand Diseases Returned to Spring" (eg, "Restored to Health")

Availability:

Cyperus & Cluster Combination (EG)
Cyperus & Cardamon Combination (KP)
Xiang Sha Yang Wei Tang (BP)
Xiang Sha Yang Wei Wan (HT, MS, PM, TL)

Ingredients: (from the standardized "*Cyperus & Cluster/Cardamon Combination*")

bái zhú (白术), Rhizoma Atractylodis Macrocephalae	11.3 %	AA
fú líng (茯苓), Poria	11.3	FC
cāng zhú (苍术), Rhizoma Atractylodis	7.8	FB
hòu pò (厚朴), Cortex Magnoliae Officinalis	7.8	FB
chén pí (陈皮), Pericarpium Citri Reticulatae	7.8	G
xiāng fù (香附), Rhizoma Cyperi	7.8	G
bái dòu kòu (白豆蔻), Fructus Amomi Kravanh	7.8	FB
rén shēn (人参), Radix Ginseng	7.8	AA
shēng jiāng (生姜), Rhizoma Zingiberis Recens	7.8	BA
mù xiāng (木香), Radix Aucklandiae	5.7	G
shā rén (砂仁), Fructus Amomi	5.7	FB
gān cǎo (甘草), Radix Glycyrrhizae	5.7	AA
dà zǎo (大枣), Fructus Jujubae	5.7	AA

Dispels damp, dissolves phlegm, harmonizes the stomach, descends stomach qi, tonifies spleen qi, soothes the liver, promotes digestion, stops nausea. Use for chronic digestive complaints characterized by poor appetite, abdominal distension, accumulation of phlegm and food matter, nausea, acid regurgitation, borborygmus (abdominal gurgling) and loose or erratic stools. Can be used for chronic acid reflux and GERDS, gastritis, duodenal ulcer and morning sickness.

Pulse: Soft, wide or excess
Tongue: Normal, or coated

Comments: This is an important formula for food stasis with accumulation of damp and *qi* stagnation overlapping a weak digestion, causing bloating and discomfort following eating. *Xiang Sha Yang Wei Wan* is similar to *Xiang Sha Liu Jun Zi Tang* (Chapter 6A), adding in *hòu pò, bái dòu kòu* and *xiāng fù* to enhance *qi* moving and *qi* descending actions. Though a larger formula, *Xiang Sha Yang Wei Tang* came first historically.

The formula equally addresses stagnation of *qi*, phlegm and damp with underlying spleen *qi* deficiency. The presentation of simultaneous excess and deficiency is quite common, and in this regard, the formula can be used for GERDS and acid reflux due to its actions of tonifying spleen *qi* while descending stomach *qi*. The formula is also helpful for chronic food stagnation, and for spleen deficiency morning sickness.

Note: Most manufacturers substitute *dǎng shēn* (党参, Radix Codonopsis) for *rén shēn.*

Further Reading:

Bensky et al, p. 312
Chen & Chen, p. 534
Ellis, p. 338

ZI SHENG WAN

Formula: *zī shēng wán* (资生丸), "Support Life Pills"
Author: Miào Xī-Yōng (缪希雍)
Source: *Xiān Xǐng Zhāi Yī Xué Guǎng Bǐ Jì* (先醒斋医学广笔记), 1613
Literal: "First Awakened Studio Medical Studies Extensive Short Notes"

Availability:

Zi Sheng Teapills (PF)
Zi Sheng Wan (GC, MS, PM)

Ingredients: (from Minshan's *"Zi Sheng Wan"*)

dǎng shēn (党参), Radix Codonopsis	11.7 %	AA
bái zhú (白术), Rhizoma Atractylodis Macrocephalae	11.7	AA
yì yǐ rén (薏苡仁), Semen Coicis	11.7	FC
shén qū (神曲), Massa Medicata Fermentata	7.8	H
jú hóng (橘红), Exocarpium Citri Rubrum	7.8	G
shān zhā (山楂), Fructus Crataegi	7.8	H
shān yào (山药), Rhizoma Dioscoreae	5.9	AA
qiàn shí (芡实), Semen Euryales	5.9	L
fú líng (茯苓), Poria	5.9	FC
mài yá (麦芽), Fructus Hordei Germinatus	5.8	H
bǎi biǎn dòu (百扁豆), Semen Dolichos/Lablab Album	3.9	DF
lián zǐ (莲子), Semen Nelumbinis	3.9	L
jié gěng (桔梗), Radix Platycodonis	2.0	CA
huò xiāng (藿香), Herba Agastachis	2.0	FB
gān cǎo (甘草), Radix Glycyrrhizae	2.0	AA
zé xiè (泽泻), Rhizoma Alismatis	1.4	FC
bái dòu kòu (白豆蔻), Fructus Amomi Kravanh	1.4	FB
huáng lián (黄连), Rhizoma Coptidis	1.4	DB

Tonifies spleen qi, dispels damp, resolves food stasis, harmonizes the stomach, counters ascent of stomach qi, increases appetite. Use for chronic digestive complaints characterized by accumulation of food matter and damp. Symptoms include poor appetite, abdominal distension and nausea. Patients particularly benefiting would include those with chronically loose stools. Also useful for acute summer damp-heat syndromes or food poisoning characterized by vomiting or diarrhea; also for morning sickness, and for poor appetite and low weight in children.

Pulse: Soft, wide, slippery or excess
Tongue: Normal, or greasy

Comments: This is an effective formula for chronic food stagnation with excessive damp, as indicated by loose or erratic stools. It is also useful in morning sickness complicated by combined excess and deficiency patterns. The formula deals with excess by removing food matter (Category H), dispelling damp (Categories FB, FC and DF) and descending stomach *qi* (Category G); tonification includes supplementing spleen *qi* (Category AA).

Caution 1: *Shén qū* contains a wheat binder and is contraindicated for people with celiac disease or gluten sensitivity.

Caution 2: *Yì yǐ rén* is contraindicated during pregnancy.

Further Reading:

Chen & Chen, p. 1278

Modern Formulas:

KANG NING WAN
CURING PILL

Formula: *kāng níng wán* (康宁丸), "Peaceful Pill"
Source: Modern patent medicine

Availability:

Culing Pills (PM)
Curing Formula (CC, K)
Curing Pills (PF, PM)
Curing Pills Formula (HS)
Dr. Shen's Stomach Curing Pill (DS)
Ease Digestion Formula (GF)
Kang Ning Pian (PIM)
Kang Ning Wan (BP, HT)

Ingredients:(from Yihetang Pharmaceutical, Guangdong *"Culing Pill"*)

fú líng (茯苓), Poria	16.8 %	FC
cāng zhú (苍术), Rhizoma Atractylodis	9.7	FB
huò xiāng (藿香), Herba Agastachis	9.6	FB
bái zhǐ (白芷), Radix Angelicae Dahuricae	9.6	BA
yì yǐ rén (薏苡仁), Semen Coicis	8.9	FC
gé gēn (葛根), Radix Puerariae Lobatae	8.8	BB
shén qū (神曲), Massa Medicata Fermentata	8.8	H
gǔ yá (谷芽), Fructus Oryzae Germinatus	6.8	H
chén pí (陈皮), Pericarpium Citri Reticulatae	6.8	G
bò hé (薄荷), Herba Menthae	5.4	BB
jú huā (菊花), Flos Chrysanthemi	4.4	BB
jú hóng (橘红), Exocarpium Citri Rubrum	4.4	G

Ingredients: (from Herbal Times *"Kang Ning Wan"*)

fú líng (茯苓), Poria	15.5 %	FC
yì yǐ rén (薏苡仁), Semen Coicis	9.0	FC
jú huā (菊花), Flos Chrysanthemi	7.3	BB
bái zhǐ (白芷), Radix Angelicae Dahuricae	7.2	BA
cāng zhú (苍术), Rhizoma Atractylodis	7.2	FB
gé gēn (葛根), Radix Puerariae Lobatae	7.2	BB

hòu pò (厚朴), Cortex Magnoliae Officinalis	7.2	FB
huò xiāng (藿香), Herba Agastachis	7.2	FB
mù xiāng (木香), Radix Aucklandiae	7.2	G
shén qū (神曲), Massa Medicata Fermentata	7.2	H
gŭ yá (谷芽), Fructus Oryzae Germinatus	5.5	H
tiān huā fĕn (天花粉), Radix Trichosanthis	5.5	CB
jú hóng (橘红), Exocarpium Citri Rubrum	3.6	G
bò hé (薄荷), Herba Menthae	3.2	BB

Resolves food stasis, harmonizes the stomach and spleen, descends stomach qi, dispels damp. Use for acute symptoms of food stagnation, including epigastric or abdominal bloating, abdominal cramps, frontal headache, belching, hiccoughs, and nausea. Symptoms include poor digestion or appetite, distension, pain or hyperacidity in the epigastrium, nausea, and poorly formed stools. Useful in morning sickness, motion sickness, hyperacidity, overeating, or to alleviate hang-over. Can be used in acute food poisoning.

Pulse: Slippery or excess
Tongue: Normal or greasy

Comments: The *Kang Ning* formulas are based on the Chinese patent medicine, *Curing Pills* (now labeled *Culing Pills*.) These come in red boxes with 10 smaller boxes, each containing vials of small pills. One whole vial is used as a single dose. Other manufacturers such as Herbal Times will use their own familiar pill size or capsule.

Kang Ning Wan is helpful in acute situations of food stagnation, epigastric distension or nausea, including morning sickness due to excess. It can also be taken with or after greasy meals to prevent boating and nausea. Although *Kang Ning* Wan is helpful in food poisoning, the formula *Huo Xiang Zheng Qi Pian* (Chapter 6D) is preferred.

Within the formula, the FB herbs descend *qi* and dampness, the FC herbs dispel dampness, the G herbs descend stomach *qi*, and the H herbs resolve food stagnation. The combination of *jú huā* and *gé gēn* address frontal headache.

The Herbal Times version follows the original formula, adding in three herbs: *hòu pò, mù xiāng* and *tiān huā fĕn.*

Caution 1: *Shén qū* contains a wheat binder and is contraindicated for people with celiac disease or gluten sensitivity.

Caution 2: *Tiān huā fĕn* and *yì yĭ rén* are contraindicated during pregnancy. Many experienced practitioners feel confident of their safety during the first trimester.

OTHER FORMULAS APPROPRIATE TO THIS CHAPTER:

Classical Formulas:

Jin Jian Fei Er Wan

Ginseng & Poria/Hoelen Formula (EG)

Ju Pi Zhu Ru Tang

Citrus & Bamboo Combination (EG)

Xuan Fu Dai Zhe Shi Tang

Inula & Hematite Combination (EG)
* Counterflow Pearls (CP)

Modern Formulas:

Chen Xiang Hua Qi Wan

Chen Xiang Hua Qi Wan (TL)

Shu Gan Wan

See Chapter 7A

Other:

Astra 18 Diet (HC)
Chzyme (HC)
Diagnostic Tablets (SF)
Disperse Qi (CMS)
Earth-Harmonizing Formula (GF)
Earth Pearls (CP)
Ease Digestion Formula (GF)
Enteromend (HC)
Escape Restraint (HC)
Gallus-Malt Tablets (SF)
Limpid Sea (TT)
Lotus Leaf Tablets (SF)
Magnolia & Ginger Formula Modified (EG)
Purge Qi (CMS)
Quiet Digestion (HC)
Shen-Chu 16 (SF)
Stomach-Harmonizing Formula (GF)

PEDIATRIC FORMULAS

Classical Formulas:

Xiao Er Qi Xing Cha

Xiao Er Qi Xing Cha (PM)

Modern Formulas:

Bo Ying Pills (PM)
Easy Going (K)
Lapis 16 (SF)
Tummy Tamer (K)
Quiet Nights (BP)

6. DIGESTIVE DISORDERS

6D. DAMP-TURBIDITY
(Abdominal Cramping and Diarrhea)

Classical Formulas:

Huo Xiang Zheng Qi San	*huò xiāng zhèng qì sǎn* (藿香正气散)
Tong Xie Yao Fang	*tòng xiè yào fāng* (痛泻药方)
Wu Mei Wan	*wū méi wán* (乌梅丸)

Modern Formulas:

Huang Lian Su Pian	*huáng lián sù pian* (黄连素片)

The formulas in this category address acute gastrointestinal disorders such as food poisoning, stomach flu and acute diarrhea. In traditional Chinese medicine, this is often a problem of damp-turbidity caused by exogenous pathogenic toxins. Otherwise, damp-turbidity can be due to a spleen-stomach disharmony aggravated by exogenous pathogenic factors, including wind-cold. It is often seen during the summer, when food has a tendency to go bad, or when one's body is overheated and consumes too much raw food or cool liquids. In this regard, the syndrome is also referred to as *summer damp-heat* or *summer heat.*

Symptoms include sudden onset headache with nausea, vomiting or diarrhea. Occasionally, symptoms of the common cold may be evident: sore throat, fever or aches. The formulas described here are effective, and relief may happen in one or two doses. Typically, dosing is continued every three hours until symptoms are gone. For chronic turbid-damp or diarrhea, they may have to be taken for a continued period of time. There are safe to do so, if necessary.

Several of the formulas are used for protozoan or bacterial infections of the gut, causing abdominal bloating erratic stools, and lowered immune response.

In general Chinese medical practitioners advise patients to discontinue spicy and greasy food during episodes of damp-turbidity.

For chronic and less severe episodes, refer to formulas in *Chapter 6C. Food Stagnation and Indigestion.*

Classical Formulas:

HUO XIANG ZHENG QI SAN

Formula: *huò xiāng zhèng qì sǎn* (藿香正气散), "Agastache Rectify Qi Powder"
Author: Imperial Medical Bureau (*tài yī jú*, 太医局); revised by Chén Shī-Wén (陈师文)
Source: *Tài Píng Huì Mín Hé Jì Jú Fāng* (太平惠民和剂局方), 1078
Literal: "(Era of) Great Peace, Benefit People Harmonious Medicines, Office (of) Formulas"

Availability:

Agastache Formula (EG)
Huo Xiang Zheng Qi Pian (PIM, PM)
Huo Xiang Zheng Qi San (BP)
Huo Xiang Zheng Qi Wan (HT, MS, TL)
* Early Comfort (K)
* Jiawei Huo Xiang Zheng Qi Formula (HS)

Ingredients: (from the standardized *"Agastache Formula"*)

huò xiāng (藿香), Herba Agastachis	10.0 %	FB
dà fù pí (大腹皮), Pericarpium Arecae	10.0	G
zǐ sū yè (紫苏叶), Folium Perillae	10.0	BA
fú líng (茯苓), Poria	10.0	FC
bái zhǐ (白芷), Radix Angelicae Dahuri	10.0	BA
shēng jiāng (生姜), Rhizoma Zingiberis Recens	10.0	BA
jié gěng (桔梗), Radix Platycodonis	6.7	CA
bái zhú (白术), Rhizoma Atractylodis Macrocephalae	6.7	AA
bàn xià (半夏), Rhizoma Pinelliae	6.7	CA
chén pí (陈皮), Pericarpium Citri Reticulatae	6.7	G
hòu pò (厚朴), Cortex Magnoliae Officinalis	6.7	FB
zhì gān cǎo (炙甘草), Radix Glycyrrhizae Praep.	3.3	AA
dà zǎo (大枣), Fructus Jujubae	3.3	AA

Dispels pathogenic factors, resolves the exterior, clears summer heat and dispels damp, dispels turbidity, descends stomach qi, harmonizes the middle jiao, relieves diarrhea. Use for early stage of summer damp-heat invasion or wind-cold invasion where there is dampness or damp-turbidity in the interior. Symptoms include fever with chills, frontal headache, loose stools or diarrhea, epigastric or abdominal bloating, abdominal pain, and vomiting or nausea. Applicable in acute gastroenteritis, food poisoning, and infections associated with stomach flu. Also useful for food stagnation, motion sickness, overeating and alcohol hangover.

Pulse: Soggy, slippery or floating
Tongue: White or yellow greasy coat

Comments: *Huo Xiang Zheng Qi San* was originally formulated for exogenous wind-cold with a concurrent stagnation of the middle *jiao*, causing headache, vomiting and diarrhea. Despite the preponderance of warming herbs, the formula was also used for acute pathogenic summer damp-heat and cholera. Modern application has it as the medicine of choice for food poisoning and stomach flu, often requiring only one or two doses. It can also be used for food stagnation due to over-eating.

Huò xiāng, the principal herb, resolves turbid damp and harmonizes stomach and spleen. It is very good for nausea and vomiting. The synergistic coupling of *huò xiāng, dà fù pí* and *zǐ sū yè* works against communicable aerobic bacteria as well as viruses triggering gastrointestinal illness. In itself, *huò xiāng* address turbid-dampness with resultant nausea and vomiting. Five groups of herbs achieve the total affect: the AA herbs strengthen spleen; the BA herbs dispel wind-cold; the CA herbs address phlegm causing nausea; the FB and FC herbs dispel and descend dampness; and finally, the G herbs descend stomach *qi*.

In acute cases of food poisioning, it is often helpful to combine *Huo Xiang Zheng Qi San* with *Huang Lian Su*, described below.

Further Reading:

Bensky et al, p. 691
Chen & Chen, p. 1079
Ellis, p. 151

TONG XIE YAO FANG

Formula: *tòng xiè yào fāng* (痛泻药方), "Painful Diarrhea Important Formula"
Author: Zhāng Jiè-Bīn (张介宾) *aka* Zhāng Jǐng-Yuè (张景岳)
Source: *Jǐng Yuè Quán Shū* (景岳全书), 1624
Literal: "Jing-Yue's Complete Writings"

also attributed to:

Author: Zhū Zhèn-Hěng (朱震亨) *aka* Zhū Dān-Xī (朱丹溪)
Source: *Dān Xī Xīn Fǎ* (丹溪心法), 1481
Literal: "Dan-Xi's Heart Method" (eg, "Personal Insights")

also attributed to:

Author: Wú Kūn (吴昆)
Source: *Yī Fāng Kǎo* (医方考), 1584
Literal: "Medical Formula Investigations"

Availability:

Calm Wind Teapills (PF)
Tong Xie Yao Fang Wan (HT)

Ingredients: (from Plum Flower *"Calm Wind Teapills"*)

chǎo bái sháo (炒白芍), Radix Paeoniae Alba	40.0 %	AB
chǎo bái zhú (炒白术), Rhizoma Atractylodis Macro.	29.9	AA
chǎo chén pí (炒陈皮), Pericarpium Citri Reticulatae	20.0	G
fáng fēng (防风), Radix Saposhnikov./Ledebouriellae	10.1	BA

Ingredients: (from Herbal Times *"Tong Xie Yao Fang Wan"*)

bái sháo (白芍), Radix Paeoniae Alba	40 %	AB
bái zhú (白术), Rhizoma Atractylodis Macro.	30	AA
chén pí (陈皮), Pericarpium Citri Reticulatae	20	G
fáng fēng (防风), Radix Saposhnikov./Ledebouriellae	10	BA

Soothes the liver, tonifies spleen, descends stomach qi, relieves diarrhea, stops pain. Use for liver-spleen imbalance causing abdominal distension with pain, indigestion, borborygmus (abdominal gurgling), diarrhea with pain, or straining during defecation. Useful in acute or chronic gastroenteritis, dysentery, irritable bowel syndrome and colitis. Useful for loose stools caused by stress or anxiety.

Pulse: Wiry, slippery, or thin
Tongue: Normal, or may be coated

Comments: This small formula treats abdominal pain or painful diarrhea whose underlying pattern is a combined spleen deficiency, liver stasis, and failure of stomach *qi* to descend. Early symptoms include abdominal distension with gradual development into abdominal pain, and later, small, unformed stools or diarrhea with pain and straining.

Bái sháo relaxes liver constraint, *bái zhú* supports spleen *qi,* and *chén pí* descends stomach *qi*. While *fáng fēng* is known for its effects in dispelling wind-cold, a secondary function is the control of diarrhea. Herbs that dispel wind go to the "exterior", which includes the epithelium of the digestive tract. Also, combined with *bái sháo*, it helps relieve cramping.

The Plum Flower version follows the classical prescription, using dry stir-frying (*chǎo,* 炒) for three of the ingredients. This enhances an astringent effect, further inhibiting diarrhea.

Further Reading:

Bensky et al, p. 125
Chen & Chen, p. 257

WU MEI WAN

Formula: *wū méi wán* (乌梅丸), "Mume Pills"
Author: Zhāng Zhòng-Jǐng (张仲景)
Source: *Shāng Hán Lùn* (伤寒论), 220
Literal: "Injury (by) Cold, Discussion"

Availability:

Wu Mei Wan (BP, HT)

Ingredients: (from Blue Poppy *"Wu Mei Wan"*)

wū méi (乌梅), Fructus Mume	20. %	L
gān jiāng (干姜), Rhizoma Zingiberis	12	E
guì zhī (桂枝), Ramulus Cinnamomi	12	BA
zhì fù zǐ (炙附子), Radix Aconiti Lateralis Praeparata	12	E
huáng bǎi (黄柏), Cortex Phellodendri	12	DB
rén shēn (人参), Radix Ginseng	12	AA
dāng guī (当归), Radix Angelicae Sinensis	12	AB
huáng lián (黄连), Rhizoma Coptidis	6	DB
huā jiāo (花椒), Pericarpium Zanthoxyli	2	E

Ingredients: (from Herbal Times *"Wu Mei Wan"*)

wū méi (乌梅), Fructus Mume	18.5 %	L
dāng guī (当归), Radix Angelicae Sinensis	11.1	AB
zhì fù zǐ (炙附子), Radix Aconiti Lateralis Praeparata	11.1	E
gān jiāng (干姜), Rhizoma Zingiberis	11.1	E
guì zhī (桂枝), Ramulus Cinnamomi	11.1	BA
huáng bǎi (黄柏), Cortex Phellodendri	11.1	DB
rén shēn (人参), Radix Ginseng	11.1	AA
huáng lián (黄连), Rhizoma Coptidis	7.4	DB
huā jiāo (花椒), Pericarpium Zanthoxyli	3.7	E
shǐ jūn zǐ (使君子), Fructus Quisqualis	3.7	Q

Warms the intestines, clears heat, resolves toxins, quiets roundworms. Use for roundworm infestation of the intestines with intermittent attacks of abdominal cramping, vomiting following eating, or vomiting of worms. Also for chronic gastrointestinal disturbances marked by diarrhea or loose stools due to cold middle *jiao* with heat in the small or large intestines. Use for roundworms, biliary worms, and chronic amebic or bacterial dysentery. Helpful for protozoan infections including Giardia and Blastocystis hominis.

Pulse: Deep, forceful, or weak
Tongue: Normal, or greasy coat

Comments: This formula has endured as a prescription for treating roundworms, with accompanying symptoms of abdominal pain and vomiting. It contains both warming and cooling herbs, which address the common presentation cold in the the middle *jiao* and heat in the lower *jiao*, found in chronic parasitic presentations. Traditionally, the herb *wū méi* kills worms, stops diarrhea, and is used in dysentery.

In the modern clinic, *Wu Mei Wan* can be used for chronic amebic or bacterial dysentery marked by diarrhea and borborygmus (abdominal gurgling), and also protozoan infections such as Giardia, Blastocystis hominis, and amebiasis. My clinical experience indicates usefulness of this formula for small intestine inflammation due to food allergies or micro-colitis with diarrhea, as found in leaky gut syndrome.

The two representative formulas use the same ingredients, except that the Herbal Times version adds Quisqualis *shǐ jūn zǐ* to further address parasites.

Caution: *Zhì fù zǐ* is used with caution during pregnancy.

Further Reading:

Bensky et al, p. 847
Chen & Chen, p. 1292
Ellis, p. 327

Modern Formulas:

HUANG LIAN SU PIAN

Formula: *huáng lián sù pian* (黄连素片), "Coptis Extract Tablet"
Source: Modern patent medicine
Manufacturer: Hubei Yichang Minkang Factory, Yichang, China

Availability:

Huang Lian Su Tablets (PM)
* Coptis Teapills (PF)

Ingredients: (from Hubei Yichang Minkang Factory *"Huang Lian Su Pian"*)

huáng lián sù (黄连素), Rhizoma Coptidis extract	100 %	DB

Clears heat, resolves toxin, relieves dysentery. Use for intestinal bacteria causing bacterial dysentery, food poisoning, gastroenteritis, abdominal pain and distension. Can be used in acute and chronic appendicitis, tooth abscess, canker sores, strep throat, and sinus infection. Can be applied topically for infections.

Pulse: Deep, forceful, or weak
Tongue: Normal, or greasy coat

Comments: *Huang Lian Su Tablets* uses a very concentrated extraction of Coptis *Huang Lian*, producing berberine hydrochloride. It comes in a red and yellow box with twelve vials, each with twelve small tablets. The therapeutic dosage is 3 tablets, taken one to three times daily.

It is commonly used in China and Southeast Asia for acute diarrhea, bacterial dysentery, and food poisoning. It can be used to successfully treat a variety of intestinal pathogens, including pathogenic bacteria (Proteus, Citrobacter, Klebsiella, Salmonella), the fungus Candida albicans, and protozoa such as Giardia, Blastocystis hominis and Toxoplasmosis. Also, the pills can be crushed into powder and mixed with water or salve to treat infected wounds topically.

As a manufactured extraction (*sù*, 素), it is significantly stronger and more concentrated than powdered *huáng lián.* Plum Blossom offers a product by the same name, which is not concentrated, but has similar applications.

Caution: *Huáng lián* is a cold herb. Prolonged use or excessive dosage may cause diarrhea, abdominal or epigastric pain, or gastric upset. Monitor and adjust dose if necessary.

OTHER PRODUCTS APPROPRIATE FOR THIS CATEGORY:

Classical Formulas:

Bai Tou Weng Tang
Anemone Combination (EG)

Ban Xia Xie Xin Tang
Ban Xia Xie Xin Tang (TZ)
Ban Xia Xie Xin Pian/Wan (GC)
Drain The Middle (K)
Pinellia Combination (EG)
Pinellia Formula to Drain the Epigastrium (HS)
* Counterflow Pearls (CP)
* One Mind (K)

Da Chai Hu Tang
See Chapter 7C

Gan Cao Xie Xin Tang
Pinellia & Licorice Combination (EG)

Ge Gen Huang Qin Huang Lian Tang
Pueraria, Coptis & Scute Combination (EG)

Liu He Tang
Cardamon Combination (EG)

Mu Xiang Bing Lang Wan
See Chapter 6E

Qing Shu Yi Qi Tang
Astragalus & Atractylodes Combination (EG)
Qing Shu Formula (K)

Shao Yao Tang
Peony Combination (EG)

Sheng Jiang Xie Xin Tang
Pinellia & Ginger Combination (EG)

Wei Ling Tang
Magnolia & Poria/Hoelen Combination (EG)

Modern Formulas:

Cinnamon Pearls (CP)
Disperse Moisture (CMS)
GI Care II (EV)
Irritease (K)
Three Kernel Decoction (AL)

6E. CONSTIPATION

Classical Formulas:

Da Cheng Qi Tang	*dà chéng qì tāng* (大承气汤)
Ma Zi Ren Wan	*má zǐ rén wán* (麻子仁丸)
Mu Xiang Bing Lang Wan	*mù xiāng bīng láng wán* (木香槟榔丸)
Run Chang Wan	*rùn cháng wán* (润肠丸)
Wu Ren Wan	*wǔ rén wán* (五仁丸)

Constipation can refer to hard dry stools, or infrequency of passing stool even if the stool appears normal. It can be due to a variety of causes, including heat, stagnation of *qi*, deficiency of *qi*, deficiency of blood or deficiency of spleen *yang*. In chronic conditions, the root patterns often needs to be addressed at the same time by combining constipation formulas with products from other chapters.

Some of the formulas in this chapter combine various therapies simultaneously, so that they tonify blood, move *qi,* clear heat and purge the bowels. Some use oily seeds in their ingredients, which lubricate the intestines and provide roughage for moving impacted stool and allowing beneficial bacteria colonies to thrive.

Taken alone, the products in this chapter are effective for inducing a bowel movement, but may not cure the problem unless the underlying cause is also addressed. Many formulas are gentle and can be used for long periods of time safely, and do not have the side effects of harsh purgatives. Other formulas are harsher and should not be used for extended periods.

Because most of the products here use downward purging herbs, they are prohibited in the second and third trimesters of pregnancy.

Classical Formulas:

DA CHENG QI TANG

Formula: *dà chéng qì tāng* (大承气汤), "Major Order (the) *Qi* Decoction"
Author: Zhāng Zhòng-Jǐng (张仲景)
Source: *Shāng Hán Lùn* (伤寒论), 220
Literal: "Injury (by) Cold, Discussion"

Availability:

Major Rhubarb Combination (EG)

Ingredients: (from the standardized *"Major Rhubarb Combination"*)

hòu pò (厚朴), Cortex Magnoliae	44.4 %	FB
dà huáng (大黄), Radix/Rhizoma Rhei	22.2	PA
máng xiāo (芒硝), Natrii Sulfas/Mirabilitum	16.7	PA
zhǐ shí (枳实), Fructus Aurantii Immaturus	16.7	G

Descends stomach qi, clears heat, unblocks the bowel and frees the stool. Use for constipation due to heat and stagnation, with symptoms of dry hard stool, abdominal distension or abdominal pain before defecation. Helpful in constipation during or following fever, and in chronic heat presentations. May also be used to clear the bowels in pathogenic diarrhea and dysentery, and can be used in acute appendicitis.

Pulse: Forceful; may be slippery, rapid or normal
Tongue: Dry with a yellow coat; body may be red

Comments: This foundation formula for constipation was recorded in the *Shang Han Lun* in the 2nd century CE, and originally applied to constipation due to fever. The purgation method was commonly employed to break a fever, as well as rid the body of toxins. It was also used for watery diarrhea due to heat-toxins, and for manic episodes accompanied by constipation.

Both *dà huáng* and *máng xiāo* are strong downward purgatives with cold properties, and are particularly useful in impaction of hard stool. *Hòu pò* and *zhǐ shí* help descend stomach *qi*, aiding the purgation method. It is particularly useful in constipation in infants and children, marked by abdominal distension, crying and hard stool. It is also helpful to lower fever by freeing the stool. This formula is only available in extracted granule form.

Caution: *Dà huáng* and *máng xiāo* are prohibited during pregnancy. Also, the formula may be too strong in weak or elderly patients. In general, because of its drastic purgative effects, use should be discontinued once stools have passed.

Further Reading:

Bensky et al, p. 63
Chen & Chen, p. 158
Ellis, p. 59

MA ZI REN WAN

Formula: *má zǐ rén wán* (麻子仁丸), "Hemp Seed Pill"
Author: Zhāng Zhòng-Jǐng (张仲景)
Source: *Shāng Hán Lùn* (伤寒论), 220
Literal: "Injury (by) Cold, Discussion"

Availability:

Apricot Seed & Hemp Seed Formula (EG)
Apricot Semen & Linum Formula (EG)
Ma Zi Ren Wan (BP, HT, TL, TZ)
Ma Zi Ren Wan Teapills (PF)

Ingredients: (from the standardized *"Apricot Seed & Hemp Seed Formula"*)

huǒ má rén (火麻仁), Semen Cannabis	33.4 %	PB
dà huáng (大黄), Radix/Rhizoma Rhei	22.2	PA
bái sháo (白芍), Radix Paeoniae Alba	11.1	AB
zhǐ shí (枳实), Fructus Aurantii Immaturus	11.1	G
hòu pò (厚朴), Cortex Magnoliae Officinalis	11.1	FB
xìng rén (杏仁), Semen Armeniacae	11.1	CC

Ingredients: (from Herbal Times *"Ma Zi Ren Wan"*)

hú má rén (胡麻仁), Semen Lini usitatissimi	37.1 %	PB
bái sháo (白芍), Radix Paeoniae Alba	18.5	AB
dà huáng (大黄), Radix/Rhizoma Rhei	11.1	PA
hòu pò (厚朴), Cortex Magnoliae Officinalis	11.1	FB
xìng rén (杏仁), Semen Armeniacae	11.1	CC
chǎo zhǐ shí (炒枳实), Fructus Aurantii Immaturus	11.1	G

Ingredients: (from Plum Flower *"Ma Zi Ren Teapills"*)

yà má zǐ (亚麻子), Semen Lini usitatissimi	20.0 %	PB
xìng rén (杏仁), Semen Armeniacae	17.4	CC
zhǐ shí (枳实), Fructus Aurantii Immaturus	17.4	G
hòu pò (厚朴), Cortex Magnoliae Officinalis	17.4	FB
bái sháo (白芍), Radix Paeoniae Alba	17.4	AB
dà huáng (大黄), Radix/Rhizoma Rhei	10.4	PA

Moistens the intestines, clears heat, descends stomach qi, unblocks the bowel and frees the stool. Use for constipation due to stagnation, dryness, and heat. Use in heat and excess conditions where the *yin* has been depleted, with symptoms of dry or hard stool, abdominal pain and dry mouth. Useful in chronic constipation, as well as constipation following fever, childbirth, or surgery. Can be used for hemorrhoid accompanying constipation.

Pulses: Deep, choppy, may be rapid
Tongue: Dry, thin coat, may be yellow

Comments: *Ma Zi Ren Wan* is suitable for constipation marked by stagnation, heat and dryness. It uses three herbs from *Da Cheng Qi Tang* (above) - *hòu pò, dà huáng* and *zhǐ shí* - adding in *huǒ má rén* and *xìng rén* to moisten the intestines. In this regard, it is more moistening and not as harsh as *Da Cheng Qi Tang*.

The original formula uses dry-fried hemp seed (*huǒ má rén*). In both the Herbal Times and Plum Flower versions, flax seed (*hú má rén,* 胡麻仁, Semen Lini usitatissimi, also known as or *yà má zǐ,* 亚麻子) is substituted. *Ma Zi Ren Tang* is suitable for impacted or dry stool due to heat, and is better tolerated than *Da Cheng Qi Tang* for elderly and weak patients, as well as constipation following surgery.

Dà huáng is the main purgative, and is tolerated to varying degrees. The 22% offered in the Taiwan extract products may be too strong for repeated use.

Caution: *Dà huáng* is prohibited during pregnancy. One can make the formula without *dà huáng* for use during pregnancy.

Further Reading:

Bensky et al, p. 81
Chen & Chen, p. 176
Ellis, p. 197

MU XIANG BING LANG WAN

Formula: *mù xiāng bīng láng wán* (木香槟榔丸), "Aucklandia, Areca Pill"
Author: Zhāng Cóng-Zhèng (张从正) *aka* Zhāng Zǐ-Hé (张子和)
Source: *Rú Mén Shì Qīn* (儒门事亲), 1228
Literal: "Confucians' Duties (to their) Parents"

also cited in:

Author: Zhū Zhèn-Hēng (朱震亨) *aka* Zhū Dān-Xī (朱丹溪)
Source: *Dān Xī Xīn Fǎ* (丹溪心法), 1481
Literal: "Dan-Xi's Heart Method" (eg, "Personal Insights")

Availability:

Mu Xiang Bing Lang Wan (HT)
Saussurea & Areca Formula (EG)
Vladimiria & Areca Seed Formula (KP)

Ingredients: (from Herbal Times *"Mu Xiang Bing Lang Wan"*)

bīng láng (槟榔), Semen Arecae	14.3 %	Q
dà huáng (大黄), Radix/Rhizoma Rhei	14.3	PA
mù xiāng (木香), Radix Aucklandiae	14.3	G
é zhú (莪术), Rhizoma Curcumae	10.7	K
qiān niú zǐ (牵牛子), Semen Pharbitidis	10.7	PC
xiāng fù (香附), Rhizoma Cyperi	10.7	G
chén pí (陈皮), Pericarpium Citri Reticulatae	7.0	G
huáng bǎi (黄柏), Cortex Phellodendri	7.0	DB
qīng pí (青皮), Pericarpium Citri Reticulatae Viride	7.0	G
huáng lián (黄连), Rhizoma Coptidis	4.0	DB

Ingredients: (from KPC *"Vladimiria & Areca Seed Formula"*)

xiāng fù (香附), Rhizoma Cyperi	23.3 %	G
dà huáng (大黄), Radix/Rhizoma Rhei	11.7	PA
máng xiāo (芒硝), Natrii Sulfas/Mirabilitum	11.7	PA
mù xiāng (木香), Radix Aucklandiae	5.9	G
bīng láng (槟榔), Semen Arecae	5.9	Q
qīng pí (青皮), Pericarpium Citri Reticulatae Viride	5.2	G
chén pí (陈皮), Pericarpium Citri Reticulatae	5.9	G
zhǐ ké (枳壳), Fructus Aurantii	5.9	G
huáng bǎi (黄柏), Cortex Phellodendri	5.9	DB
huáng lián (黄连), Rhizoma Coptidis	5.9	DB
sān léng (三棱), Rhizoma Sparganii	5.9	K
é zhú (莪术), Rhizoma Curcumae	5.9	K

Frees the stool, harmonizes liver and stomach, descends stomach qi, dispels damp-heat, descends turbidity, kills worms and expels parasites. Use for abdominal distension with pain or cramping, constipation or inability to pass stool, or damp-heat diarrhea including dysentery; also frontal headache, belching, nausea or vomiting. Applicable in acute constipation due to food poisoning or enteritis. Also applicable in mucus diarrhea due to parasites, dysentery or microbial colitis.

Pulse: Deep and excess
Tongue: Yellow greasy coat with a red tongue

Comments: *Mu Xiang Bing Lan Wan* uses the traditional purgation method to treat acute abdominal distress, and should be used in cases of excess, not deficiency. It can be used for constipation with tight abdomen and prolonged abdominal pain or discomfort; it can also be used for damp-heat or pathogenic diarrhea.

The original formula relies on strong amounts of *dà huáng, bīng láng* and *qiān niú zǐ* to unblock acute obstruction in the digestive tract. These herbs also attack parasitic infections causing straining, and stool with small broken pieces and mucus. This includes Giardia and other protozoan causes of diarrhea. It can also be used for chronic diarrhea due to microbial colitis.

The Herbal Times formula contains all of the ingredients of the original prescription. In the KPC version, *qiān niú zǐ* is missing, while *sān léng, máng xiāo* and *zhǐ ké* are added. *Sān léng* helps resolve abdominal hardness, while *máng xiāo* reinforces the purgative effect of *dà huáng.*

Caution: Due to the inclusion of *dà huáng, sān léng, máng xiāo, é zhú* or *qiān niú zǐ*, these formulas are contraindicated during pregnancy. *Sān léng* (in the KPC version) is contraindicated for patients taking Coumadin.

Further Reading:

Bensky et al, p. 831
Chen & Chen, p. 1272
Ellis, p. 202

RUN CHANG WAN

Formula: *rùn cháng wán* (润肠丸), "Moisten Intestines Pill"
Author: Lĭ Găo (李杲) *aka* Lĭ Dōng-Yuán (李东垣)
Source: *Pí Wèi Lùn* (脾胃论), 1249
Literal: "Spleen, Stomach Discussion"

Availability:

Hemp Seed & Rhubarb Formula (KP)
Linum & Rhubarb Formula (EG)
Peach Kernel Pills (MS)
Peach Kernel Teapills (PF)
Run Chang Wan (BP, PM, TL)
Smooth Response (K)

Ingredients: (from Plum Flower "*Peach Kernel Teapills*")

táo rén (桃仁), Semen Persicae	28.6 %	K
yà má zĭ (亚麻子), Semen Lini usitatissimi	28.5	AD
dà huáng (大黄), Radix/Rhizoma Rhei	14.3	PA
qiāng huó (羌活), Radix Notopterygii	14.3	BA
dāng guī (当归), Radix Angelicae Sinensis	14.3	AB

Ingredients: (fromthe standardized *"Linum/Hemp Seed & Rhubarb Formula"*)

táo rén (桃仁), Semen Persicae	28.6 %	K
huŏ má rén (火麻仁), Fructus Cannabis	28.6	AD
dà huáng (大黄), Radix/Rhizoma Rhei	14.3	PA
dāng guī (当归), Radix Angelicae Sinensis	14.3	AB
qiāng huó (羌活), Radix Notopterygii	14.2	BA

Moistens the intestines, clears heat, tonifies blood, unblocks the bowel and frees the stool. Use for chronic constipation due to heat, deficiency of fluid and deficiency of blood. Helpful in chronic constipation due to older age, postpartum, during a fever, or following a chronic illness.

Pulses: Normal, or thin or deep
Tongue: Dry with a yellow coat

Comments: This is a popular prescription for treating chronic constipation due to heat and dryness. Li Gao's original formula uses *táo rén* (peach seed) and *huǒ má rén* (hemp seed), seeds that contain up to 30% essential oils that lubricate the intestines. *Dāng guī* tonifies blood and helps moistening. *Dà huáng* is a purgative and treats constipation due to heat.

Several companies make substitutions for *huǒ má rén*. The Herbal Times version substitutes *hēi zhī ma* (黑芝麻, Semen Sesami Nigrum, black sesame seed) and the Plum Flower version, *Peach Kernel Teapills*, substitutes *yà má zǐ* (亚麻子, Semen Lini) - flax seed/ linseed.

Caution: Both *táo rén* and *dà huáng* are contraindicated during pregnancy. *Táo rén* is contraindicated for patients taking blood thinners such as Coumadin.

Further Reading:

Bensky et al, p. 80
Chen & Chen, p. 177
Ellis, p. 243

WU REN WAN

Formula: *wǔ rén wán* (五仁丸), "Five Seed Pill"
Author: Wēi Yì-Lín (危亦林)
Source: *Shì Yī Dé Xiào Fāng* (世医得效方), 1345
Literal: "Generations (of) Physicians Obtained Effective Formulas"

Availability:

Five Seed Teapills (PF)
Wu Ren Tang (PM)

Ingredients: (from Plum Flower *"Five Seed Teapills"*)

chén pí (陈皮), Pericarpium Citri Reticulatae	25.7 %	G
xìng rén (杏仁), Semen Armeniacae	25.7	CC
táo rén (桃仁), Semen Persicae	15.2	K
bǎi zǐ rén (柏子仁), Semen Platycladi/Biotae	15.2	N
yù lǐ rén (郁李仁), Semen Pruni	10.2	PB
sōng zǐ rén (松子仁), Semen Pini Koraiensis	8.0	PB

Moistens the intestines, descends qi, frees the stool. Use for chronic deficiency constipation due to dryness or deficiency of fluid and blood. Helpful in constipation in the elderly, or with weakness, postpartum and post-surgery.

Pulses: Thin, rough
Tongue: Dry

Comments: This is a gentle formula for constipation due to dryness. The oils of the five seeds act to lubricate the intestines, and the crushed seeds provide roughage that can score into impacted stool and provide insoluble fibers for probiotic growth. The formula is useful in constipation in the aged and following childbirth. The five seeds (*rén,* 仁) that are used are almond (*xìng rén*), peach (*táo rén*), pine (*sōng zǐ rén*), bush cherry (*yù lǐ rén*) and thuja (*bǎi zǐ rén*). *Chén pí* moves and descends stomach *qi*.

Caution: *Táo rén* is contraindicated during pregnancy.

Further Reading:

Bensky et al, p. 78
Chen & Chen, p. 176

OTHER PRODUCTS APPROPRIATE FOR THIS CATEGORY:

Classical Formulas:

Da Chai Hu Tang

See Chapter 7C

Da Huang Mu Dan Pi Tang

See Chapter 2A

Fang Feng Tong Sheng Wan

See Chapter 2C

Tao He Cheng Qi Tang

Peach Pit Formula To Order The Qi (HS)
Tao He Cheng Qi Tang (TZ)
* Jade Disperse 1 (JW)

Modern Formulas:

Aquilaria Pills (MS)
Belly Binder (GW)
Dr. Shen's Rhubarb Rx For Constipation (DS)
Free The Flow (BP)
Gentle Lax-Deficient (EV)
Gentle Lax-Excess (EV)
Gentle Senna (HC)
Persica and Cistanches Formula (GF)
Rhubarb 17 (SF)
Rhubarb Teapills (PF)
Tiger Pearls (CP)
Tong Bian Pian/Wan (GC)
Xiao Cheng Qi Pian/Wan (GC)

6. DIGESTIVE DISORDERS

6F. HEMORRHOID

Classical Formulas:

Huai Jiao Wan (Fructus Sophora) *huái jiăo wán* (槐角丸)

Modern Formulas:

Hua Zhi Ling (Fargelin)	*huà zhì líng* (化痔灵)
Zhi Bao	*zhì băo* (痔宝)

Hemorrhoids are highly vascularized structures in the anus that normally aid with stool control. When inflamed, they become enlarged and can cause pain, itching, or localized bleeding. Hemorrhoids present either externally or internally. They can develop from prolonged sitting, prolonged standing, or walking long distances while carrying heavy loads. They can also develop from overeating spicy or rich, sweet foods, from chronic constipation, from overexertion, or following pregnancy and childbirth. Obesity can also be a factor.

In Chinese medicine, hemorrhoids form as a result of stagnation of *qi* and blood with production of damp-heat. The herbal formulas in this chapter act by invigorating blood, breaking blood stasis, dispelling damp-heat, and stopping bleeding. The products described here are taken internally, but Chinese herbal topical ointments can also be found. Chinese herbal medicine is very effective for treatment and control of hemorrhoids.

Caution is advised during pregnancy, and some formulas are prohibited. Hemorrhoids unresponsive to herbal therapy may require surgery.

Classical Formulas:

HUAI JIAO WAN
FRUCTUS SOPHORA

Formula: *huái jiăo wán* (槐角丸), "Sophora Pill"
Author: Imperial Medical Bureau (*tài yī jú*, 太医局); revised by Chén Shī-Wén (陈师文)

Source: *Tài Píng Huì Mín Hé Jì Jú Fāng* (太平惠民和剂局方), 1078
Literal: "(Era of) Great Peace, Benefit People Harmonious Medicines, Office (of) Formulas"
also attributed to:
Author: Zhū Zhèn-Hěng (朱震亨) *aka* Zhū Dān-Xī (朱丹溪)
Source: *Dān Xī Xīn Fǎ* (丹溪心法), 1481
Literal: "Dan-xi's Heart Method" (eg, "Personal Insights")

Availability:

Fructus Sophorae Concentrated (PM)

Ingredients: (from Minkang Factory, Yichang *"Fructus Sophorae Concentrated"*)

huái jiǎo (槐角), Fructus Sophorae	28.5 %	J
zhǐ ké (枳壳), Fructus Aurantii	14.3	G
dāng guī (当归), Radix Angelicae Sinensis	14.3	AB
dì yú (地榆), Radix Sanguisorbae	14.3	J
fáng fēng (防风), Radix Saposhnikov./Ledebouriellae	14.3	BA
huáng qín (黄芩), Radix Scutellariae	14.3	DB

Stops bleeding, disperses swelling, dispels heat, relieves itching, descends qi, frees the stool, relieves pain. Use to stop hemorrhoid swelling, with or without bleeding, and to control symptoms of pain, bleeding, swelling, and itchiness. Can be used to treat intestinal bleeding, rectal prolapse, burning anus, anal fissure and constipation.

Pulse: Normal, or slippery or wiry
Tongue: Normal, or reddish with a yellow coat

Comments: This formula treats hemorrhoid swelling with bleeding. *Huái jiǎo*, the fruit, is the main ingredient, having both astringent and hemostatic effects. *Dì yú* stops hemorrhoidal bleeding. This product may only require one or two doses for acute presentations, or require continued treatment in chronic cases. The classical formula used *chǎo huái jiǎo* (炒槐角, dry-fried), to aid the astringing effect.

Caution: *Huái jiǎo* is used with caution during pregnancy.

Further Reading:

Bensky et al, p. 606

Modern Formulas:

HUA ZHI LING
FARGELIN

Formula: *huà zhì líng* (化痔灵), "Transform Hemorrhoids Effective-Remedy"
Source: Modern patent medicine

Availability:

Fargelin (PF, PM)
High Strength Fargelin (PM)
Hua Zhi Ling (PIM)

Ingredients: (from Yang Cheng Brand *"High Strength Fargelin"*)

tián qī (田七), Radix/Rhizoma Notoginseng	20. %	J
huáng qín (黄芩), Radix Scutellariae	15	DB
huái huā (槐花), Flos Sophorae	15	J
zǐ zhū yè (紫珠叶), Folium Callicarpae Pedunculatae	15	J
hǔ pò (琥珀), Succinum	15	N
dì yú (地榆), Radix Sanguisorbae	10	J
zhū dǎn fěn (猪胆粉), Pulvis Fellis Suis	5	CB
yán hú suǒ (延胡索), Rhizoma Corydalis	5	K

Ingredients: (from Plum Flower *"Fargelin"*)

shí liú pí (石榴皮), Pericarpium Granati	30. %	L
hǎi gé ké (海蛤壳), Concha Meretricis seu Cyclinae	30	CB
tián qī (田七), Radix/Rhizoma Notoginseng	17	J
huáng lián (黄连), Rhizoma Coptidis	10	DB
hǔ pò (琥珀), Succinum	10	N
zhū dǎn fěn (猪胆粉), Pulvis Fellis Suis Zhi	3	CB

Clears heat, dispels damp-heat, disperses swelling, relieves itching, invigorates blood, stops bleeding, relieves pain. Use to treat hemorrhoids with symptoms of pain, bleeding, inflammation, swelling and itchiness.

Pulse: Slippery or wiry, may be rapid
Tongue: Normal, or yellow coat

Comments: The *Hua Zhi Ling* formulas are known as the *Fargelin* formulas, and come from a variety of manufacturers with various ingredients. In the main, they all contain *tián qī, hŭ pò, dì yú, huái jiăo* (or *huái huā*), and either *huáng qín* or *huáng lián* as their foundation. *Tián qī, dì yú* and *huái huā* stop bleeding, while *hŭ pò* breaks up stasis, and *huáng qín* or *huáng lián* clears damp-heat.

The product, *High Strength Fargelin*, is better for stopping bleeding due to hemorrhoid. The Plum Flower version adds to the basic formula *shí liú pí* (pomegranate rind) and *hăi gé ké* (clam shell); both herbs astringe swelling. *High Strength Fargelin* and the Plum Flower version both use *zhū dăn fĕn* (pig bile powder) to address swelling.

Caution: *Tián qī* and *huái jiăo* are used with caution during pregnancy.

ZHI BAO

Formula: *zhì bǎo* (痔宝), "Hemorrhoid Treasure"
Source: Modern patent medicine

Availability:

Zhi Bao (HT)

Ingredients: (from Herbal Times *"Zhi Bao"*)

mǔ lì (牡蛎), Concha Ostreae	17.2 %	N
huáng qín (黄芩), Radix Scutellariae	17.2	DB
huái jiǎo (槐角), Fructus Sophorae	17.2	J
pú gōng yīng (蒲公英), Herba Taraxaci	10.3	DD
jīn yín huā (金银花), Flos Lonicerae Japonicae	10.3	DD
zhǐ shí (枳实), Fructus Aurantii Immaturus	6.9	G
dà huáng (大黄), Radix/Rhizoma Rhei	6.9	PA
dì yú (地榆), Radix Sanguisorbae	6.9	J
dāng guī (当归), Radix Angelicae Sinensis	6.9	AB

Clears heat, disperses swelling, relieves itching, stops bleeding, relieves pain. Use to stop hemorrhoid bleeding, to shrink hemorrhoids, and to stop the symptoms of pain, bleeding, swelling, and itchiness. Also used for intestinal bleeding, burning anus and constipation. Can also be used for anal herpes simplex.

Pulse: Slippery or wiry, may be rapid
Tongue: Normal, or yellow coat

Comments: This formula contains several herbs used in the *Hua Zhi Ling* (Fargelin) formulas, including *huáng qín*, *huái jiǎo*, and *dì yú*. To this is added *mǔ lì* (oyster shell), a salty medicine that breaks hardened masses. *Jīn yín huā and pú gōng yīng* clears heat, while *dà huáng* breaks up masses and clears heat. In the main, it is preferred for swelling with itching, with or without bleeding. Given its composition, it would also be appropriate for anal herpes simplex.

Caution: *Dà huáng* is contraindicated during pregnancy. Also, regulate dosage if diarrhea develops.

OTHER PRODUCTS APPROPRIATE FOR THIS CATEGORY:

Classical Formulas:

Yi Zi Tang

Cimicifuga Formula (EG, HS)

Modern Formulas:

Formula H (HC)
Hua Zhi Pian - Hemmoroff (GC)
Sophora Support - Hemorrease (K)

Topical Application:

Hemorrhoid Ointment (BP)
Ma Ying Long Hemorrhoid Ointment (GC)

7. LIVER AND GALLBLADDER DISORDERS

7A. LIVER STAGNATION

Classical formulas:

Chai Hu Shu Gan San	*chái hú shū gān sǎn* (柴胡疏肝散)
Ge Xia Zhu Yu Tang	*gé xià zhú yū tāng* (膈下逐瘀汤)
Tian Tai Wu Yao San	*tiān tái wū yào sǎn* (天台乌药散)
Xiao Chai Hu Tang	*xiǎo chái hú tāng* (小柴胡汤)
Xiao Yao San	*xiāo yáo sǎn* (逍遥散)
Yi Guan Jian	*yī guàn jiān* (一贯煎)

Modern formulas:

Shu Gan Wan	*shū gān wán* (舒肝丸)

Liver stagnation refers to stagnation of liver *qi* and/or liver blood. It is difficult, and clinically unreasonable, to separate the functions of liver *qi* and blood. When one is deficient, the other is deficient, and when one is stagnant, the other is stagnant. Benefiting one is often required to benefit the other. However, different herbs are used to affect liver *qi* than liver blood. In the formulas, one may find that herbs for *qi* and blood are often combined.

In Chinese medicine, the liver has the function of moving and storing *qi* and blood. In its moving function, the liver smoothly distributes *qi* and blood to the tendons, muscles and flesh through the microcirculation. It also smoothes and regulates the flow of *qi* and blood through the acupuncture channels and the blood vessels. In its function of storing blood, which happens in the early morning hours of 1 to 3 am, the liver cleanses and detoxifies the blood.

There are two TCM terms to describe the correction or adjustment of liver stagnation. The main one is *shū gān* (疏肝), which has been translated as "soothe, course, spread, or dredge the liver". Here, the idea is to pull or push out liver stasis, which is seen as sludge. The second term has the same *pinyin* name and tone, but uses a different Chinese character: *shū gān* (舒肝), which translates as "relax the liver".

Stagnation of liver *qi* and blood is a common clinical presentation when a patient arrives showing numerous symptoms attributable to both excess and deficiency. Clincally, it is best to move liver *qi* and blood first, before applying any tonifying formula, and the formulas in this chapter offer choices for that first visit.

Liver stagnation can affect both the *zang* organ and the liver channel. The liver organ has a direct impact on the functioning of stomach and spleen, the uterus and the lymphatic system, and thereby can be involved in disorders of digestion, menstruation, fertility and pregnancy, as well as immunity and infection.

The liver channel distributes through the genital region, including the scrotum, testicles, and vagina, to the breast and on to the lips, eyes, and head. In this regard, stagnation of *qi* in the liver channel commonly causes breast or costal distension. When combined with cold in the channel, it can lead to scrotal swelling, inguinal pain, or inguinal hernia. When the liver or gallbladder channels heat up excessively, it lays the foundation for outbreaks of herpes simplex along the liver channel, or herpes zoster/shingles, along the gallbladder channel. Liver fire or *yang* rising can cause headaches and migraines. (See Chapters 7B and 7C).

Etiology. Stagnation of liver occurs for a variety of reasons. Historically, TCM held that internalization of emotions, particularly anger and depression, could stagnate the movement of *qi* and blood. In this regard, internalization of emotional factors can lead to menstrual disorders such as dysmenorrhea and irregular menses; digestive disorders such as irritable bowel syndrome, gastric reflux and esophageal constriction; and channel syndromes including headache, anxiety, insomnia and inhibited sex drive.

Second, internal heat can lead to and aggravate liver stasis. This can develop from overconsumption of fatty foods, affecting both liver and gallbladder, or an overconsumption of refined carbohydrates, including sugars and alcohol.

The liver can also heat up due to environmental toxins in the air, food or water, as well as pharmaceutical drugs. These chemicals require liver enzymatic activity to metabolize, which can release heat, or cause direct inflammation. Heat can also develop due to a deficiency of liver *yin* or blood, both of which are necessary to cool the liver: *yin* by moistening and cooling the liver, and blood, which absorbs liver heat to help warm blood for distribution around the body.

Also, a woman's body increases in temperature between ovulation and menstruation, and this heat will aggravate any existing liver stasis. This is the etiology behind premenstrual syndrome, and formulas that address this directly are also included in *Chapter 8B. Premenstrual Tension*.

The third etiological factor behind liver stagnation involves its interrelationship with both stomach and spleen. One can imagine a vertical wheel consisting of spleen *qi* going upwards, with stomach *qi* going downwards. A horizontal axis also exists between liver and stomach-spleen, and all three of the these movements influence each other. If spleen *qi* is weak, or stomach loses its ability to descend downwards, these wheels can stop or slow down, and inhibit the smooth flowing of liver *qi* and blood. Conversely, if liver is stagnant, it can affect the movement of spleen, stomach or both. Stagnation of liver *qi*, failure of stomach *qi* to descend, and deficiency of spleen *qi* can combine as one, two or three patterns. Symptoms of liver and stomach stagnation include bloating, epigastric or abdominal distension, esophageal reflux or constriction, nausea, vomiting and pain.

Liver *qi* stagnation easily transforms into liver blood stagnation. When the *qi* and blood do not move smoothly, muscles and tendons become tight or tense. This is the mechanism responsible for irritability and headache, including symptoms found in premenstrual tension. If the liver cannot smoothly deliver blood to the uterus, dysmenorrhea (menstrual cramping) and uterine fibroids can develop, as well as menstrual irregularity. Blood stagnation is the energetic etiology of cirrhosis (liver scarring), hepatomegaly (liver swelling) and splenomegaly (spleen swelling), which can follow the introduction of exogenous heat-toxins.

Other products for liver stagnation can be found in Chapter *8B. Premenstrual Tension*. Liver stagnation that leads to liver *yang* flourishing upwards, with formula descriptions, are described in *Chapter 7B. Liver Yang and Internal Wind.* Liver stagnation that leads to liver fire or damp-heat are found in *Chapter 7C. Liver-Gallbladder Damp-Heat.*

FORMULA QUICK REFERENCE:

Chai Hu Shu Gan San	Liver *qi* stagnation
Ge Xia Zhu Yu Tang	Liver blood stagnation
Tian Tai Wu Yao San	Cold in the liver channel
Xiao Chai Hu Tang	Liver *qi* stasis with spleen deficiency
Xiao Yao San	Liver *qi* stasis with *qi* & blood deficiency
Yi Guan Jian	Liver *yin* deficiency
Shu Gan Wan	Liver overacting on stomach

Classical Formulas:

CHAI HU SHU GAN SAN

Formula: *chái hú shū gān săn* (柴胡疏肝散), "Bupleurum Soothe Liver Powder"
Author: Zhāng Jiè-Bīn (张介宾) *aka* Zhāng Jĭng-Yuè (张景岳)
Source: *Jĭng Yuè Quán Shū* (景岳全书), 1624
Literal: "Jing-Yue's Complete Writings"

Availability:

Bupleurum & Cyperus Combination (EG)
Bupleurum Shu Gan Teapills (PF)
Bupleurum Soothe The Liver Formula (HS)
Bupleurum Soothing Liver Formula (K)
Chai Hu Shu Gan San (BP)
Chai Hu Shu Gan Wan (GC, HT, PM, TL)

Ingredients: (from Herbal Times *"Chai Hu Shu Gan Wan"*)

chái hú (柴胡), Radix Bupleuri	25. %	BB
bái sháo (白芍), Radix Paeoniae Alba	19	AB
xiāng fù (香附), Rhizoma Cyperi	19	G
zhĭ ké (枳壳), Fructus Aurantii	19	G
chuān xiōng (川芎), Rhizoma Ligustici Chuanxiong	12	K
gān căo (甘草), Radix Glycyrrhizae	6	AA

Ingredients: (from standardized *"Bupleurum & Cyperus Combination"*)

chái hú (柴胡), Radix Bupleuri	19.0 %	BB
chén pí (陈皮), Pericarpium Citri Reticulatae	19.0	G
chuān xiōng (川芎), Rhizoma Ligustici Chuanxiong	14.3	K
bái sháo (白芍), Radix Paeoniae Alba	14.3	AB
zhĭ ké (枳壳), Fructus Aurantii	14.3	G
xiāng fù (香附), Rhizoma Cyperi	14.3	G
gān căo (甘草), Radix Glycyrrhizae	4.8	AA

Soothes the liver, activates the qi, invigorates blood, harmonizes spleen and liver, stops pain. Use for stagnation of liver *qi* and blood causing costal fullness, abdominal pain or distension, poor circulation, cold feet and hands, belching, nausea, gastritis, premenstrual syndrome, morning sickness, dysmenorrhea and hepatomegaly. Also useful for depression and anxiety. Can be used adjunctively in cases of chronic hepatitis, mastitis, fibrocystic breasts and gallstone.

Pulses: Normal, or wiry in wood position
Tongue: Normal, or slightly dark

Comments: *Chai Hu Shu Gan Wan* is an elaboration of Zhong Zhong-Jing's *Sì Nì Săn* (四逆散; 220), which contained *chái hú* to move liver *qi*, *bái sháo* to move liver blood, *zhǐ ké* to descend stomach *qi*, and *gān căo* to boost spleen *qi*. In the newer formula, *xiāng fù* is added to reinforce the movement of *qi,* and *chuān xiōng* to reinforce the movement of blood.

The formula was originally created to address hypochondriac pain and costal distension. (*Formulas and Strategies* attributes its creation to a doctor Ye Wen-Ling, with Zhang Jie-Bin recording it in his book.) In the modern clinic, it is excellent for excess patterns of liver *qi* and blood stasis affecting digestion and menstruation, as well as emotional disorders such as anxiety, depression and insomnia. It can also be an effective formula for premenstrual syndrome.

Chai Hu Shu Gan San is useful when a patient first comes to the clinic showing combined symptoms of excess and deficiency, because it clears underlying stagnation first. Due to its ability to move liver *qi* and blood, it facilitates detoxification of the liver and lymphatic system, and helps regulate blood sugar.

Chai Hu Shu Gan San should not be confused with *Shu Gan Wan*,described below.

Further Reading:

Bensky et al, p. 512
Chen & Chen, p. 238
Ellis, p. 50.

GE XIA ZHU YU TANG

Formula: *gé xià zhú yū tāng* (膈下逐瘀汤)
"Diaphragm, Below, Drive-Out Stasis Decoction"
Author: Wáng Qīng-Rèn (王清任)
Source: *Yī Lín Gǎi Cuò* (医林改错), 1830
Literal: "Physicians' Circle, Correction (of) Errors"

Availability:

Ge Xia Zhu Yu Tang (BP, PM)
Stasis In The Lower Chamber Teapills (PF)
Tangkuei & Corydalis Combination (EG)

Ingredients: (from the standardized *"Tangkuei & Corydalis Combination")*

dāng guī (当归), Radix Angelicae Sinensis	11.5 %	AB
táo rén (桃仁), Semen Persicae	11.5	K
hóng huā (红花), Flos Carthami	11.5	K
gān cǎo (甘草), Radix Glycyrrhizae	11.5	AA
wǔ líng zhī (五灵脂), Faeces Trogopterori	7.7	K
chì sháo (赤芍), Radix Paeoniae Rubra	7.7	K
chuān xiōng (川芎), Rhizoma Ligustici Chuanxiong	7.7	K
mǔ dān pí (牡丹皮), Cortex Mouta	7.7	DC
wū yào (乌药), Radix Linderae	7.7	G
xiāng fù (香附), Rhizoma Cyperi	5.8	G
zhǐ ké (枳壳), Fructus Aurantii	5.8	G
yán hú suǒ (延胡索), Rhizoma Corydalis	3.9	K

Ingredients: (from Plum Flower's *"Stasis in the Lower Chamber Teapills"*)

dāng guī (当归), Radix Angelicae Sinensis	11.5 %	AB
táo rén (桃仁), Semen Persicae	11.5	K
hóng huā (红花), Flos Carthami	11.4	K
wū yào (乌药), Radix Linderae	11.4	G
chuān xiōng (川芎), Rhizoma Ligustici Chuanxiong	7.5	K
mǔ dān pí (牡丹皮), Cortex Mouta	7.5	DC
chì sháo (赤芍), Radix Paeoniae Rubra	7.5	K
xiāng fù (香附), Rhizoma Cyperi	6.1	G
zhǐ ké (枳壳), Fructus Aurantii	6.1	G
rǔ xiāng (乳香), Olibanum/Boswelliae	5.8	K
mò yào (没药), Myrrha	5.7	K
yán hú suǒ (延胡索), Rhizoma Corydalis	4.0	K
gān cǎo (甘草), Radix Glycyrrhizae	4.0	AA

Invigorates blood, breaks blood stasis, soothes the liver, relieves pain, dissipates masses. Use for blood stagnation in the liver or spleen, causing distending pain or pain upon palpation in costal region or epigastrium. Applicable in liver cirrhosis, hepatomegaly, and splenomegaly. Can be used for uterine blood stagnation causing dysmenorrhea or uterine fibroids.

Pulse: Wiry, deep, choppy
Tongue: Normal, or dark or purple, perhaps with dark spots

Comments: In the early 19th century, Wang Qing-Ren developed numerous formulas to address blood stasis, including *Ge Xia Zhu Yu Tang* for the middle *jiao*, *Shao Fu Zhu Yu Tang* (lower *jiao*, Chapter 8C), *Shen Tong Zhu Yu Tang* (*bi* syndrome, Chapter 4B), and *Xue Fu Zhu Yu Tang* and *Tong Qiao Huo Xue Tang* (upper *jiao,* Chapter 10).

Ge Xia Zhu Yu Tang is an effective formula for blood stasis causing enlarged liver (hepatomegaly) or spleen (splenomegaly), and is used in acute and chronic hepatitis, cirrhosis, pancreatitis, and splenomegaly due to AIDS. The strong effort to move *qi* and blood is helpful in reducing elevated liver enzymes. Wang Qing-Ren recommended this formula for any mass below the diaphragm, and it is also useful for treating menstrual cramps and reducing small uterine fibroids.

The original formula uses *wǔ líng zhī,* which is included by the Taiwan granule manufacturers. Other companies may make substitutions; Plum Flower, for example, uses a combination of *rǔ xiāng* and *mò yào.*

Caution: Due to the inclusion of *táo rén, wǔ líng zhī, hóng huā, rǔ xiāng* and *mò yào,* this formula is prohibited during pregnancy, and for patients taking blood thinners such as Coumadin.

Further Reading:

Bensky et al, p. 567
Chen & Chen, p. 885
Ellis, p. 112

TIAN TAI WU YAO SAN

Formula: *tiān tái wū yào sǎn* (天台乌药散)
"Tian Tai (Mountain) Lindera Powder"
Author: Anonymous, Song Imperial Court
Source: *Zhèng Hé Shèng Jì Zông Lù* (政和圣济总录), 1117
Literal: "(Era of) Political Harmony, Sagely Assistance, Comprehensive Recording"

Availability:

Lindera Combination Teapills (PF)
Tian Tai Wu Yao Wan (HT)

Ingredients: (from Plum Flower *"Lindera Combination Teapills"*)

wū yào (乌药), Radix Linderae	18.4 %	G
xiǎo huí xiāng (小茴香), Fructus Foeniculi	12.6	E
gāo liáng jiāng (高良姜), Rhizoma Alpiniae Offic.	12.6	E
mù xiāng (木香), Radix Aucklandiae	12.5	G
qīng pí (青皮), Pericarpium Citri Reticulatae Viride	12.5	G
chuān liàn zǐ (川楝子), Fructus Meliae Toosenda	12.5	G
bīng láng (槟榔), Semen Arecae	12.5	Q
wú zhū yú (吴茱萸), Fructus Evodiae	6.4	E

Ingredients: (from Herbal Times *"Tian Tai Wu Yao Wan"*)

bīng láng (槟榔), Semen Arecae	13. %	Q
chuān liàn zǐ (川楝子), Fructus Meliae Toosenda	13	G
gāo liáng jiāng (高良姜), Rhizoma Alpiniae Offic.	13	E
mù xiāng (木香), Radix Aucklandiae	13	G
qīng pí (青皮), Pericarpium Citri Reticulatae Viride	13	G
wū yào (乌药), Radix Linderae	13	G
xiǎo huí xiāng (小茴香), Fructus Foeniculi	13	E
ròu guì (肉桂), Cortex Cinnamomi	5	E
wú zhū yú (吴茱萸), Fructus Evodiae	4	E

Soothes the liver, warms the liver channel, dissipates cold, relieves pain. Use for stagnation of liver qi with cold in the liver channel causing inguinal pain, hernia or testicular swelling. Also useful for liver stagnation due to cold causing costal distension, menstrual cramps or menstrual irregularities. Helpful for warming the uterus.

Pulse: Normal, or deep, slow, wiry or tight
Tongue: Normal, or pale

Comments: *Tian Tai Wu Yao San* primarily addresses invasion of cold into the liver channel leading to *qi* stagnation, and causing inguinal or testicular pain. It can be helpful for treatment of hernia, if it has not progressed too far, and can be used following hernia surgery to correct the underlying weakness in the inguinal area. It also dispels exogenous cold from the uterus, following exposure during the menses or post-partum. Traditionally, it is recommended that the formula be taken with alcohol, to increase the warming and dispersing actions.

Lindera *wū yào* and Areca *bīng láng* are the principal herbs to warm the channel, activate the *qi,* and bring the formula to the lower *jiao*. Other warming herbs include *gāo liáng jiāng, xiǎo huí xiāng,* and *wú zhū yú*. Herbal Times also adds Cinnamomum *ròu guì*. Herbs that open the liver channel include *chuān liàn zǐ, qīng pí* and *wū yào.*

The original formula contained *bā dòu* (巴豆, Fructus Crotonis), which purges cold accumulation. It is not included by either of the modern manufacturers.

Caution: *Bīng láng* is used with caution during pregnancy. In the Herbal Times version, *ròu guì* is contraindicated during pregnancy.

Further Reading:

Bensky et al, p. 527
Chen & Chen, p. 835

XIAO CHAI HU TANG

Formula: *xiǎo chái hú tāng* (小柴胡汤),"Minor Bupleurum Decoction"
Author: Zhāng Zhòng-Jǐng (张仲景)
Source: *Shāng Hán Lùn* (伤寒论), 220
Literal: "Injury (by) Cold, Discussion"s

Availability:

Minor Bupleurum Combination (EG, PIM)
Minor Bupleurum Formula (CC, GF, HS)
Minor Bupleurum (K)
Xiao Chai Hu Tang (BP, TZ)
Xiao Chai Hu Tang Wan (GC, MS, TL)
Xiao Chai Hu Wan (HT, PM)
* Calm (EV)

Ingredients: (from the standardized *"Minor Bupleurum Combination"*)

chái hú (柴胡), Radix Bupleuri	25.8 %	BB
bàn xià (半夏), Rhizoma Pinelliae	25.8	CA
huáng qín (黄芩), Radix Scutellariae	9.7	DB
rén shēn (人参), Radix Ginseng	9.7	AA
zhì gān cǎo (炙甘草), Radix Glycyrrhizae Praep.	9.7	AA
shēng jiāng (生姜), Rhizoma Zingiberis Recens	9.7	BA
dà zǎo (大枣), Fructus Jujubae	9.6	AA

Ingredients: (from Herbal Times *"Xiao Chai Hu Wan"*)

chái hú (柴胡), Radix Bupleuri	28. %	BB
jiāng bàn xià (姜半夏), Rhizoma Pinelliae Praep.	14	CA
dà zǎo (大枣), Fructus Jujubae	14	AA
dǎng shēn (党参), Radix Codonopsis	14	AA
huáng qín (黄芩), Radix Scutellariae	14	DB
gān cǎo (甘草), Radix Glycyrrhizae	9	AA
shēng jiāng (生姜), Rhizoma Zingiberis Recens	7	BA

Soothes the liver, dispels liver heat, harmonizes and resolves half exterior-half interior, transforms phlegm, tonifies spleen qi. Use for various applications: 1) harmonizes and resolves *shaoyang* syndrome (half exterior-half interior syndromes), including exogenous heat-toxins that have moved in towards the interior, causing costal distension, lymphatic congestion, alternating chills and fever, bitter taste in mouth, nausea, and lingering illness; 2) congestion of liver *qi* with spleen *qi* deficiency causing digestive disturbance, including nausea, poor appetite, epigastric or costal distension, blood sugar imbalance, fatigue, irritability, and chronic hepatitis; 3) menstrual disorders due to liver *qi* stagnation, including irregular periods and premenstrual tension. The formula is also helpful for wind-cold attacking the uterus after childbirth or menses.

Pulse: Wiry in liver/gallbladder position and soft in spleen position
Tongue: Normal, or white coat

Comments: This historic formula addresses deficiency of liver stasis with deficiency of spleen *qi* and accumulation of phlegm. It is applied to three distinct presentations: *shaoyang* fevers with chills, including malaria; liver-spleen disharmony affecting digestion; and liver-spleen disharmony affecting menses. From a physiological perspective, it also facilitates detoxification of the liver and lymphatic system, and helps regulate blood sugar.

Bupleurum *chái hú* is the principal herb for moving liver *qi*. When combined with *huáng qín,* it clears liver heat. *Dǎng shēn, dà zǎo* and *gān cǎo* boost spleen *qi* sand harmonize liver and spleens. *Bàn xià* with *shēng jiāng* clears phlegm, harmonize the stomach and gallbladder, and lower rebellious *qi*.

Caution: Do not use in cases of hyperactive liver *yang*.

Further Reading:

Bensky et al, p. 104
Chen & Chen, p. 206
Ellis, p. 344

XIAO YAO SAN

Formula: *xiāo yáo sǎn* (逍遥散), "Free Wanderer Powder"
Author: Imperial Medical Bureau (*tài yī jú*, 太医局);
revised by Chén Shī-Wén (陈师文)
Source: *Tài Píng Huì Mín Hé Jì Jú Fāng* (太平惠民和剂局方), 1078
Literal: "(Era of) Heavenly Peace, Benefit People (with) Harmonious Medicines, Office (of) Formulas"

Availability:

Bupleurum & Tang Kuei Formula (GF)
Bupleurum & Dong Quai Formula (CC)
Dr. Shen's Free & Easy Pill (DS)
Free & Easy Wanderer Teapills (PF)
Free And Easy Wanderer (K)
Tangkuei & Bupleurum Formula (EG)
Xiao Yao San (BP)
Xiao Yao Wan (GC, HT, JD, MS, PIM, PM, TL)
* Freeing The Moon (TT)
* Jade Fluid (JW)

Ingredients: (from the standardized *"Tangkuei and Bupleurum Formula"*)

chái hú (柴胡), Radix Bupleuri	14.3 %	BB
bái zhú (白术), Rhizoma Atractylodis Macrocephalae	14.3	AA
bái sháo (白芍), Radix Paeoniae Alba	14.3	AB
fú líng (茯苓), Poria	14.3	FC
dāng guī (当归), Radix Angelicae Sinensis	14.3	AB
gān jiāng (干姜), Rhizoma Zingiberis	14.3	E
bò hé (薄荷), Herba Menthae	7.1	BB
zhì gān cǎo (炙甘草), Radix Glycyrrhizae Praep.	7.1	AA

Soothes the liver, moves liver blood, harmonizes liver and spleen, tonifies spleen qi, tonifies blood. Use for stagnation of liver *qi* and blood with blood deficiency causing irritability, anxiety, depression, headache, or breast distension. Also used for digestive symptoms including poor digestion, costal distension or pain, poor appetite and loose stools. Can be used for premenstrual tension, irregular menses, elevated liver enzymes, and chronic hepatitis.

Pulses: Wiry, thin
Tongue: Normal, or pale

Comments: This formula addresses liver stagnation with *qi* and blood deficiency, and is useful for both gynecological and digestive complaints. Although *Jia Wei Xiao Yao San* (see Chapter 8B) is preferred for premenstrual tension due to its heat dispersing qualities, *Xiao Yao San* can be used throughout the cycle to keep liver *qi* and blood moving. It also is useful for liver stasis with spleen *qi* deficiency, affecting digestion or blood sugar regulation. By moving liver *qi* and blood, the formula also helps the liver detoxify, and can normalize elevated liver enzymes.

Chái hú moves *qi* and *bái sháo* moves blood; *dāng guī* tonifies blood, while *bái zhú*, *fú líng*, *gān jiāng* and *gān cǎo* benefit the spleen. *Bò hé* clears liver heat due to stagnation, and helps to spread liver *qi*.

Further Reading:

Bensky et al, p. 120
Chen & Chen, p. 247
Ellis, p. 356

YI GUAN JIAN

Formula: *yī guàn jiān* (一贯煎),"Single Linking Water-Decoction"
Author: Wèi Zhī-Xiù (魏之琇)
Source: *Xù Míng Yī Lèi Àn* (续名医类案), 1770
Literal: "Continuation (of) Famous Doctors' Categorized Cases"

Availability:

Linking Decoction (EG)
Linking Decoction Teapills (PF)
Linking Formula (GF)
Yi Guan Jian (BP, TZ)
Yi Guan Jian Wan (HT, TL)
* Fertile Garden (HC)
* Gracious Power (K)
* Linking Decoction (AL)

Ingredients: (from the standardized *"Linking Decoction"*)

shēng dì huáng (生地黄), Radix Rehmanniae	30.8 %	DC
gǒu qǐ zǐ (枸杞子), Fructus Lycii	15.4	AB
běi shā shēn (北沙参), Radix Glehniae	15.4	AD
mài mén dōng (麦门冬), Radix Ophiopogonis	15.4	AD
dāng guī (当归), Radix Angelicae Sinensis	15.4	AB
chuān liàn zǐ (川楝子), Fructus Meliae Toosenda	7.6	G

Ingredients: (from Herbal Times *"Yi Guan Jian Wan"*)

shēng dì huáng (生地黄), Radix Rehmanniae	25. %	DC
gǒu qǐ zǐ (枸杞子), Fructus Lycii	16	AB
běi shā shēn (北沙参), Radix Glehniae	16	AD
mài mén dōng (麦门冬), Radix Ophiopogonis	16	AD
dāng guī (当归), Radix Angelicae Sinensis	16	AB
chuān liàn zǐ (川楝子), Fructus Meliae Toosenda	11	G

Nourishes liver yin and blood, soothes the liver, moistens the tendons, supports kidney yin. Use for deficiency of liver *yin* and blood with some *qi* stasis. Symptoms include dry eyes, dry hair and skin, dry or stiff tendons, or amenorrhea. Other symptoms can include acid regurgitation or dry mouth, Useful for repairing liver tissue with elevated liver enzymes found in chronic hepatitis. Also for *yin* and blood deficiency failing to moisten the tendons causing joint or tendon pain, due to aging or chronic diabetes. Can also be used for *yin* deficiency of the stomach, manifesting as dry throat or acid regurgitation.

Pulse: Thin, slightly weak, especially in liver position; perhaps wiry
Tongue: Normal or pale, with a thin body; may be reddish

Comments: *Yi Guan Jian* treats deficiency of liver *yin* and blood leading to liver stagnation. Only *chuān liàn zǐ* soothes the liver (11%) while the rest of the formula focuses on nourishing liver *yin* and blood. Rehmannia *shēng dì huáng* is the herb with the largest dosage, benefiting both *yin* and blood. In this it is supported by *gǒu qǐ zǐ. Běi shā shēn* and *mài mén dōng* further nourish *yin*, while *dāng guī* nourishes blood.

Altogether, the formula acts as a liver tonic, excellent at repairing liver tissue following inflammation. Dr. Wu Boping, the famous Beijing liver specialist, used it for middle stage presentations of Hepatitis C, both to lower liver enzymes and to rebuild damaged liver cells. It can be used to repair the liver following inflammation due to pharmaceuticals, such as acetaminophen or statins, or to chemical and environmental toxins.

The formulas can also used in premenstrual syndrome due to liver *yin* deficiency, and to prevent or treat tight stiff tendons in people as they age.

Caution: Do not use in cases with phlegm and damp, or liver fire without deficiency.

Further Reading:

Bensky et al, p. 381
Chen & Chen, p. 657
Ellis, p. 378

Modern Formulas:

SHU GAN WAN

Formula: *shū gān wán* (舒肝丸), "Relax (the) Liver Pill"
Source: Modern patent medicine

Availability:

Liver Flow (K)
Shu Gan (HC)
Shu Gan Formula (GF)
Shu Gan Wan (GC, HT, MS, PIM, TL)
Shu Kan Formula (CC)
Soothe Liver Teapills (PF)

Ingredients: (from Plum Flower *"Soothe Liver Teapills"*; also Minshan "*Shu Gan Wan*")

xiāng fù (香附), Rhizoma Cyperi	10.6 %	G
bái sháo (白芍), Radix Paeoniae Alba	10.6	AB
chái hú (柴胡), Radix Bupleuri	7.1	BB
zhǐ ké (枳壳), Fructus Aurantii	7.1	G
qīng pí (青皮), Pericarpium Citri Reticulatae Viride	7.1	G
chén pí (陈皮), Pericarpium Citri Reticulatae	7.1	G
shā rén (砂仁), Fructus Amomi	7.1	FB
hòu pò (厚朴), Cortex Magnoliae	7.1	FB
yán hú suǒ (延胡索), Rhizoma Corydalis	7.1	K
mǔ dān pí (牡丹皮), Cortex Moutan	7.1	DC
xiāng yuán (香橼), Fructus Citri	3.5	G
gān cǎo (甘草), Radix Glycyrrhizae	3.5	AA
mù xiāng (木香), Radix Aucklandiae	3.5	G
jiāng huáng (姜黄), Rhizoma Curcumae Longae	2.6	K
fó shǒu (佛手), Fructus Citri Sarcodactylis	2.6	G
chén xiāng (沉香), Lignum Aquilariae Resinatum	2.2	G
bái dòu kòu (白豆蔻), Fructus Amomi Kravanh	2.2	FB
tán xiāng (檀香), Lignum Santali Albi	1.8	G

Ingredients: (from Herbal Times *"Shu Gan Wan"*)

chuān liàn zǐ (川楝子), Fructus Meliae Toosenda	13.0 %	G
bái sháo (白芍), Radix Paeoniae Alba	10.4	AB
chén xiāng (沉香), Lignum Aquilariae Resinatum	8.6	G
fú líng (茯苓), Poria	8.6	FC
jiāng huáng (姜黄), Rhizoma Curcumae Longae	8.6	K
yán hú suǒ (延胡索), Rhizoma Corydalis	8.6	K
zhǐ ké (枳壳), Fructus Aurantii	8.6	G
chén pí (陈皮), Pericarpium Citri Reticulatae	6.9	G
mù xiāng (木香), Radix Aucklandiae	6.9	G
shā rén (砂仁), Fructus Amomi	6.9	FB
bái dòu kòu (白豆蔻), Fructus Amomi Kravanh	5.3	FB
hòu pò (厚朴), Cortex Magnoliae Officinalis	5.3	FB
yù jīn (郁金), Radix Curcumae	2.3	K

Soothes liver qi, moves liver blood, cools liver heat, harmonizes liver and stomach, descends stomach qi, relieves pain. Use for liver *qi* stagnation overacting on stomach and spleen, causing epigastric distension or pain, costal distension, indigestion, poor appetite, belching, nausea, or hiccups. Other symptoms may include esophageal spasm, vomiting, ulcer and irritability. Also used in esophageal reflux, gastritis, duodenal ulcer, chronic pancreatitis, chronic hepatitis and postoperative gastrointestinal dysfunction.

Pulses: Wiry in liver and stomach positions
Tongue: Normal; may be coated

Comments: *Shu Gan Wan* should not be confused with *Chai Hu Shu Gan Wan* (above). This modern formula addresses stagnation of both liver *qi* and stomach *qi*, whereas *Chai Hu Shu Gan* Tang is for stagnation of liver *qi* and blood. *Shu Gan Wan* is used for abdominal distension, bloating after eating and esophageal reflux. It can also be used in excess presentations of irritable bowel syndrome (IBS).

In the original 18 herb formula represented by Plum Flower and Minshan, 45% of the formula is used to soothe liver *qi: xiāng fù, bái sháo, chái hú, qīng pí, jiāng huáng* and *yán hú suǒ.* Herbs that help descend stomach *qi* make up 42% of the formula: *shā rén, hòu pò, zhǐ ké, chén pí,xiāng yuán, mù xiāng, fó shǒu, chén xiāng* and *bái dòu kòu.*

The Herbal Times version has reduced the formula to 13 herbs, with 43% dredging liver *qi* and 48% descending stomach *qi*.

Caution: Both *jiāng huáng* and *yù jīn* are contraindicated during pregnancy, although experienced practitioners often use this formula to treat first semester morning sickness due to excess stagnation. The formula should not be used for digestive problems due to deficiency.

Note: The modern *Shu Gan Wan* should not be confused with the classical formula, *Shu Gan Tang:*

Formula: *shū gān tāng* (疏肝汤), "Soothe Liver Decoction"
Author: Gōng Tíng-Xián (龚廷贤)
Source: *Wàn Bìng Huí Chūn* (万病回春), 1587

Availability:

Bupleurum & Evodia Combination (EG)
Shu Gan Tang (BP)

Further Reading:

Bensky et al, p. 513
Chen & Chen, p. 241
Ellis, p. 286

OTHER FORMULAS APPROPRIATE TO THIS CATEGORY:

1) LIVER QI STAGNATION:

Classical Formulas:

Si Ni San

Bupleurum & Aurantium Immaturus Formula (EG)
Four Pillars Teapills (PF)

Modern Formulas:

Break Into A Smile (TT)
Cyperus 18 (SF)
Ease Pearls (CP)
Strengthen Liver (CMS)

2) LIVER QI STAGNATION WITH SPLEEN DEFICIENCY:

Classical Formulas:

Dang Gui Shao Yao San

See Chapter 8C

Chai Hu Gui Zhi Tang

Bupleurum & Cinnamon Combination (EG)
Bupleurum And Cinnamon Formula (GF)
Chai Hu Gui Zhi Tang (TZ)
Ease 2 (HC)
* Bupleurum 12 (SF)

Chai Hu Gui Zhi Gan Jiang Tang

Bupleurum, Cinnamon And Ginger Formula (HS)

Modern Formulas:

Remission Pills (SF)

OTHER FORMULAS APPROPRIATE TO THIS CATEGORY:

3) LIVER-STOMACH-SPLEEN DISHARMONY:

Classical Formulas:

Shu Gan Wan (classical)
Bupleurum & Evodia Combination (EG)
Shu Gan Tang (BP)

Xiang Su San
Cyperus & Perilla Formula (EG)
Xiang Su San (TZ)

Modern Formulas:

Bupleurum-S (SF)
Gastroquell (BP)
Harmonize Liver & Spleen (CMS)
Peony 9 (SF)
Qi Rectifying Decoction (AL)
Release Restraint (K)
Salvia Ten Formula (GF)
Remission Pills (SF)

4) LIVER BLOOD STAGNATION

Classical Formulas:

Dang Gui Shao Yao San
See Chapter 8C

Shao Fu Zhu Yu Wan
See Chapter 8C

Tao Hong Si Wu Tang
See Chapter 8C

Modern Formulas:

Jade Disperse 2 (JW)

5) LIVER DEPRESSION/ANXIETY

Classical Formulas:

Jia Wei Xiao Yao San

See Chapter 8B

Yi Gan San

Bupleurum Formula (EG)

Modern Formulas:

Albizzia 9 (SF)
Aspiration (HC)
Cystiquell (BP)
Cyperus 18 (SF)
Ease Pearls (CP)
Qi Rectifying Decoction (AL)
Salvia Ten Formula (GF)
Shine (EV)

6) SYSTEMIC DETOXIFICATION

Modern Formulas:

Herbal DTX (EV)
Liver DTX (EV)

7B. LIVER YANG AND ENDOGENOUS WIND
(Dizziness, Ear Ringing, Headache, Hypertension)

Classical Formulas:

Ban Xia Bai Zhu Tian Ma Tang	*bàn xià bái zhú tiān má tang* (半夏白术天麻汤)
Chai Hu Jia Long Gu Mu Li Tang	*chái hú jiā lóng gŭ mŭ lì tāng* (柴胡加龙骨牡蛎汤)
Er Long Zuo Ci Wan	*ĕr lóng zuŏ cí wán* (耳聋左慈丸)
Tian Ma Gou Teng Yin	*tiān má gōu téng yĭn* (天麻钩藤饮)
Zhen Gan Xi Feng Tang	*zhèn gān xī fēng tāng* (镇肝息风汤)

Modern Formulas:

Jiang Ya Wan	*jiàng yā wán* (降压丸)
Tian Ma Qu Feng Wan	*tiān má qū fēng bŭ wán* (天麻祛风补丸)
/ Tian Ma Wan	*tiān má wán* (天麻丸)

Ascendant hyperactivity of liver *yang* can cause a variety of disorders, including hypertension, headache and tinnitus (ear ringing). In prolonged cases, it can stir endogenous liver wind with symptoms of dizziness or vertigo, unsteady gait, trembling, spasm or convulsion. The nature of liver *yang* is to rise, but this is generally rooted by the presence of liver *yin* and blood. Therefore, ascendant liver *yang* often has its root in deficiency of blood or deficiency of *yin* (kidney-liver).

The formulas listed here combine herbs to nourish *yin* while subduing *yang.* They are used to control hypertension and associated symptoms of headache, dizziness, flushed face, pressure behind the eyes and irritability. They are also useful for insomnia, anxiety, and headache unrelated to blood pressure. Medicinals to subdue *yang* may be plant source, or may use heavy substances such as seashells, bones or rocks.

The effectiveness of Chinese herbal products for hypertension is mixed. For 50% of patients they offer an effective control, especially when combined with acupuncture. These are patients who tend to have, without pharmaceutical medication, fluctuating blood pressures. For patients with consistently elevated blood pressure, pharmaceutical medicine is often required. Hypertension can damage the kidneys and heart when higher than 165/95 mm Hg, and needs to be controlled by either modern or herbal medicine. It should not be ignored.

Classical Formulas:

BAN XIA BAI ZHU TIAN MA TANG

Formula: *bàn xià bái zhú tiān má tang* (半夏白术天麻汤)
"Pinellia, Atractylodes, Gastrodia Decoction"

First version:

Author: Lǐ Gǎo (李杲) *aka* Lǐ Dōng-Yuán (李东垣)
Source: *Pí Wèi Lùn* (脾胃论), 1249
Literal: "Spleen, Stomach Discussion"

Availability:

Ban Xia Bai Zhu Tian Ma Wan (GC, PM)
Pinellia & Gastrodia Combination (EG)
* Clear Yang (TT)

Ingredients: (from the standardized *"Pinellia & Gastrodia Combination"*)

bàn xià (半夏), Rhizoma Pinelliae	16.8 %	CA
mài yá (麦芽), Fructus Hordei Germinatus	16.8	H
bái zhú (白术), Rhizoma Atractylodis Macrocephalae	10.8	AA
shén qū (神曲), Massa Medicata Fermentata	10.8	H
tiān má (天麻), Rhizoma Gastrodiae	5.6	O
rén shēn (人参), Radix Ginseng	5.6	AA
cāng zhú (苍术), Rhizoma Atractylodis	5.6	FB
huáng qí (黄芪), Radix Astragali	5.6	AA
zé xiè (泽泻), Rhizoma Alismatis	5.6	FC
chén pí (陈皮), Pericarpium Citri Reticulatae	5.6	G
fú líng (茯苓), Poria	5.6	FC
gān jiāng (干姜), Rhizoma Zingiberis	3.4	E
huáng bǎi (黄柏), Cortex Phellodendri	2.2	DB

Further Reading:

Bensky et al, p. 812
Chen & Chen, p. 1250
Ellis, p. 21

Second version:

Author: Chéng Guó-Péng (程国彭)
Source: *Yī Xué Xīn Wù* (医学心悟), 1732
Literal: "Medical Studies Mind Awakening (eg, Insights)"

Availability:

Ascending Clarity (K)
Ban Xia Bai Zhu Tian Ma San (PF)
Ban Xia Bai Zhu Tian Ma Tang (BP)
Ban Xia Bai Zhu Tian Ma Wan (TL)
Pinellia, Atractylodes & Gastrodia (CC)

Ingredients: (from Tanglong *"Ban Xia Bai Zhu Tian Ma Wan"*)

fú líng (茯苓), Poria	21.0 %	FC
bàn xià (半夏), Rhizoma Pinelliae	15.8	CA
bái zhú (白术), Rhizoma Atractylodis Macrocephalae	15.8	AA
dà zǎo (大枣), Fructus Jujubae	15.8	AA
tiān má (天麻), Rhizoma Gastrodiae	10.5	O
jú hóng (橘红), Exocarpium Citri Rubrum	10.5	G
gān cǎo (甘草), Radix Glycyrrhizae	5.3	AA
shēng jiāng (生姜), Rhizoma Zingiberis Recens	5.3	BA

Further Reading:

Bensky et al, p. 811
Chen & Chen, p. 1247

Soothes the liver to extinguish internal wind, dissolves phlegm, dries dampness, dispels wind-cold, subdues yang, boosts qi, calms vertigo. Use for dizziness, vertigo or headache due to wind-phlegm accumulation and following a wind-cold attack. Accompanying symptoms may include nausea, poor appetite, thirst, cloudy or muddled thinking. Applicable for vertigo, Meniere's disease, dizziness due to common cold, and acute nausea with diarrhea. Can be used for dizziness during pregnancy.

Pulse: Wiry or slippery
Tongue: White, greasy coat

Comments: This formula addresses dizziness, vertigo and headache. The etiology is complex. There is an underlying accumulation of spleen damp and stomach phlegm. Heat is generated in the liver, leading to endogenous *yang* and wind, causing vertigo. It also may be triggered by a wind-cold attack, combining both hot and cold aspects. In either case, the head feels heavy, as if surrounded by a damp heavy cloth, or there may be a spinning sensation.

There are two versions of the formula available. The larger (13 herbs) dates back to 1249, and is based on *Er Chen Tang* (see Chapter 3C). The second smaller formula (8 herbs) shares six of the ingredients from the first formula: *fú líng*, *bàn xià, bái zhú, tiān má, chén pí/jú hóng* and *gān jiāng/shēng jiāng*. Both formulas address accumulation of phlegm and dampness, and *tiān má* acts as the primary herb to settle ascendant *yang*.

The first formula is stronger for accumulation of phlegm-dampness and food stasis, containing *mài yá, shén qū, and zé xiè.* It also addresses spleen *qi* deficiency, employing *rén shēn* and *huáng qí.*

In chronic cases, either formula will need to be taken for a prolonged period of time. In acute cases, effects may be felt immediately.

CHAI HU JIA LONG GU MU LI TANG

Formula: *chái hú jiā lóng gŭ mŭ lì tāng* (柴胡加龙骨牡蛎汤)
"Bupleurum with Draconis, Ostrea Decoction"
Author: Zhāng Zhòng-Jǐng (张仲景)
Source: *Shāng Hán Lùn* (伤寒论), 220
Literal: "Injury (by) Cold, Discussion"

Availability:

Bupleurum & Dragon Bone (CC)
Bupleurum & Dragon Bone Combination (EG)
Bupleurum Dragon Bone Oyster Shell Teapills (PF)
Bupleurum Plus Dragon Bone And Oyster Shell Formula (HS)
Calm Dragon Formula (K)
Chai Hu Jia Long Gu Mu Li Tang (BP, TZ)
Chai Hu Long Gu Mu Li Wan (GC, HT, PM)
Ease Plus (HC)
* Ardisia 16 (SF)
* Bupleurum D Formula (GF)

Ingredients: (from the standardized *"Bupleurum & Dragon Bone Combination"*)

chái hú (柴胡), Radix Bupleuri	10. %	BB
bàn xià (半夏), Rhizoma Pinelliae	10	CA
guì zhī (桂枝), Ramulus Cinnamomi	10	BA
fú ling (茯苓), Poria	10	FC
rén shēn (人参), Radix Ginseng	10	AA
huáng qín (黄芩), Radix Scutellariae	10	DB
lóng gŭ (龙骨), Os Draconis	10	
mŭ lì (牡蛎), Concha Ostreae	10	N
dà zăo (大枣), Fructus Jujubae	10	AA
gān jiāng (干姜), Rhizoma Zingiberis	10	E

Ingredients: (from the Herbal Times *"Chai Hu Long Gu Mu Li Wan"*)

chái hú (柴胡), Radix Bupleuri	17.5 %	BB
jiāng bàn xià (姜半夏), Rhizoma Pinelliae Praep.	14.0	CA
guì zhī (桂枝), Ramulus Cinnamomi	10.5	BA
fú ling (茯苓), Poria	10.5	FC
rén shēn (人参), Radix Ginseng	8.7	AA
huáng qín (黄芩), Radix Scutellariae	8.7	DB

lóng gǔ (龙骨), Os Draconis	8.7	N
mǔ lì (牡蛎), Concha Ostreae	8.7	N
dà zǎo (大枣), Fructus Jujubae	8.7	AA
shēng jiāng (生姜), Rhizoma Zingiberis Recens	4.0	E

Soothes liver qi, cools liver heat, subdues yang, releases excess from the taiyang, shaoyang and yangming, transforms phlegm, tonifies qi. Use for stagnant liver *qi* with ascendant *yang* causing chest oppression, palpitations, irritability, dizziness, insomnia, anxiety or fright. Applicable in neurotic disorders due to fright, hysteria or insomnia, and is also used for drug withdrawal. The formula can be used for irregular heartbeat that is worse with rest. Also used for hypertension, hyperthyroid, premenstrual tension and menopausal disorder.

Pulse: Wiry, floating
Tongue: Normal, or coated

Comments: Zhang Zhong-Jing's formula is an elaboration of his own *Xiao Chai Hu Tang* (Chapter 7A), adding four herbs: *guì zhī, fú ling, lóng gǔ,* and *mǔ lì*. The original application for *Chai Hu Jia Long Gu Mu Li Tang* addressed exogenous invasions that had gone into the interior and were then inappropriately treated with purgatives, driving the problem deeper while developing ascendant liver *yang*. In modern times, it is used when liver *qi* stagnation progresses to the rising of liver *yang*, causing headache, insomnia, irritability, palpitations and mania.

Lóng gǔ and *mǔ lì* are heavy mineral substances that settle and subdue ascendant *yang. Guì zhī* may help to distribute *yang* more equitably. The original formula contained *dà huáng* (大黄, Radix/Rhizoma Rhei), which is still retained by Plum Flower (3.5%), Honso (3.4%) and Golden Flower (6.7%). Other manufacturers may omit this ingredient.

Caution: *Dà huáng* is prohibited during pregnancy, and may cause loose stools. Heavy mineral substances such as *lóng gǔ* and *mǔ lì* can cause digestive upset if overused. Monitor and reduce dosage if necessary.

Further Reading:

Bensky et al, p. 113
Chen & Chen, p. 715
Ellis, p. 47

ER LONG ZUO CI WAN

Formula: *ěr lóng zuŏ cí wán* (耳聋左慈丸)
"Ear Deafness, Left Kindness (to Kidney) Pill"
aka *ěr míng zuŏ cí wán* (耳鸣左慈丸)
"Ear Buzzing (Tinnitus) Left Kindness (to Kidney) Pill"
Author: Dài Tiān-Zhāng (戴天章)
Source: *Guăng Wēn Yì Lùn* (广温疫论), 1774
Literal: "Widespread Warm Epidemic Discussion"

Availability:

Er Long Zuo Ci Teapills (PF)
Er Long Zuo Ci Wan (MS, PM, TL)
Er Ming Zuo Ci Pian (GC)
Er Ming Zuo Ci Wan (HT, PM)
* Morus Fruit Tablets (SF)

Ingredients: (from Herbal Times "*Er Ming Zuo Ci Wan*")

shú dì huáng (熟地黄), Radix Rehmanniae Praep.	30.0 %	AB
shān yào (山药), Rhizoma Dioscoreae	15.0	AA
shān zhū yú (山茱萸), Fructus Corni	15.0	L
zé xiè (泽泻), Rhizoma Alismatis	11.0	FC
fú líng (茯苓), Poria	11.0	FC
mŭ dān pí (牡丹皮), Cortex Mouta	11.0	DC
cí shí (磁石), Magnetitum	3.5	N
chái hú (柴胡), Radix Bupleuri	3.5	BB

Nourishes kidney yin, clears deficiency heat, settles the liver, subdues yang. Use for deficiency of kidney and liver *yin* with ascendant liver *yang*, causing ear ringing or tinnitus, especially in the elderly. Other symptoms include dizziness, headache, insomnia, or anxiety. May be appropriate for hypertension due to kidney *yin* deficiency.

Pulse: Thin; may be wiry or rapid
Tongue: Normal, may be thin or reddish

Comments: This formula, a variation of *Liu Wei Di Huang Wan* (Chapter 17A), has been modified to address loss of hearing or chronic ear ringing associated with weakened kidney *qi*, particularly as people age. In China, it is a popular kidney *yin* tonic used by the elderly. The foundation formula (*Liu Wei Di Huang Wan*) nourishes kidney *yin*. The addition of *chái hú* opens the *shaoyang* channels around the ear, and helps to soothe liver *qi*. *Cí shí*, a heavy mineral (magnetite) leads ascendant *yang* back to the kidneys, reducing ear ringing. The formula is not particularly helpful for ear ringing due to trauma or nerve damage.

The prescriptions from Minshan and Plum Flower are virtually identical to the listed formula from Herbal Times.

Further Reading:

Bensky et al, p. 369
Chen & Chen, p. 633

TIAN MA GOU TENG YIN

Formula: *tiān má gōu téng yǐn* (天麻钩藤饮)
"Gastrodia, Uncaria Cool-Decoction"
Author: Hú Guāng-Cí (胡光慈)
Source: *Zá Bìng Zhèng Zhì Xīn Yì* (杂病证治新义), 1958
Literal: "Miscellaneous Disorders Patterns (and) Treatment New Significance"

Availability:

Calm Liver Wind Formula (JD)
Gastrodia & Gambir Combination (EG)
Gastrodia & Uncaria Formula (CC)
Gastrodia & Uncaria Wind Relief (K)
Gastrodia And Uncaria Extract (PM)
Gastrodia And Uncaria Formula (GF)
Gastrodia And Uncaria Wind Relief (K)
Tian Ma Gou Teng Pian (GC, PIM)
Tian Ma Gou Teng Yin (BP, HT, TZ)
Tian Ma Gou Teng Yin Teapills (PF)
Tian Ma Gou Teng Yin Wan (TL, PM)
* Gastrodia 9 (SF)
* Gastrodia Relieve Wind (HC)

Ingredients: (from the standardized *"Gastrodia and Gambir Combination"*)

yè jiāo téng (夜交藤), Caulis Polygoni Multiflori	16.8 %	N
shí jué míng (石决明), Concha Haliotidis	16.8	O
sāng jì shēng (桑寄生), Herba Taxilli/Loranthi	13.6	AD
gōu téng (钩藤), Ramulus Uncariae Cum Uncis	8.4	O
fú shen (茯神), Sclerotium Poriae Pararadicis	8.4	N
yì mǔ cǎo (益母草), Herba Leonuri	8.4	K
chuān niú xī (川牛膝), Radix Cyathulae	6.8	K
dù zhòng (杜仲), Cortex Eucommiae	5.2	AC
tiān má (天麻), Rhizoma Gastrodiae	5.2	O
zhī zǐ (栀子), Fructus Gardeniae	5.2	DA
huáng qín (黄芩), Radix Scutellariae	5.2	DB

Subdues liver yang, calms the liver and extinguishes wind, clears heat, invigorates blood, boosts yin, tonifies kidney, nourishes liver. Use for ascendant *yang* with deficiency of *qi* and blood causing dizziness or vertigo, headache, blurry vision or trembling, irritability, anxiety and insomnia. Applicable in hypertension, facial paralysis, deficiency *bi* arthritis, deficiency *wei* syndromes (flaccid paralysis), trembling or twitching of limbs, and following stroke. May be useful in Bell's palsy, and pre-eclampsia.

Pulse: Wiry and floating; may be rapid; excess or deficient
Tongue: Reddish; may be trembling

Comments: A modern "classical" formula*, Tian Ma Gou Teng Yin* was originally developed for headaches due to hypertension, and is now commonly used for general cases of headaches or dizziness. It is also used for trembling disorders, including early stage Parkinson's disease and hemiplegia.

Shí jué míng, yè jiāo téng, tiān má and *gōu téng* subdue ascendant *yang*. *Dù zhòng, sāng jì shēng* and *chuān niú xī* work together to strengthen kidney *qi*, further helping to root *yang*. *Zhī zǐ* and *huáng qín* clear liver heat, the source of ascending *yang*.

The formula is considered mild to moderate, and can be used for prolonged periods. In China, it is popular as a geriatric tonic to control trembling and enhance memory.

Caution: *Chuān niú xī* is contraindicated during pregnancy, although experienced practitioners can modify the formula for pre-eclampsia. Long-term use of *shí jué míng* (abalone shell) can damage stomach and spleen *qi.* Reduce dosage or discontinue with epigastric pain or poor digestion.

Further Reading:

Bensky et al, p. 647
Chen & Chen, p. 1004
Ellis, p. 306

ZHEN GAN XI FENG TANG

Formula: *zhèn gān xī fēng tāng* (镇肝息风汤)
"Pacify Liver, Extinguish Wind Decoction"

Author: Zhāng Xī-Chún (张锡纯)

Source: *Yī Xué Zhōng Zhōng Cān Xī Lù* (医学衷中参西录), 1918-1934
Literal: "Medical Studies Heartfelt (towards) Chinese, Respecting Western, Records"

Availability:

Hematite & Scrophularia Combination (EG)
Zhen Gan Xi Feng Tang (BP)
Zhen Gan Xi Feng Teapills (PF)
Zhen Gan Xi Feng Wan (HT)

Ingredients: (from the standardized *"Hematite & Scrophularia Combination"*)

dài zhě shí (代赭石), Haematitum	19.1 %	N
huái niú xī (怀牛膝), Radix Achyranthis Bidentatae	19.1	N
tiān mén dōng (天门冬), Radix Asparagi	9.5	AD
lóng gŭ (龙骨), Os Draconis	9.5	N
mŭ lì (牡蛎), Concha Ostreae	9.5	N
bái sháo (白芍), Radix Paeoniae Alba	9.5	AB
xuán shēn (玄参), Radix Scrophulariae	9.5	DC
chuān liàn zĭ (川楝子), Fructus Meliae Toosenda	3.8	G
mài yá (麦芽), Fructus Hordei Germinatus	3.8	H
yīn chén hāo (茵陈蒿), Herba Artemisiae Scopariae	3.8	FC
gān căo (甘草), Radix Glycyrrhizae	2.9	AA

Subdues liver yang, soothes the liver, extinguishes wind, opens the channels and collaterals, nourishes yin, clears heat. Use for ascendant *yang* with deficiency of *yin* causing headache, dizziness, vertigo, eye pressure, tinnitus, or cloudy consciousness. Other symptoms may include flushed face or belching. Applicable for preventing stroke or following stroke, with symptoms of hypertension, facial paralysis, aphasia (inability to speak), confusion, and trembling or twitching of limbs. Can be used in hyperthyroid.

Pulse: Wiry, forceful, floating
Tongue: Normal, or red on sides, stiff or trembling

Comments: This 20th century formula is for acute presentations of ascendant liver *yang* with liver *yin* deficiency. It was developed to address patients with the risk of stroke due to hypertension, especially with early signs of headache or loss of balance when walking. It is also given following a stroke, with drooping mouth or face, slurred speech, etc. It can be used to control hypertension, with symptoms of chronic headache, irritability and mental confusion, and has also been used for ascendant stomach *qi* causing belching or flushed face.

Heavy mineral substances that sedate *yang* (*dài zhě shí, lóng gŭ, mŭ lì*) comprise 38% of the formula, and *huái niú xī*, which leads the *yang* downwards, is another 19%.

Caution: *Huái niú xī* is contraindicated during pregnancy, although experienced practitioners can modify this formula for pre-eclampsia. Use of *dài zhě shí* is cautioned during pregnancy.

Further Reading:

Bensky et al, p. 644
Chen & Chen, p. 999
Ellis, p. 400

Modern Formulas:

JIANG YA WAN / JIANG PING WAN

Formula: *jiàng yā wán* (降压丸), "Lower Pressure Pill"
jiàng píng wán (降平丸), "Lower (and) Equalize Pill"
Source: Modern patent medicine

Availability:

Anchor The Yang (K)
Jiang Ping Wan (HT)
Jiang Ya Pian (GC, PF, PM)
Jiang Ya Wan (TL)

Ingredients: (From Plum Flower *"Jiang Ya Pian"* and Herbal Times *"Jiang Ping Wan"*)

chōng wèi zǐ (茺蔚子), Fructus Leonuri	15. %	K
huái niú xī (怀牛膝), Radix Achyranthis Bidentatae	13	K
shēng dì huáng (生地黄), Radix Rehmanniae	10	DC
ē jiāo (阿胶), Colla Corii Asini	10	AB
dāng guī (当归), Radix Angelicae Sinensis	8	AB
gōu téng (钩藤), Ramulus Uncariae cum Uncis	7	O
chén xiāng (沉香), Lignum Aquilariae Resinatum	5	G
chuān xiōng (川芎), Rhizoma Ligustici Chuanxiong	5	K
mŭ dān pí (牡丹皮), Cortex Mouta	5	DC
xià kū căo (夏枯草), Spica Prunellae	5	DA
dà huáng (大黄), Radix/Rhizoma Rhei	4	PA
tiān má (天麻), Rhizoma Gastrodiae	4	O
hŭ pò (琥珀), Succinum	3	N
huáng lián (黄连), Rhizoma Coptidis	3	DB
shuĭ niú jiao (水牛角), Cornu Bubali	3	DC

Clears liver heat, settles the liver, subdues yang, tonifies blood. Use for hypertension due to liver heat with ascendant liver *yang*, with symptoms of dizziness or vertigo, headache, elevated blood pressure, flushed or red face, pressure behind the eyes or red eyes, tinnitus, irritability, stiff neck, insomnia or restlessness. Can be used for headache and migraine unrelated to blood pressure.

Pulse: Wiry, floating, possibly rapid
Tongue: Red or red on sides, yellow coat

Comments: The various *Jiang Ya Wan* formulas treat elevated blood pressure due to liver heat with ascendant liver *yang*. They can be successful for blood pressure that varies throughout the day, rather than consistently elevated.

The version offered by Herbal Times, Plum Flower and Kan are based on the original *Jiang Ya Wan* from Beijing Tong Ren Factory. The first two herbs *chōng wèi zǐ* and *huái niú xī* (28%), lead the yang downwards towards the kidney. *Chōng wèi zǐ*, the seed of the plant that gives us *yì mǔ cǎo* (益母草, Herba Leonuri), cools liver heat and settles *yang*. It's clinical use is unique to this formula, developed in modern clinical practice. Another 19% of the formula settles ascendant *yang* (*xià kū cǎo, hǔ pò, gōu téng, tiān má*), while 18% clears blood heat (*shēng dì huáng, mǔ dān pí*, and *shuǐ niú jiao*, water buffalo horn). The remaining herbs nourish blood (*dāng guī* and *ē jiāo*) and further clear heat (*huáng lián, dà huáng*). It should be seen as a cooling formula for liver heat leading to ascendant liver *yang.*

There are other *Jiang Ya* formulas that follow the same principles but with smaller prescriptions from Guang Ci Tang and Tanglong.

Caution: *Huái niú xī* is contraindicated during pregnancy, although experienced practitioners can modify this formula for pre-eclampsia.

TIAN MA QU FENG BU WAN / TIAN MA WAN

Formula: *tiān má qū fēng bǔ wán* (天麻祛风补丸) / *tiān má wán* (天麻丸)
"Gastrodia Disperse Wind Tonifying Pill" / "Gastrodia Pills"

Source: Song dynasty (960-1279), source unknown.
Revived as a modern patent medicine.

Availability:

Circulex (PM)
Tian Ma Qu Feng Bu Wan (HT)
Tian Ma Teapills (PF)
Tian Ma Wan (MS, TL)
Tienma Chu Feng Pien (PM)
Tienma Qufengbu Tablets (PM)

Ingredients: (From Herbal Times *"Tian Ma Qu Feng Bu Wan"*)

shēng dì huáng (生地黄), Radix Rehmanniae	22.0 %	DC
dāng guī (当归), Radix Angelicae Sinensis	14.0	AB
qiāng huó (羌活), Radix Notopterygii	14.0	BA
dù zhòng (杜仲), Cortex Eucommiae	9.5	AC
bì xiè (萆薢), Rhizoma Dioscoreae Hypoglaucae	8.0	FC
huái niú xī (怀牛膝), Radix Achyranthis Bidentatae	8.0	K
xuán shēn (玄参), Radix Scrophulariae	8.0	DC
tiān má (天麻), Rhizoma Gastrodiae	8.0	O
dú huó (独活), Radix Angelicae Pubescentis	7.0	FA
zhì fù zǐ (炙附子), Radix Aconiti Lateralis Praeparata	1.5	E

Ingredients: (From Minshan *"Tian Ma Wan"* and Plum Flower *"Tian Ma Teapills"*)

shēng dì huáng (生地黄), Radix Rehmanniae	21.4 %	DC
dāng guī (当归), Radix Angelicae Sinensis	14.4	AB
qiāng huó (羌活), Radix Notopterygii	14.4	BA
dù zhòng (杜仲), Cortex Eucommiae	9.3	AC
tiān má (天麻), Rhizoma Gastrodiae	8.4	O
xuán shēn (玄参), Radix Scrophulariae	8.4	DC
huái niú xī (怀牛膝), Radix Achyranthis Bidentatae	8.4	K
bì xiè (萆薢), Rhizoma Dioscoreae Hypoglaucae	8.4	FC
dú huó (独活), Radix Angelicae Pubescentis	6.0	FA
xiāng fù (香附), Rhizoma Cyperi	0.9	G

Subdues liver yang, nourishes yin and blood, extinguishes wind. Use for dizziness or headache due to ascendant yang with deficiency of *yin* and blood. Applicable in hypertensive symptoms including headache, with tension in shoulders and neck. Also used for facial paralysis, deficiency *bi* syndromes (arthritis), deficiency *wei* syndromes (flaccid paralysis), poor memory and as a general tonic.

Pulse: Thin, wiry, occasionally rapid
Tongue: Normal, or slight red

Comments: This formula is used for elevated blood pressure, as well as deficiency headaches and dizziness. It can be successful for blood pressure that varies throughout the day, rather than consistently elevated. The formula uses *shēng dì huáng* and *dāng guī* as its foundation, to nourish *yin* and blood. *Qiāng huó* and *dú huó* distribute the formula through the limbs, helping control mild trembling in early stage Parkinson's disease. *Tiān má* is a valuable herb for subduing *yang*, and *dù zhòng* and *huái niú xī* work together to strengthen kidney *qi*, further helping to root *yang*.

The formulas listed above are virtually identical. Herbal Times follows the original patent medicine formula, while Minshan and Plum Flower substitute *xiāng fù* for *zhì fù zǐ*. The percentage of these ingredients is so small (<1.5%) that the difference is insignificant.

Caution: *Zhì fù zǐ* is used with caution during pregnancy.

OTHER FORMULAS APPROPRIATE FOR THIS CATEGORY:

Classical Formulas:

Du Zhong Pian

Compound Cortex Eucommia Tablets (PM)
Eucommia Combination (PF)

Luo Bu Ma Pian

Luo Bu Ma Pian (PF)
Luo Bu Ma Formula (GF)

Jian Ling Tang

Dioscorea & Achyranthes Combination (EG)

Modern Formulas:

Albizzia 9 (SF)
Anchor the Yang (K)
Gastrodia & Succinum Combination (EG)
Gastrodia Complex (EV)
Hyperquell (BP)
Purge Internal Wind (CMS)
Sea Ace (HC)
Sedate Liver Yang & Nourish Yin Pill (TL)
Stabilizing Tablets (SF)
Tian Ma Mi Huan Su (PF)
Uncaria 6 (SF)

HEADACHE

Classical Formulas:

Chuan Xiong Cha Tiao San

See *Chapter 1A*

Modern Formulas:

Angelica 14 (SF)
Angelica And Chuanxiong (HS)
Cnidium 9 (SF)
Corydalin (EV)
Head Relief Tablets (GF)
Head-Q (HC)
Migratrol (EV)
Pian Tou Tong (PM)

TREMOR AND SPASM

Classical Formulas:

Ding Xian Wan

Gastrodia & Succinum Combination (EG)

Modern Formulas:

Otolith Tablets (SF)

s

7. LIVER AND GALLBLADDER DISORDERS

7C. LIVER-GALLBLADDER DAMP-HEAT AND FIRE

Classical formulas:

Da Chai Hu Tang	*dà chái hú tāng* (大柴胡汤)
Long Dan Xie Gan Tang	*lóng dǎn xiè gān tāng* (龙胆泻肝汤)
Wen Dan Tang	*wēn dǎn tāng* (温胆汤)

Modern Formulas:

Ji Gu Cao Pian	*jī gǔ cǎo piàn* (鸡骨草片)

In both damp-heat and fire affecting the liver or gallbladder, heat is the common factor; it can be due to exogenous or endogenous factors. Exogenous factors include pathogenic heat-toxins, especially viruses found in hepatitis, AIDS, mononucleosis, and viral pancreatitis. Exogenous factors also include chemical toxins and parasites such as worms. Endogenous sources of heat develop with stagnation of liver *qi* due to internalized emotions or overindulgence of spicy and fatty foods. Heat can turn to damp-heat when there is pre-existing spleen dampness, or when heat-toxins attack the gallbladder, affecting the bile.

Both exogenous and endogenous etiologies can affect the *zang-fu* organs liver and gallbladder or their associated channels. When the organs are affected, symptoms include poor appetite, nausea or vomiting, erratic stools, and costal distension. When the channels are affected, symptoms include red eye, stye, temporal or vertex headache, ear ringing, dizziness, irritability, and high blood pressure. Gallbladder channel fire can also contribute to mania, nightmares, insomnia and obsessive-compulsive behavior.

Damp-heat tends to include nausea, while fire symptoms extend along the channel, causing red eye or headache. If heat or damp-heat extends downwards along the liver channel, symptoms can include vaginal discharge, redness or irritation of the vulva and vagina, painful scrotum, swollen testicle, urinary tract infections, painful urination, or painful ejaculations.

Liver and gallbladder fire or damp-heat can exacerbate herpes outbreaks, both herpes simplex and herpes zoster (shingles). In herpes simplex, eruptions along the liver channel are apparent, including the eyes, lips, or genitalia. Herpes zoster (shingles) manifests along the gallbladder channel, including the temporal aspects of the head, costal regions and the buttocks.

Besides herbal products, Chinese medical practitioners advise patients with liver-gallbladder damp-heat to discontinue spicy, greasy and fatty food.

When prolonged damp-heat congeals the bile, it causes gallstone or gallbladder congestion. Formulas can be found in *Chapter 7D. Gallstones.*

Classical formulas:

DA CHAI HU TANG

Formula: *dà chái hú tāng* (大柴胡汤), "Major Bupleurum Decoction"
Author: Zhāng Zhòng-Jǐng (张仲景)
Source: *Shāng Hán Lùn* (伤寒论), 220
Literal: "Injury (by) Cold, Discussion"

Availability:

Major Bupleurum Combination (EG)
Major Bupleurum Formula (HS)
Major Bupleurum Teapills (PF)

Ingredients: (from the standardized *"Major Bupleurum Combination"*)

chái hú (柴胡), Radix Bupleuri	22.8 %	BB
bàn xià (半夏), Rhizoma Pinelliae	22.8	CA
shēng jiāng (生姜), Rhizoma Zingiberis Recens	14.3	BA
huáng qín (黄芩), Radix Scutellariae	8.6	DB
bái sháo (白芍), Radix Paeoniae Alba	8.6	AB
zhǐ shí (枳实), Fructus Aurantii Immaturus	8.6	G
dà zǎo (大枣), Fructus Jujubae	8.6	AA
dà huáng (大黄), Radix/Rhizoma Rhei	5.7	PA

Ingredients: (from Plum Flower *"Major Bupleurum Teapills"*)

shēng jiāng (生姜), Rhizoma Zingiberis Recens	19.3 %	BA
chái hú (柴胡), Radix Bupleuri	12.3	BB
bàn xià (半夏), Rhizoma Pinelliae	12.3	CA
huáng qín (黄芩), Radix Scutellariae	12.3	DB
zhǐ shí (枳实), Fructus Aurantii Immaturus	12.3	G
bái sháo (白芍), Radix Paeoniae Alba	12.3	AB
dà zǎo (大枣), Fructus Jujubae	10.3	AA
dà huáng (大黄), Radix/Rhizoma Rhei	8.9	PA

Soothes the liver, cools liver and gallbladder heat, harmonizes and resolves half exterior, half interior, harmonizes liver and spleen, transforms phlegm, stems counterflow ascent of stomach qi, stops vomiting. Use for combined *shaoyang* and *yangming* stage illness with alternating fever and chills, costal or epigastric pain, nausea and vomiting, constipation and irritability. Useful in acute gastroenteritis, gastrointestinal flu, acute food poisoning, acute cholecystitis or pancreatitis, hepatitis, chronic gallbladder congestion, and the fever stage of malaria. Can also be used for liver-stomach-spleen disharmony causing abdominal fullness.

Pulses: Wiry, forceful
Tongue: Yellow coat

Comments: *Da Chai Hu Tang* is used for liver-gallbladder heat invading the stomach causing nausea or vomiting, abdominal pain, fever and irregular stool (diarrhea or constipation). As a foundation, the formula uses five herbs from Zhang Zhong-Jing's *Xiao Chai Hu Tang* (Chapter 7A): *chái hú, bàn xià, shēng jiāng, huáng qín* and *dà zǎo*. It adds in *zhǐ shí, bái sháo* and *dà huáng.*

Chái hú and *bàn xià* harmonize liver and spleen; *bái sháo* and *zhǐ shí* relieve abdominal pain; and *dà huáng* and *huáng qín* clear heat. *Dà huáng*, a cool and bitter herb, helps descend stomach *qi* and clear toxin.

The formula can be used in fever with constipation or diarrhea, to help purge pathogens through the stool. Besides acute abdominal distress, it can be used for chronic gallbladder inflammation.

Caution: *Dà huáng* is prohibited during pregnancy. Also, it can cause loose stools; reduce dosage if necessary.

Further Reading:

Bensky et al, p. 286
Chen & Chen, p. 283
Ellis, p. 57-58

LONG DAN XIE GAN TANG

Formula: *lóng dăn xiè gān tāng* (龙胆泻肝汤), "Gentiana Drain Liver Decoction"
Author: Wāng Áng (汪昂)
Source: *Yī Fāng Jí Jiě* (医方集解), 1682
Literal: "Medical Formulas Collected, Explained"

Antecedents found in:
Author: Qián Yĭ (钱乙)
Source: *Qián Shì Xiăo Ér Yào Zhèng Zhí Jué* (钱氏小儿药证直), 1119
Literal: "Qian's Children's Medical Patterns, Straight Secrets"

and
Author: Luó Tiān-Yì (羅天益)
Source: *Wèi Shēng Bǎo Jiàn* (卫生宝鉴), 1281
Literal: "Protect Life Precious Mirror"

Availability:

Cool Liver Fire Formula (JD)
Gentiana Combination (EG)
Gentiana Drain Fire Formula (GF)
Gentiana Formula (CC)
Long Dan Xie Gan Tang (BP, TZ)
Long Dan Xie Gan Wan (GC, HT, MS, PIM, PM, TL)
Quell Fire (K)
The Snake & The Dragon (PF)
* Coptis Purge Fire (HC)
* Gentiana 12 (SF)
* Gentiana Complex (EV)

Ingredients: (from the standardized *"Gentiana Combination"*)

lóng dăn căo (龙胆草), Radix/Rhizoma Gentianae	15.4 %	DA
chái hú (柴胡), Radix Bupleuri	15.4	BB
zé xiè (泽泻), Rhizoma Alismatis	15.3	FC
chē qián căo (车前草), Herba Plantaginis	7.7	FC
chuān mù tōng (川木通), Caulis Clematidis Armandii	7.7	FC
shēng dì huáng (生地黄), Radix Rehmanniae	7.7	DC
dāng guī (当归), Radix Angelicae Sinensis*Wei*	7.7	AB
zhī zĭ (栀子), Fructus Gardeniae	7.7	DA
huáng qín (黄芩), Radix Scutellariae	7.7	DB
gān căo (甘草), Radix Glycyrrhizae	7.7	AA

Drains liver and gallbladder heat, dispels damp, soothes the liver, tonifies blood, benefits the movement of urine. Use for heat in the liver or gall bladder channel causing symptoms that can affect any of the three *jiao.* Upper *jiao* symptoms include headache or migraine, red eye, conjunctivitis, earache or infection, irritability, insomnia or dizziness. Middle *jiao* symptoms include liver and gallbladder inflammation, costal distension or pain, or jaundice. Lower *jiao* symptoms include scanty or difficult urination, vaginal discharge and leukorrhea, swelling of the vulva, pruritus vulvae, urinary infection, acute prostatitis and chronic pelvic inflammatory disease. Helpful in oral or genital herpes simplex, and herpes zoster (shingles). Also used for hypertension or hyperthyroidism due to liver fire.

Pulses: Wiry, rapid, forceful
Tongue: Red on sides, possible yellow coat

Comments: This formula has a multitude of applications for problems due to liver or gallbladder fire or damp-heat. Symptoms can develop anywhere along the liver or gallbladder channels, from the eyes to the genitalia. Liver fire can affect the emotional and mental as well as the physical. Most common applications are headache, insomnia, red eye, and vaginal burning. It is an effective treatment for herpes simplex or zoster when combined with *Chuan Xin Lian* (Chapter 2A).

Caution: Prolonged use of cold and bitter herbs can injure spleen *yang*, affecting digestion.

Further Reading:

Bensky et al, p. 199
Chen & Chen, p. 371
Ellis, p. 191

WEN DAN TANG

Formula: *wēn dǎn tāng* (温胆汤), "Warm (the) Gallbladder Decoction"
Author: Chén Yán (陈言) *aka* Chén Wú-Zé (陈无择)
Source: *Sān Yīn Jí Yī Bìng Zhèng Fāng Lùn* (三因极一病证方论), 1174
Literal: "Three Etiologies Unification (of) Illness, Patterns (and) Formulas Discussion"

Antecedent found in:
Formula: *wēn dǎn tāng* (温胆汤), "Warm (the) Gallbladder Decoction"
Author: Sūn Sī-Miǎo (孙思邈)
Source: *Qiān Jīn Yào Fāng* (千金要方), 652
Literal: "Thousand Gold (Pieces) Important Formulas"

Availability:

Hoelen & Bamboo Combination (EG)
Poria & Bamboo Formula (GF, KP)
Rising Courage Teapills (PF)
Wen Dan Tang/Wan (BP, GC, HT, TL)
* Clear Phlegm (HC)
* Peaceful Shen (K)

Ingredients: (from the standardized *"Poria/Hoelen & Bamboo Formula"*)

chén pí (陈皮), Pericarpium Citri Reticulatae	24.0 %	G
bàn xià (半夏), Rhizoma Pinelliae	15.9	CA
zhǐ shí (枳实), Fructus Aurantii Immaturus	15.9	G
zhú rú (竹茹), Caulis Bambusae in Taenia	15.9	CB
fú líng (茯苓), Poria	11.1	FC
gān cǎo (甘草), Radix Glycyrrhizae	6.2	AA
shēng jiāng (生姜), Rhizoma Zingiberis Recens	6.2	BA
dà zǎo (大枣), Fructus Jujubae	4.8	AA

Ingredients: (from Herbal Times *"Wen Dan Wan"*)

fú líng (茯苓), Poria	20 %	FC
jiāng bàn xià (姜半夏), Rhizoma Pinelliae Praep	15	CA
chén pí (陈皮), Pericarpium Citri Reticulatae	15	G
chǎo zhǐ shí (炒枳实), Fructus Aurantii Immaturus	15	G
zhú rú (竹茹), Caulis Bambusae in Taenia	15	CB
dà zǎo (大枣), Fructus Jujubae	10	AA
gān cǎo (甘草), Radix Glycyrrhizae	5	AA
shēng jiāng (生姜), Rhizoma Zingiberis Recens	5	BA

Normalizes qi, dissolves phlegm, harmonizes gallbladder and stomach. Use for disharmony between gallbladder and stomach allowing accumulation of phlegm-heat in the interior. Symptoms are diverse, and include insomnia, dizziness, vertigo, headache, nausea, vomiting, poor appetite or digestion, chest or costal oppression, and palpitation. Emotional and mental symptoms can include depression, anxiety, irritability and disturbing dreams. Useful for gastritis, digestive fullness, chronic gallbladder congestion, and in the treatment of obesity. Also for morning sickness due to phlegm accumulation.

Pulse: Normal, or slippery, wiry or rapid
Tongue: Yellow coat

Comments: This formula is for chronic gallbladder damp-heat with accumulation of phlegm. There is often a bitter taste in the mouth with abdominal distension and discomfort after eating. It is useful in gallbladder congestion prior to the formation of gallstones with accompanying symptoms of weight gain, tension in the neck and shoulders, headache, and irritability. It is also appropriate for insomnia, and is frequently used to address mental disturbance (irritability, anxiety, confusion) due to phlegm accumulation.

The foundation formula uses the herbs of *Er Chen Tang* (see Chapter 3C), to dissolve phlegm: *chén pí, bàn xià, fú ling* and *gān cǎo*. Sun Simiao's original formula (652 CE) contained a large amount of the warming herb *shēng jiāng* (生姜, Rhizoma Zingiberis Recens); hence the name "Warm the Gallbladder Decoction". The later formulation by Chen Yan is not warming, and the addition of *zhú rú* further addresses phlegm-heat.

Further Reading:

Bensky et al, p. 786
Chen & Chen, p. 1213
Ellis, p. 318

Modern Formulas

JI GU CAO WAN

Formula: *jī gŭ căo wán* (鸡骨草丸), "Abrus Pills"
Source: Modern patent medicine
Availability:
Ji Gu Cao Wan (PF, PM)
Jigucao Jiannang (PM)

Ingredients: (from Plum Flower's *"Ji Gu Cao Pian"*. The current formula is proprietary. Ingredient percentages listed are from an earlier version, and may be the same.)

jī gŭ căo (鸡骨草), Herba Abri	40. %	K
shé dăn (蛇胆), Fel Serpentis	15	CB
dān shēn (丹参), Radix/Rhiz. Salviae Miltiorrhizae	15	K
rén gōng niú huáng (人工牛黄), Calculus Bovis Synth.	10	M
dāng guī (当归), Radix Angelicae Sinensis	10	AB
gŏu qĭ zĭ (枸杞子), Fructus Lycii	7	AB
zhēn zhū (珍珠), Margarita	3	N

Ingredients: (from Solstice Medicine Company, Guangxi Yulin Pharmaceutical Factory *"Jigucao Wan"*)

jī gŭ căo (鸡骨草), Herba Abri	42.5 %	K
dān shēn (丹参), Radix/Rhiz. Salviae Miltiorrhizae	20.5	K
gŏu qĭ zĭ (枸杞子), Fructus Lycii	19.5	AB
yīn chén hāo (茵陈蒿), Herba Artemisiae Scopariae	17.5	FC

Ingredients: (from Yulin Pharmaceutical Factory *"Jigucao Jiaonang"*. Ingredient percentages not listed.)

jī gŭ căo (鸡骨草), Herba Abri	K
yīn chén hāo (茵陈蒿), Herba Artemisiae Scopariae	FC
zhī zĭ (栀子), Fructus Gardeniae	DA
tián qī (田七), Radix/Rhizoma Notoginseng	J
rén gōng niú huáng (人工牛黄), Calculus Bovis Synth.	M
zhū dăn fĕn (猪胆粉), Pulvis Fellis Suis	CB
bái sháo (白芍), Radix Paeoniae Alba	AB
niú zhì (牛至), Herba Origanum vulgare	Q
gŏu qĭ zĭ (枸杞子), Fructus Lycii	AB
dà zăo (大枣), Fructus Jujubae	AA

Clears damp-heat, clears liver heat, subdues liver yang, invigorates and nourishes liver blood, opens the orifices, dispels jaundice, relieves pain. Use for acute damp-heat in the liver and gallbladder causing jaundice, costal pain and distension, and nausea or vomiting. Useful in acute viral Hepatitis A, with symptoms of yellow sclera and skin. Can also be used in gallbladder inflammation or congestion, chronic hepatitis and symptoms due to liver heat or fire, including vertigo, tinnitus, red eye, ear pain, and burning urination.

Pulse: Slippery, wiry, forceful or rapid
Tongue: Yellow greasy coat

Comments: There are various formulas using the name *Ji Gu Cao Wan/Pian*. The original patent medicine from Yulin Pharmaceutical Factory has been discontinued, but is reproduced in the Plum Flower version. Currently, two alternative versions exist from the Yulin Pharmaceutical factory (listed above).

The formula is indicated for acute jaundice due to viral hepatitis or other inflammatory factors, and can be used for any inflammatory condition of the liver or gallbladder. The principal herb is *jī gŭ căo,* a recently utilized herb from Guangxi province that has not been described in the regular *materia medica*. It comprises over 40% of the formula, and is effective for clearing liver damp-heat and moving liver blood, both factors in jaundice. Supportive herbs clear liver damp-heat (*yīn chén hāo, zhī zǐ*), move blood (*dān shēn*), and nourish liver blood and *yin* (*dāng guī, gǒu qǐ zǐ*).

OTHER FORMULAS APPROPRIATE FOR THIS CATEGORY:

FORMULAS FOR GALLBLADDER CONGESTION

Classical Formulas:

Chai Hu Qing Gan Tang

Bupleurum & Rehmannia Combination (EG)
Chai Hu Qing Gan Tang (TZ)

Zhu Ru Wen Dan Tang

Bamboo & Ginseng Combination (EG)

Modern Formulas:

GB-6 (HC)
Purge Damp-Heat (CMS)
Wei Bao (HT)

FORMULAS FOR ACUTE HEPATITIS AND JAUNDICE

Classical Formulas:

Yin Chen Hao Tang

Capillaris Combination (EG)
Yin Chen Hao Pian/Wan (GC)
Yin Chen Hao Tang (TZ)

Yin Chen Wu Ling San

Capillaris & Poria/Hoelen Five Formula (EG)

FORMULAS FOR CHRONIC HEPATITIS AND LIVER TOXICITY

Modern Formulas:

Bupleurum Gardenia Tablets (SF)
Da Bu Gan Pian/Wan (GC)
Eclipta Tablets (SF)
Ecliptex (HC)
Gan Bing Zhi Ben Wan (GC, TL)
Hepatoplex One (HC)
Hepatoplex Two (HC)
Liver C Formula (GF)
Liver DTX (EV)
Milk Thistle 80 (HC)
Salvia/Ligustrum Tablets (SF)

7. LIVER AND GALLBLADDER DISORDERS

7D. GALLSTONES AND GALLBLADDER CONGESTION

Modern Formulas:

Li Dan Pai Shi Wan	*lǐ dǎn pái shí wán* (利胆排石丸)
Li Dan Wan	*lǐ dǎn piàn* (理胆片)

Gallbladder congestion involves a progressive thickening of bile. Over time, gallstones can develop in the gallbladder, the biliary tree (common bile duct and bile ducts within the liver) or the ampulla of Vater (leading to the pancreas). Stones can be grain size or as large as a golf ball. In chronic conditions, large stones can literally fill the whole of the gallbladder.

In modern medicine, the development of gallstones is called cholelithiasis; stones are composed of cholesterol, thickened bile, calcium carbonate, and bile pigments. They may develop as a result of poor cholesterol metabolism. Demographically, gallstones start at age 40, with women just prior to menopause at the highest risk.

When gallstones migrate to the bile ducts, it is called choledocholithiasis. Obstruction of the ampulla of Vater can cause pancreatitis. Cholecystitis is a chronic inflammatory condition with secondary bacterial infection, and may or may not involve obstruction. Obstructions of bile or pancreatic ducts by stones are considered surgical emergencies. In an acute obstruction, costal pain is intense, with possible jaundice of the skin or eyes.

In Chinese medicine, gallstones and gallbladder congestion develop due to prolonged heat or damp-heat in the liver and gallbladder, leading to stasis and inflammation. Causative factors include an overly rich diet, especially spicy and fatty foods. Obesity and chronically elevated cholesterol are also considered risk factors. Perimenopausal heat can also lead to liver and gallbladder heat.

In the absence of an ultrasound or other imaging diagnosis, both gallbladder congestion and the presence of gallstones share clinical manifestations, including costal pain, nausea or vomiting, and discomfort following fatty or greasy meals, as well as symptoms along the *shaoyang* channels affecting the neck and shoulder, and temporal headache.

When stones are absent on imagery, Western medicine has little to offer. If stones are present, it is considered a surgical situation. In both cases, Chinese herbal medicine can be very helpful. The formulas can thin and soften bile stasis, and reduce or dissolve gallstones enough to prevent surgery.

The formulas discussed here are modern, using newer herbal combinations. The most effective and important herb is *jīn qián cǎo* (金钱草, Herba Lysimachiae), which can actually dissolve stones. It is combined with *yīn chén hāo* (茵陈蒿, Herba Artemisiae Scopariae) for gallstones, as well as supportive herbs to clear gallbladder damp-heat, move liver *qi* and blood, purge stool to stimulate the release of bile, and clear local inflammation and infection.

Modern Formulas:

LI DAN PAI SHI WAN

Formula: *lǐ dǎn pái shí wán* (利胆排石丸), "Benefit Gallbladder Expel Stone Pill"
Source: Modern patent medicine

Availability:

Li Dan Hua Shi Wan (TL)
Li Dan Pai Shi Wan (HT, PM)
Qing Dan Hua Shi Pian/Wan (GC)

Ingredients: (from Herbal Times *"Li Dan Pai Shi Wan"*)

jīn qián cǎo (金钱草), Herba Lysimachiae	23.0 %	FC
yīn chén hāo (茵陈蒿), Herba Artemisiae Scopariae	23.0	FC
bīng láng (槟榔), Semen Arecae	11.0	Q
dà huáng (大黄), Radix/Rhizoma Rhei	11.0	PA
huáng qín (黄芩), Radix Scutellariae	7.0	DB
mù xiāng (木香), Radix Aucklandiae	7.0	G
yù jīn (郁金), Radix Curcumae	7.0	K
hòu pò (厚朴), Cortex Magnoliae	4.5	FB
zhǐ shí (枳实), Fructus Aurantii Immaturus	4.5	G
máng xiāo (芒硝), Natrii Sulfas	2.0	PA

Clears damp-heat, soothes liver qi, benefits gallbladder, expels stones, frees the stool, relieves pain. Use for dissolution and expulsion of gallstones, with accompanying symptoms of costal pain, jaundice, trapezius muscle tension or headache. Can be used in chronic gallbladder congestion or inflammation, and in acute or chronic hepatitis.

Pulse: Slippery, wiry, forceful, possibly rapid
Tongue: Red on sides with a yellow greasy coat

Comments: *Li Dan Pai Shi Wan* formulas follow a prescription first offered by Qingdao Drug Works and based on hospital clinical experience; it is successful in reducing the size of gallstones so that they can be expelled. The key herbal combination for doing this uses *jīn qián cǎo* with *yīn chén hāo*, and in the Herbal Times version, this accounts for 46% of the formula. It is reinforced with herbs to clear heat (*dà huáng, huáng qín*) and herbs to purge congealed bile through the stool (*dà huáng, bīng láng, máng xiāo*). *Yù jīn* moves liver blood, while *hòu pò* and *mù xiāng* help descend the *qi*. While reducing the size of the stone, the formula gently dilates the common biliary duct to expel the stones.

The formula can also soften thick bile found in gallbladder congestion, thereby preventing stone formation.

Caution 1: Obstruction of ducts within the biliary tree is considered a surgical emergency.

Caution 2: *Dà huáng* and *máng xiāo* are prohibited during pregnancy; *bīng láng* and *yù jīn* are used with caution during pregnancy. Also, reduce dosage or discontinue if diarrhea develops.

LI DAN PIAN

Formula: *lǐ dǎn piàn* (理胆片), "Benefit Gallbladder Tablets"
Source: Modern patent medicine

Availability:

Li Dan Pian (PF)
Li Dan Support (K)
Li Dan Tablets (PM)
Li Dan Wan (HT)

Ingredients: (from Plum Flower *"Li Dan Pian"*)

huáng qín (黄芩), Radix Scutellariae	30. %	DB
tǔ mù xiāng (土木香), Radix Inulae	16	G
jīn qián cǎo (金钱草), Herba Lysimachiae	10	FC
jīn yín huā (金银花), Flos Lonicerae Japonicae	10	DD
yīn chén hāo (茵陈蒿), Herba Artemisiae Scopariae	10	FC
chái hú (柴胡), Radix Bupleuri	10	BB
dà qīng yè (大青叶), Folium Isatidis	10	DD
dà huáng (大黄), Radix/Rhizoma Rhei	4	PA

Ingredients: (from Herbal Times *"Li Dan Wan"*)

mù xiāng (木香), Radix Aucklandiae	16.0 %	G
bái sháo (白芍), Radix Paeoniae Alba	9.5	AB
jīn yín huā (金银花), Flos Lonicerae Japonicae	9.5	DD
zhī mǔ (知母), Rhizoma Anemarrhenae	9.5	DA
dà qīng yè (大青叶), Folium Isatidis	9.5	DD
chái hú (柴胡), Radix Bupleuri	9.5	BB
yīn chén hāo (茵陈蒿), Herba Artemisiae Scopariae	9.5	FC
jīn qián cǎo (金钱草), Herba Lysimachiae	9.5	FC
dà huáng (大黄), Radix/Rhizoma Rhei	9.5	PA
huáng qín (黄芩), Radix Scutellariae	5.0	DB
máng xiāo (芒硝), Natrii Sulfas/Mirabilitum	3.0	PA

Clears damp-heat, soothes the liver, clears heat and resolves toxin, benefits gallbladder, expels stones, frees the stool, relieves pain. Use for gallbladder inflammation causing thickened and congealed bile with accompanying symptoms of costal pain, jaundice, muscle tension, or headache. Can be used to reduce gallstones. Useful in chronic gallbladder inflammation, and acute or chronic hepatitis.

Pulse: Slippery, wiry, forceful, possibly rapid
Tongue: Red on sides with a yellow greasy coat

Comments: *Li Dan Pian* is similar to *Li Dan Pai Shi Wan* (above), but uses smaller amounts of *jīn qián cǎo* and *yīn chén hāo*. It is preferred for gallbladder congestion or inflammation before stones are formed. The formula can be used for extended periods of time, until symptoms of gallbladder congestion (costal distension and pain) are relieved. It can also be taken periodically to reduce the formation of gallstones. The formulas can also be used to treat acute hepatitis. (For viral hepatitis, combine with *Chuan Xin Lian,* Chapter 2A).

The Plum Flower version follows the original *Li Dan Pian* formula from Qingdao Pharmaceutical. The Herbal Times version adds *bái sháo, zhī mǔ* and *máng xiāo* to the original formula.

Caution: *Dà huáng* and *máng xiāo* are prohibited during pregnancy. Also, reduce dosage or discontinue if diarrhea develops.

OTHER FORMULAS APPROPRIATE FOR THIS CATEGORY:

Modern Formulas:

Dissolve GS (EV)
Lysimachia 3 (SF)
Lysimachia GB Formula (GF)
Zhu Dan Tablets (SF)

8. GYNECOLOGICAL DISORDERS

8A. GYNECOLOGICAL TONICS
(Amenorrhea, Infertility, Pregnancy, Postpartum)

Classical Formulas:

Fu Ke Zhong Zi Wan	*fù kē zhǒng zǐ wán* (妇科种子丸)
Jiao Ai Tang	*jiāo ài tāng* (胶艾汤)
Wen Jing Tang	*wēn jīng tāng* (温经汤)
Wu Ji Bai Feng Wan (White Phoenix Pills)	*wū jī bái fèng wán* (乌鸡白凤丸)

Modern Formulas:

Bu Xue Tiao Jing Wan	*bǔ xuè tiáo jīng wán* (补血调经丸)
Yang Rong Tang	*yǎng róng tāng* (养荣汤)
Zhong Zi Wan	*zhǒng zǐ wán* (种子丸)

Although three other sections of this book describe various tonic formulas (Groups 16, 17, 18), we have devoted this chapter to gynecological tonics. Most of these formulas nourish blood at their core; some also boost kidney *qi* and *yang,* and others move *qi* and blood or break blood stasis. The formulas in this chapter are used for habitual miscarriage, light or scanty periods, amenorrhea (the absence of menses), and postmenstrual or menopausal fatigue. They are also useful as pregnancy tonics during the first trimester, for postpartum fatigue, and to treat infertility. Accompanying signs and symptoms of blood deficiency include dry hair or skin, brittle nails, light-headedness, poor memory or concentration, stiff tendons and joints, and a pale tongue with a thin, weak pulse.

Formulas in this chapter that tonify kidney *yang* and blood may also be helpful for hypothyroid. Blood tonics are also found in chapters *16B. Blood Tonics* and *16C. Qi and Blood Tonics* are also useful for gynecological problems due to deficiency, including the well-known *Ba Zhen Wan.*

It is recommended that the formulas in this chapter be discontinued during menses in cases of excessive menstrual bleeding. As with all tonics, it is best to discontinued during the early stages of common cold or flu, as they may draw pathogenic factors deeper into the body. Also, use may lead to loose stools; in these cases reduce the dosage.

Infertility in Chinese medicine is usually due to weak kidney *qi* combined with blood deficiency or blood stasis, and most of the formulas described here boost kidney as well as blood. These deficiencies can lower progesterone, complicating fertility or allowing miscarriage, and the formulas are known to boost progesterone levels. They are not helpful for infertility due to fallopian blockage or scarring. In cases of infertility, the formulas in this category should be continued for at least six months, as well as taken the first trimester of pregnancy.

For infertility cases due to liver stagnation, combine formulas in this chapter with those from *Chapter 7A. Liver Stagnation*. Sometimes it is necessary to treat liver stasis first, followed by tonification of kidney and blood. Other cases of infertility, particularly in obese women, may be complicated with accumulation of phlegm and damp.

Most of the Chinese herbal tonics in this chapter can be used as **pregnancy** tonics, as **post-partum** tonics, and to treat or prevent **threatened miscarriage**, including spotting. First trimester miscarriage is often due to progesterone deficiency, and these formulas are effective at boosting and maintaining progesterone levels. The formulas may not be able to prevent miscarriage due to genetic defect or fragility of the egg due to aging, nor are they meant to deal with emergency miscarriage (spontaneous abortion). For second or third trimester spotting and cramping, Chinese herbal medicine can be helpful, but these cases will need individual prescribing by a competent practitioner.

For treatment of **morning sickness**, refer to formulas listed in *Chapter 6A. Spleen Qi Deficiency; 6C. Food Stagnation and 7A. Liver Stagnation.*

The products included here are safe during pregnancy. However, qualified herbal practitioners (such as those with NCCAOM CH or OM certification) should give treatment during pregnancy.

Classical Formulas:

FU KE ZHONG ZI WAN

Formula: *fù kē zhǒng zǐ wán* (妇科种子丸), "Gynecology Seed Pill"
Author: Xiāng Tīan-Ruì (项天瑞)
Source: *Tóng Shòu Lù* (同寿录), 1762
Literal: "Common Longevity Records"

Availability:

Fertile Fields Teapills (PF)
Fu Ke Zhong Zi Wan (MS, PM)
Nuan Gong Yun Zi Wan (TL)
* Jade Pearl 2 (JW)

Ingredients: (from Minshan *"Fu Ke Zhong Zi Wan"*)

shú dì huáng (熟地黄), Radix Rehmanniae Praep.	23.5 %	AB
dù zhòng (杜仲), Cortex Eucommiae	11.8	AC
xiāng fù (香附), Rhizoma Cyperi	11.8	G
chuān xiōng (川芎), Rhizoma Ligustici Chuanxiong	8.8	K
dāng guī (当归), Radix Angelicae Sinensis	8.8	AB
xù duàn (续断), Radix Dipsaci	8.8	AC
ài yè (艾叶), Folium Artemisiae Argyi	8.8	J
huáng qín (黄芩), Radix Scutellariae	5.9	DB
ē jiāo (阿胶), Colla Corii Asini	5.9	AB
bái sháo (白芍), Radix Paeoniae Alba	5.9	AB

Nourishes and invigorates blood, strengthens kidney, warms the uterus, soothes the liver, calms the fetus. Use for female infertility caused by blood deficiency with deficiency of kidney *yang,* accompanied by stagnation of liver *qi.* Also applicable for threatened miscarriage, amenorrhea, scanty or spotty menses, irregular periods, and post-menstrual blood deficiency. Can be used as a post-partum tonic. Symptoms may also include weak lower back, cold limbs, dry hair and skin, or light leukorrhea.

Pulse: Thin, occasionally weak, or wiry
Tongue: Normal or pale

Comments: This formula addresses infertility due to deficiency of blood and *yang*, with stagnation of liver *qi*. This pattern combination often leads to hormonal infertility, including lowered levels of progesterone. Signs may include a separation of *yang* and *yin*, with heat in the face and cold abdomen or feet. It is also a good tonic for first semester pregnancy, amenorrhea and post-partum blood loss, and it may be beneficial in low female libido. Also applicable for irregular periods due to blood deficiency.

The ingredient percentages listed above for the Minshan version are probably the same as Plum Flower's *Fertile Fields Teapills.*

JIAO AI TANG

Formula: *jiāo ài tāng* (胶艾汤), "*E Jiao* and *Ai Ye* Decoction"
Author: Zhāng Zhòng-jǐng (张仲景)
Source: *Jīn Guì Yào Lüè* (金匮要略), 220
Literal: "Golden Cabinet Essential Summary"

Availability:

Chuan Xiong Jiao Ai Tang (PM)
Harmonize The Vessels (K)
Jiao Ai Wan (HT)
Tang Kuei & Gelatin Combination (EG)

Ingredients: (from Herbal Times *"Jiao Ai Wan"*)

shú dì huáng (熟地黄), Radix Rehmanniae Praep.	20. %	AB
ài yè (艾叶), Folium Artemisiae Argyi	15	J
bái sháo (白芍), Radix Paeoniae Alba	15	AB
dāng guī (当归), Radix Angelicae Sinensis	15	AB
ē jiāo (阿胶), Colla Corii Asini	15	AB
chuān xiōng (川芎), Rhizoma Ligustici Chuanxiong	10	K
gān cǎo (甘草), Radix Glycyrrhizae	10	AA

Tonifies, warms and invigorates blood, stops bleeding, regulates menses, calms the fetus. Use for bleeding or spotting during pregnancy with abdominal cramping due to blood deficiency with cold in the abdomen. Use for threatened miscarriage or restless fetus, and for menstrual disorders marked by heavy bleeding, prolonged spotting, and abdominal cramps.

Pulse: Thin, weak
Tongue: Normal, or pale

***Comments*:** This formula is used for threatened miscarriage due to cold uterus with blood deficiency. It is also helpful in non-pregnancy patients with prolonged menstrual bleeding or spotting, as well as cramps due to cold and blood deficiency. Using *Si Wu Tang* (chapter 16B) as its foundation, the blood building and warming aspect is reinforced with *ē jiāo*, the fatty tallow below the skin from horses or donkeys. *Ài yè* stops bleeding; *bái sháo* and *gān cǎo* help stop abdominal cramping.

Further Reading:

Bensky et al, p. 610
Chen & Chen, p. 950

WEN JING TANG

Formula: *wēn jīng tāng* (温经汤), "Warm (the) Menses Decoction"
Author: Zhāng Zhòng-Jǐng (张仲景)
Source: *Jīn Guì Yào Lüè* (金匮要略), 220
Literal: "Golden Cabinet Essential Summary"

Availability:

Tangkuei & Evodia Combination (EG)
Warm Cycle Teapills (PF)
Wen Jing Tang (TZ)
Wen Jing Tang Wan (TL)
Wen Jing Wan (HT)

Ingredients: (from the standardized *"Tangkuei & Evodia Combination"*)

bàn xià (半夏), Rhizoma Pinelliae	13.2 %	CA
mài mén dōng (麦门冬), Radix Ophiopogonis	13.2	AD
wú zhū yú (吴茱萸), Fructus Evodiae	10.0	E
gān jiāng (干姜), Rhizoma Zingiberis	10.0	E
dāng guī (当归), Radix Angelicae Sinensis	6.7	AB
chuān xiōng (川芎), Rhizoma Ligustici Chuanxiong	6.7	K
bái sháo (白芍), Radix Paeoniae Alba	6.7	AB
rén shēn (人参), Radix Ginseng	6.7	AA
guì zhī (桂枝), Ramulus Cinnamomi	6.7	BA
mŭ dān pí (牡丹皮), Cortex Moutan	6.7	DC
gān cǎo (甘草), Radix Glycyrrhizae	6.7	AA
ē jiāo (阿胶), Colla Corii Asini	6.7	AB

Ingredients: (from Herbal Times *"Wen Jing Wan"*)

bái sháo (白芍), Radix Paeoniae Alba	10. %	AB
chuān xiōng (川芎), Rhizoma Ligustici Chuanxiong	10	K
dāng guī (当归), Radix Angelicae Sinensis	10	AB
ē jiāo (阿胶), Colla Corii Asini	10	AB
mài mén dōng (麦门冬), Radix Ophiopogonis	10	AD
mŭ dān pí (牡丹皮), Cortex Mouta	10	DC
bàn xià (半夏), Rhizoma Pinelliae	8	CA
shēng jiāng (生姜), Rhizoma Zingiberis Recens	8	BA
wú zhū yú (吴茱萸), Fructus Evodiae	8	E
guì zhī (桂枝), Ramulus Cinnamomi	6	BA
rén shēn (人参), Radix Ginseng	6	AA
gān cǎo (甘草), Radix Glycyrrhizae	4	AA

Warms the uterus, dispels cold, tonifies qi, nourishes blood, nourishes yin, benefits yang, invigorates blood. Use for deficiency cold in the uterus, causing infertility, amenorrhea, scanty and prolonged menstrual bleeding, or irregular menstruation. Useful for chronic mild dysmenorrhea due to deficiency cold. Also applicable for post-partum spotting, and for leukorrhea due to deficiency-cold. Secondary symptoms can include fatigue, dry skin or hair, weak or cold limbs, or dry lips and mouth.

Pulse: Normal, or weak, thin or deep or rough
Tongue: Normal, or pale or dark

Comments: *Wen Jing Tang* addresses infertility and menstrual disorders due to chronic deficiency cold in the uterus, leading to mild cramping, spotting, light periods, or irregularity. This can be due to either a pre-existing weakness of *mingmen* fire/kidney *yang*, or accumulated wind-cold in the uterus following exposure to cold and damp during menses or childbirth. Symptoms invariably include coldness in the lower abdomen with cold feet prior to or during menses. The formula is also appropriate for clear vaginal discharge and leukorrhea due to cold, and can also be used as a tonic during first semester pregnancy.

Warming herbs in the formula include *wú zhū yú, guì zhī, gān jiāng, ē jiāo* and *rén shēn*. The combination of *bàn xià* and *mài mén dong* helps resolve sticky vaginal mucus. The Herbal Times version adheres to the original formula, while the Plum Flower version substitutes *shú dì huáng* (熟地黄, Radix Rehmanniae Praep.) for *ē jiāo*.

Further Reading:

Bensky et al, p. 577, 589
Chen & Chen, p. 919
Ellis, p. 320

WU JI BAI FENG WAN
WHITE PHOENIX PILLS

Formula: *wū jī bái fèng wán* (乌鸡白凤丸), "Black Chicken, White Phoenix Pill"
Author: Gōng Tíng-Xián (龚廷贤)
Source: *Shòu Shì Bǎo Yuán* (寿世保元), 1615
Literal: "Long Life Protect (the) Source"

Availability:

White Phoenix Formula (PM)
White Phoenix Teapills (PM)
Wu Chi Pai Feng Wan (PM)
Wu Ji Bai Feng Wan (HT, PM)

Ingredients: (From Tientsin Drug Manufactory; Tianjin *"Wu Chi Pai Feng Wan"*)

wū jī (乌鸡), Galli Nigroscei	33.9 %	AB
shú dì huáng (熟地黄), Radix Rehmanniae Praep.	12.9	AB
shēng dì huáng (生地黄), Radix Rehmanniae	12.9	DC
lù jiǎo shuāng (鹿角霜), Cornu Cervi Degelatinatum	6.5	AC
dāng guī (当归), Radix Angelicae Sinensis	6.4	AB
bái sháo (白芍), Radix Paeoniae Alba	6.4	AB
rén shēn (人参), Radix Ginseng	6.4	AA
bái zhú (白术), Rhizoma Atractylodis Macrocephalae	6.4	AA
xiāng fù (香附), Rhizoma Cyperi	6.4	G
huáng qí (黄芪), Radix Astragali	1.6	AA

Ingredients: (from Herbal Times *"Wu Ji Bai Feng Wan"*)

wū jī (乌鸡), Galli Nigroscei	25.1 %	AB
shēng dì huáng (生地黄), Radix Rehmanniae	10.1	DC
shú dì huáng (熟地黄), Radix Rehmanniae Praep.	10.1	AB
dāng guī (当归), Radix Angelicae Sinensis	5.6	AB
bái sháo (白芍), Radix Paeoniae Alba	5.0	AB
dān shēn (丹参), Radix/Rhiz. Salviae Miltiorrhizae	5.0	K
shān yào (山药), Rhizoma Dioscoreae	5.0	AA
lù jiǎo jiāo (鹿角胶), Colla Cornus Cervi	5.0	AC
rén shēn (人参), Radix Ginseng	5.0	AA
xiāng fù (香附), Rhizoma Cyperi	5.0	G
biē jiǎ (鳖甲), Carapax Trionycis/Amydae	2.5	AD
chuān xiōng (川芎), Rhizoma Ligustici Chuanxiong	2.5	K

qiàn shí (芡实), Semen Euryales	2.5	L
tiān mén dōng (天门冬), Radix Asparagi	2.5	AD
jīn yīng zǐ (金樱子), Fructus Rosae Laevigatae	1.9	L
lù jiǎo shuāng (鹿角霜), Cornu Cervi Degelatinatum	1.9	AC
mǔ lì (牡蛎), Concha Ostreae	1.9	N
gān cǎo (甘草), Radix Glycyrrhizae	1.2	AA
huáng qí (黄芪), Radix Astragali	1.2	AA
yín chái hú (银柴胡), Radix Stellariae	1.0	DE

Nourishes blood, tonifies qi, moves qi and invigorates blood, warms the uterus, regulates menses. Use for chronic blood deficiency affecting the menses, including amenorrhea, light or scanty periods, irregular menses due to deficiency, and protracted spotting. Also for infertility, postpartum or post-menstrual fatigue, and blood deficiency following illness or injury. Useful for other blood deficiency symptoms, including dizziness, poor memory, dry hair, hair loss, dry skin, cracked skin or fingernails, and stiff tendons.

Pulse: Normal, or weak, thin or deep
Tongue: Normal or pale

Comments: The popular *Wu Ji Bai Feng* products are routinely used in China by women as a post-menstrual tonic and for irregular menses due to blood deficiency. It is also used as a post-partum tonic. The main ingredient is *wū jī,* the black rooster. This fowl has black skin and beak with white feathers, and the Chinese call it "Black Chicken, White Phoenix". The whole chicken is considered an excellent blood tonic; here, it is reinforced with medicinals to boost blood, including *dì huáng, dāng guī* and *lù jiǎo jiāo*. Because of its animal source foundation, it is considered one of the stronger blood-building products. The formula can also be used as a general warming blood tonic for non-gynecological conditions, including post surgery, post bone marrow transplantation, or post radiation therapy.

Both the Tianjin and Herbal Times versions contain significant amounts of *wū jī* and *dì huáng* (combined 60% and 45%, respectively), although the Herbal Times version contains 19 herbs compared with Tianjin's 10 herbs. Ingredients of the Plum Flower version, *White Phoenix Teapills*, is similar to the Herbal Times formula.

The Tianjin formula comes as 10 boxes, each with a plastic "egg". Contents of the egg are split into two doses, to be taken in one day.

Modern Formulas:

BU XUE TIAO JING WAN

Formula: *bŭ xuè tiáo jīng wán* (补血调经丸)
"Tonify Blood, Regulate Menses Pill"
Source: Modern patent medicine

Availability:

Bu Xue Tiao Jing Wan (HT)

Ingredients: (from Herbal Times *"Bu Xue Tiao Jing Wan"*)

dāng guī (当归), Radix Angelicae Sinensis	28.6 %	AB
shú dì huáng (熟地黄), Radix Rehmanniae Praep.	28.6	AB
yì mŭ căo (益母草), Herba Leonuri	28.6	K
bái sháo (白芍), Radix Paeoniae Alba	7.1	AB
chuān xiōng (川芎), Rhizoma Ligustici Chuanxiong	7.1	K

Nourishes blood, invigorates blood, regulates menses. Use for menstrual disorders due to deficiency of blood, including mild menstrual cramping or irregular periods. Symptoms may include light or delayed menses, prolonged spotting or bleeding, and lower abdominal pain preceding menses. Also for postpartum abdominal pain, retention of lochia, and infertility due to blood deficiency and stagnation. Can be used as a general blood tonic.

Pulse: Normal, or weak, thin or deep
Tongue: Normal or pale

Comments: This is a good formula for menstrual disorders due to blood deficiency including mild menstrual cramps, amenorrhea, and delayed or irregular periods. It is basically *Si Wu Tang* (Chapter 16B) with the addition of *yì mŭ căo* ("Benefit Mother Herb"). Blood tonification is prioritized with *shú dì huáng* and *dāng guī,* while *yì mŭ căo* moves blood and breaks clots. Besides regulating menses, the formula is good following childbirth to replenish blood as well as discharging lochia and remaining blood in the uterus.

Note: A product with the same Chinese name (*bŭ xuè tiáo jīng wán*, 补血调经丸), exists as *Butiao Tablets*, from Yihetang Herbal Manufactory, Guangdong. It is a complex formula, using 17 herbs, with a different application.

YANG RONG WAN

Formula: *yǎng róng wán* (养荣丸), "Cultivate Flourishing Decoction"
Source: Modern patent medicine

Availability:

Cultivate Splendor Teapills (PF)
Fu Ke Yang Rong Wan (TL)
Yang Rong Wan (MS)

Ingredients: (from Minshan *"Yang Rong Wan"* and Plum Flower *"Cultivate Splendor Teapills"*)

dāng guī (当归), Radix Angelicae Sinensis	11.4 %	AB
shú dì huáng (熟地黄), Radix Rehmanniae Praep.	11.4	AB
bái zhú (白术), Rhizoma Atractylodis Macrocephalae	11.4	AA
bái sháo (白芍), Radix Paeoniae Alba	8.5	AB
chuān xiōng (川芎), Rhizoma Ligustici Chuanxiong	8.5	K
xiāng fù (香附), Rhizoma Cyperi	8.5	G
yì mǔ cǎo (益母草), Herba Leonuri	8.5	K
dù zhòng (杜仲), Cortex Eucommiae	5.7	AC
huáng qí (黄芪), Radix Astragali	5.7	AA
ài yè (艾叶), Folium Artemisiae Argyi	5.7	J
fú líng (茯苓), Poria	2.9	FC
mài mén dōng (麦门冬), Radix Ophiopogonis	2.8	AD
gān cǎo (炙甘草), Radix Glycyrrhizae	2.8	AA
chén pí (陈皮), Pericarpium Citri Reticulatae	2.8	G
ē jiāo (阿胶), Colla Corii Asini	2.8	AB
shā rén (砂仁), Fructus Amomi	.6	FB

Nourishes blood, tonifies qi, invigorates blood, dredges liver qi, boosts yang, stops bleeding, regulates chong and ren channels. Use for deficiencies of *qi* and blood affecting the *chong* and *ren* channels and the uterus. Symptoms include infertility, recurrent miscarriage, menstrual irregularity, amenorrhea, and prolonged spotting or bleeding. Other symptoms may include fatigue, poor concentration, insomnia and cold limbs. Can be used as a general tonic following childbirth or illness.

Pulse: Normal, or weak, thin, or choppy
Tongue: Normal or pale or dark

Comments: *Yang Rong Wan* is a 16 herb gynecological tonic, using *Ba Zhen Tang* (Chapter 16C) as a foundation. 34% of the formula nourishes blood, while 20% tonifies *qi*, 17% moves blood and breaks stasis, and 11% regulates liver *qi*. As such, it is used for infertility due to blood deficiency, and can also be used as a first semester pregnancy tonic which may help maintain progesterone levels, and as a postpartum blood tonic. The formula can also be used to treat irregular menses, amenorrhea and spotty prolonged menses.

Note: *Yang Rong Tang* has a similar name but different presciption to the classical formula *Ren Shen Yang Rong Tang* (also available as *Yang Ying Wan*). See *Chapter 16C.*

ZHONG ZI WAN

Formula: *zhǒng zǐ wán* (种子丸), "Seed Pill"
Source: Modern patent medicine

Availability:

Zhong Zi Wan (HT)

Ingredients: (from Herbal Times' *"Zhong Zi Wan"*)

shān yào (山药), Rhizoma Dioscoreae	12.5 %	AA
jī xuè téng (鸡血藤), Caulis Spatholobi/Millettiae	12.5	K
bái sháo (白芍), Radix Paeoniae Alba	6.3	AB
chì sháo (赤芍), Radix Paeoniae Rubra	6.3	K
dān shēn (丹参), Radix/Rhiz. Salviae Miltiorrhizae	6.3	K
fú líng (茯苓), Poria	6.3	FC
tù sī zǐ (菟丝子), Semen Cuscutae	6.3	AC
fù pén zǐ (覆盆子), Fructus Rubi	4.2	L
gǒu qǐ zǐ (枸杞子), Fructus Lycii	4.2	AB
gōu téng (钩藤), Ramulus Uncariae cum Uncis	4.2	O
huáng qí (黄芪), Radix Astragali	4.2	AA
lián zǐ (莲子), Semen Nelumbinis	4.2	L
sāng jì shēng (桑寄生), Herba Taxilli/Loranthi	4.2	AD
suān zǎo rén (酸枣仁), Semen Ziziphi Spinosae	4.2	N
xiān máo (仙茅), Rhizoma Curculiginis	4.2	AC
xù duàn (续断), Radix Dipsaci	4.2	AC
yín yáng huò (淫羊藿), Herba Epimedii	4.2	AC
lù róng (鹿茸), Cornu Cervi Pantotrichum	2.0	AC

Moves blood, warms kidney yang, tonifies kidney qi, nourishes blood. Use for infertility and menstrual problems due to blood stagnation with deficiencies of kidney *yang* and *qi* and blood. Applicable for threatened miscarriage, habitual miscarriage, dysmenorrhea, amenorrhea, scanty or spotty menses, or post-menstrual blood stagnation. Symptoms can include weak lower back, cold limbs and fatigue.

Pulse: Normal, or weak, thin, and choppy
Tongue: Normal or pale or dark

Comments: Although having a similar name to *Fu Ke Zhong Zi* Wan (above), this formula from Herbal Times is different. A large formula (18 herbs), it addresses infertility due to blood stasis with deficiency of kidney *yang* or cold in the uterus. 25% of the formula moves blood (*jī xuè téng, chì sháo* and *dān shēn*), while 21% tonifies kidney *yang* and *qi* and warms the uterus (*tù sī zǐ, xiān máo, xù duàn, yín yáng huò* and *lù róng*). The use of *shān yào* as the lead herb may help promote progesterone production. It is related to the Mexican yam that is currently being used for similar purposes.

This formula, while addressing deficiency of kidney *qi*, is unique for infertility in that it concentrates on moving blood rather than tonifying blood. It would be appropriate in cases marked by chronic menstrual cramping. It should not be confused with *Fu Ke Zhong Zi Wan* (above), which is more of a blood tonic.

Caution: *Jī xuè téng* is contraindicated during pregnancy in the second or third trimesters, and for patients taking Coumadin or other blood thinners.

OTHER FORMULAS IN THIS CATEGORY:

Single herb:

dāng guī (当归), Radix Angelicae Sinensis
See Chapter 16B

hé shǒu wū (何首乌), Radix Polygoni Multiflori
See Chapter 16B

Classical Formulas:

Ai Fu Nuan Gong Wan
Mugwort & Cyperus Combination (EG)

Bao Chan Wu You Fang
Tangkuei & Parsley Combination (EG)

Ba Zhen Tang
See Chapter 16C

Dang Gui Bu Xue Tang
See Chapter 16C

Huan Shao Dan
See Chapter 18A

Sheng Hua Tang
Sheng Hua Tang (BP)
Sheng Hua Tang Wan (TL)
Tangkuei & Ginger Combination (EG)

Si Wu Tang
See Chapter 16B

Shi Quan Da Bu Tang
See Chapter 18A

Tao Hong Si Wu Tang
See Chapter 8C

Wu Zi Yan Zong Wan
See Chapter 17B

Modern Formulas:

Dang Gui Jing – Tang Kwei Gin

See Chapter 16B

Ren Shen Bu Wan - Ginseng Tonic Capsules

See Chapter 18A

Ren Shen Lu Rong Wan - Ginseng Antler Pills

See Chapter 18A

Other:

Added Flavors Supplement The Center (BP)
Antai Wan (PM)
Balance-Cold (EV)
Butiao Tablets (PM)
Fertile Garden (HC)
Jade Moon Cool (JW)
Jade Moon Passage (JW)
Jade Moon Phase 1 (JW)
Jade Moon Phase 2 (JW)
Jade Pearl 1 (JW)
Jade Pearl 2 (JW)
Maternal Herbal (HC)
Menotrol (EV)
Mobilize Essence Formula (GF)
Moon Pearls (CP)
Nourish Jade Yin (K)
Nourish Ren and Chong Formula (GF)
Postpartum (HC)
Wise Woman's Well (CMS)
Woman's Treasure (SF)
Yuan Support Formula (GF)

8. GYNECOLOGICAL DISORDERS

8B. PREMENSTRUAL TENSION

Classical Formulas:

Jia Wei Xiao Yao San *jiā wèi xiāo yáo săn* (加味逍遥散)

Chinese doctors refer to premenstrual syndrome (PMS) as premenstrual tension, based on its key manifestation. The difference reflects an understanding of energetic etiology. In Chinese medicine, the liver is responsible for smoothing the distribution of *qi* and blood into the flesh and muscle. When liver *qi* and blood stagnate, tension in the muscles follows, particularly along the liver and gallbladder channels. This leads to the common PMS symptoms of irritability, headache, neck tension, breast distension and abdominal distension.

Liver stagnation that leads to premenstrual tension has various causes. Historically, the Chinese have pointed to internalized emotions inhibiting the free flow of *qi* and blood from the liver. Modern stressors also include the burden of environmental toxins in the food, air and water as well as infiltration of intestinal toxins through an irritated or inflamed small intestine. The over-processing of pharmaceuticals and exogenous hormones can also lead to liver stasis.

Liver *qi* stagnation can be caused or aggravated by heat. This follows deficiency of *yin* or blood, or occur naturally with women's basal temperature rhythms. Body temperature normally rises between ovulation and menstruation, and the rise in temperature exacerbates pre-existing liver *qi* stagnation.

The goal of the Chinese herbal approach is to soothe liver *qi*, tonify blood and *yin,* and clear heat from the liver. Chinese herbal formulas are very effective for PMS, and successful therapy is usually achieved in one to four months. It is best to take the medicine between ovulation and menstruation. Patients may also require a formula for dysmenorrhea during the period (see Chapter 8C) or blood tonics following menses (see Chapter 8A).

Rarely, PMS symptoms may be aggravated with herbal treatment; this is due to too strong a dosage, and satisfactory results can be obtained by reducing the dosage.

While the formula in this chapter is most commonly used for premenstrual tension, it can also be applied to a variety of presentations due to stagnation of liver *qi* and blood, including digestive disturbance, irregular periods, infertility and chronic hepatitis or cirrhosis. The formula is also appropriate for irritability during menopause, when due to heat aggravating liver stasis. Conversely, several of the formulas found in Chapter 7A. *Liver Stagnation* are also be used for premenstrual tension.

Classical Formulas:

JIA WEI XIAO YAO SAN

Formula: *jiā wèi xiāo yáo sǎn* (加味逍遥散)
"Added Ingredients Free Wanderer Powder"
Author: Xuē Jǐ (薛己) *aka* Xuē Xīn-Fǔ (薛新甫) *aka* Xuē Lì-Zhāi (薛立斋)
Source: *Nèi Kē Zhāi Yào* (内科摘要), circa 1530
Literal: "Internal (Medicine) Department Selected Essentials"

Availability:

Augmented Rambling Formula (HS)
Bupleurum & Peony Formula (CC, EG)
Dan Zhi Xiao Yao San (BP)
Easy Wanderer Plus Formula (JD)
Free & Easy Wanderer Plus Teaplls (PF)
Free and Easy Wanderer Plus Formula (GF)
Jia Wei Xiao Yao Wan (HT, PM, TL)
Relaxed Wanderer (PM)
Woman's Balance (HC)
* Freeing The Sun (TT)
* Jade Calm (JW)
* Relaxed Wanderer (K)

Ingredients: (from the standardized *"Bupleurum & Peony Formula"*)

dāng guī (当归), Radix Angelicae Sinensis	12.1 %	AB
bái sháo (白芍), Radix Paeoniae Alba	12.1	AB
fú líng (茯苓), Poria	12.1	FC
bái zhú (白术), Rhizoma Atractylodis Macrocephalae	12.1	AA
chái hú (柴胡), Radix Bupleuri	12.1	BB
gān jiāng (干姜), Rhizoma Zingiberis	12.1	E
mǔ dān pí (牡丹皮), Cortex Moutan	7.6	DC
zhī zǐ (栀子), Fructus Gardeniae	7.6	DA
zhì gān cǎo (炙甘草), Radix Glycyrrhizae Praep.	6.1	AA
bò hé (薄荷), Herba Menthae	6.1	BB

Ingredients: (from Herbal Times *"Jia Wei Xiao Yao Wan"*)

mǔ dān pí (牡丹皮), Cortex Moutan	16.7 %	DC
zhī zǐ (栀子), Fructus Gardeniae	16.7	DA
bái sháo (白芍), Radix Paeoniae Alba	11.1	AB
bái zhú (白术), Rhizoma Atractylodis Macrocephalae	11.2	AA
chái hú (柴胡), Radix Bupleuri	11.2	BB
dāng guī (当归), Radix Angelicae Sinensis	11.2	AB
fú líng (茯苓), Poria	11.2	FC
gān cǎo (甘草), Radix Glycyrrhizae	7.8	AA
bò hé (薄荷), Herba Menthae	2.9	BB

Soothes the liver, dispels liver stasis, clears heat, harmonizes liver and spleen, moves qi, invigorates blood, tonifies spleen qi, tonifies blood, regulates menses. Use for stagnation of liver *qi* with blood deficiency and heat, causing premenstrual tension or irregular menses. Symptoms include irritability, anxiety, depression, headache, breast distension or water retention. Other applications include irregular menses, infertility and symptoms associated with menopause including irritability, dizziness and fatigue. Also can be used for liver-spleen disharmony causing poor digestion or costal distension, and symptoms accompanying chronic hepatitis.

Pulse: Wiry, thin, possibly rapid
Tongue: Normal, or reddish on the sides

Comments: This formula is an enhancement of *Xiao Yao San* (see Chapter 7A), which moves liver *qi* and blood (*chái hú* and *bái sháo*), while tonifying *qi* (*bái zhú, fú líng, gān cǎo*) and blood (*dāng guī*). Dr. Xue Ji modified the formula by adding *zhī zǐ* and *mǔ dān pí* to clear liver heat. This approach is clinically more successful for the treatment of premenstrual syndrome (PMS), where liver *qi* stagnation is particularly aggravated by liver heat. In *Jia Wei Xiao Yao San*, the standardized version uses a combined 15% for these two herbs, while the Herbal Times version boosts that to 33%.

Recommended dosing is given between ovulation and the first day of the period. A course of treatment may take four to five months. The formula is also useful for liver stasis aggravated by systemic heat during menopause, causing irritability and anxiety.

Further Reading:

Bensky et al, p. 124
Chen & Chen, p. 254
Ellis, p. 159

OTHER FORMULAS APPROPRIATE FOR THIS CHAPTER:

Classical Formulas:

Chai Hu Shu Gan Tang

See Chapter 7A

Xiao Yao San

See Chapter 7A

Modern Formulas:

Ease Pearls (CP)
Nuphar 14 (SF)
Heavenly Water (HC)

8C. UTERINE BLOOD STASIS
(Menstrual Cramps, Uterine Fibroids, Ovarian Cysts, Endometriosis)

Classical Formulas:

Dang Gui Shao Yao San	*dāng guī sháo yào sǎn* (当归芍药散)
Gui Zhi Fu Ling Wan	*guì zhī fú líng wán* (桂枝茯苓丸)
Shao Fu Zhu Yu Tang	*shào fǔ zhú yū tāng* (少腹逐瘀汤)
Tao Hong Si Wu Tang	*táo hóng sì wù tāng* (桃红四物汤)

Modern Formulas:

Tong Jing Wan	*tòng jīng wán* (痛经丸)

Uterine blood stasis is the basis for conditions that include menstrual cramps, uterine fibroids, ovarian cysts, and endometriosis. Symptoms for **menstrual cramps** (dysmenorrhea) involve pain in the lower abdomen proceeding, during, or following menstruation. Clots may accompany cramps and the severity can be marked by the degree of pain, the number of days involved, and also by the number and size of clots. Most cases of dysmenorrhea have their origin in stagnation of liver *qi* and blood affecting the menses, and may be compounded by aspects of cold, heat, dampness, or deficiency of *yin* or blood. Many of the formulas listed here act by moving liver *qi*, invigorating blood, breaking blood stasis, warming the uterus, and tonifying *yin* and blood.

Uterine fibroids are treated with similar formulas as those for menstrual cramps. Certain products are available that specifically address uterine fibroids, and are listed at the end of this chapter. Generally, fibroids that are smaller than 5 cm respond to herbal formulas, but this needs to be done consistently for many months. Fibroids larger than 8 cm are not satisfactorily treated by herbs, although they should stop growing after menopause. Fibroids causing constant bleeding require surgery, either by cauterization, myomectomy, or hysterectomy.

Ovarian cysts require formulas that address fluid accumulation as well as blood invigoration. These respond well to Chinese herbal therapy, and several specific formulas are listed at the end of the chapter. One can also combine a formula in this chapter with a formula from *Chapter 12. Water Retention and Edema.*

Endometriosis involves formulas that address both blood stagnation and accumulation of damp-heat. This condition is quite stubborn, and may have its origins in embryological development. Herbs are not particularly successful except when formulated as custom prescriptions by experienced practitioners. However, certain formulas in this chapter may help reduce endometrial pain occurring during ovulation.

Most of the formulas described in this chapter are used for **menstrual cramps** (dysmenorrhea). There are several options for taking these medicines. They can be taken as an analgesic during the worst moments of pain; taken for three to ten days prior to menses; or in difficult cases, taken throughout the month. During menses, once clots have been discharged or the pain has subsided, it is best to discontinue the medicine so as not to cause excessive menstrual bleeding.

For menstrual cramps due to or accompanied by liver *qi* stagnation, supportive formulas can be found in Chapter 7A*, Liver Qi Stagnation*. For example, *Ge Xia Zhu Yu Tang* can treat menstrual cramps directly.

In complex gynecological disorders, 3 different types of formulas may be necessary: one during the pre-menstrual phase (Chapter 8B), one during menses (this chapter), and one following menses (Chapter 8A).

Cautions:

1. Many of the herbs found in dysmenorrhea formulas are strong blood invigorators and should not be used during the second and third trimester of pregnancy.

2. During menstruation, these formulas should be discontinued once cramps and clotting have stopped, so as not to cause excessive menstrual bleeding.

3. These formulas may cause loose stool or diarrhea, and in such cases dosing should be reduced.

4. Certain herbs are contraindicated for patients on blood thinners such as Coumadin.

Classical Formulas:

DANG GUI SHAO YAO SAN

Formula: *dāng guī sháo yào sǎn* (当归芍药散)
"Angelica *Dang Gui*, Paeonia Powder"
Author: Zhāng Zhòng-Jǐng (张仲景)
Source: *Jīn Guì Yào Lüè* (金匮要略), 220
Literal: "Golden Cabinet Essential Summary"

Availability:

Dang Gui and Peony Formula (HS)
Dang Gui Shao Yao San (BP, TZ)
Tang Kuei & Peony Formula (GF)
Tangkuei & Peony Formula (EG)

Ingredients: (from the standardized *"Tangkuei & Peony Formula"*)

bái sháo (白芍), Radix Paeoniae Alba	31.1 %	AB
zé xiè (泽泻), Rhizoma Alismatis	24.9	FC
fú líng (茯苓), Poria	12.5	FC
bái zhú (白术), Rhizoma Atractylodis Macrocephalae	12.5	AA
dāng guī (当归), Radix Angelicae Sinensis	9.5	AB
chuān xiōng (川芎), Rhizoma Ligustici Chuanxiong	9.5	AB

Ingredients: (from Golden Flower *"Tang Kuei & Peony Formula"*)

bái sháo (白芍), Radix Paeoniae Alba	25.0 %	AB
zé xiè (泽泻), Rhizoma Alismatis	16.7	FC
fú líng (茯苓), Poria	16.7	FC
bái zhú (白术), Rhizoma Atractylodis Macrocephalae	16.7	AA
dāng guī (当归), Radix Angelicae Sinensis	12.5	AB
chuān xiōng (川芎), Rhizoma Ligustici Chuanxiong	12.4	AB

Nourishes blood, invigorates blood, strengthens spleen, spreads liver qi, resolves dampness. Use for mild but persistent abdominal cramping with abdominal water retention found in dysmenorrhea, premenstrual syndrome, and edema. Also used for infertility, malposition of fetus, pain or bleeding during pregnancy, irregular menses and ovarian cyst. Can be used for edema in the limbs, or for scrotal hydrocele.

Pulse: Wiry, wide or soft
Tongue: Normal, or swollen with a wet coat

Comments: This formula address liver stasis with accumulation of damp in the lower abdomen. The original application was for cramping during any phase of pregnancy, or cramping with water retention during pregnancy. Currently, it is also used for non-pregnancy conditions showing abdominal pain, dysmenorrhea or premenstrual tension with accumulation of water in the lower abdomen or waist, and for ovarian cyst. Here, cramping is mild but persistent.

Bái sháo, the lead herb, moves liver blood stasis while nourishing liver blood, and is supported by *dāng guī* and *chuān xiōng. Zé xiè* and *fú líng* dispel accumulated dampness, and *bái zhú* tonifies spleen *qi*.

Caution: Herbal formulas used during pregnancy should be reserved for experienced TCM practitioners.

Further Reading:

Bensky et al, p. 587
Chen & Chen, p. 594
Ellis, p. 75

GUI ZHI FU LING WAN

Formula: *guì zhī fú líng wán* (桂枝茯苓丸), "Cinnamon Twig, Poria Pill"
Author: Zhāng Zhòng-Jǐng (张仲景)
Source: *Jīn Guì Yào Lüè* (金匮要略), 220
Literal: "Golden Cabinet Essential Summary"

Availability:

Cinnamon & Hoelen Formula (EG, HS)
Cinnamon & Poria Formula (KP)
Cinnamon And Poria Formula (GF)
Cinnamon & Poria Teapills (PF)
Gui Zhi Fu Ling Tang (TZ)
Gui Zhi Fu Ling Wan (BP, HT, PM, TL)
* Jade Control (JW)
* Women's Chamber (K)

Ingredients: (from the standardized *"Cinnamon & Poria/Hoelen Formula"*)

guì zhī (桂枝), Ramulus Cinnamomi	20. %	BA
fú líng (茯苓), Poria	20	FC
chì sháo (赤芍), Radix Paeoniae Rubra	20	K
táo rén (桃仁), Semen Persicae	20	K
mŭ dān pí (牡丹皮), Cortex Moutan	20	DC

Invigorates blood, breaks blood stasis, warms the uterus, dissipates masses, stops bleeding. Use for blood stasis causing menstrual cramps, uterine masses, endometriosis, irregular periods, ovarian cysts, or amenorrhea. Also for mild persistent bleeding during pregnancy, or retention of lochia. The formula is also used for prostate swelling, hepatomegaly, splenomegaly and hepatitis.

Pulse: Choppy, slippery or wiry
Tongue: Normal or dark

Comments: This formula was originally designed for episodes of mild bleeding or spotting during pregnancy, known in TCM as Restless Fetus Syndrome. Today it is commonly use for menstrual cramping due to cold in the uterus. It is a popular formula in the Japanese *kanpo* tradition for spotting following a period, ovarian cysts, endometriosis, and retention of lochia following childbirth.

Caution: *Táo rén* is prohibited during second and third trimesters of pregnancy, and with patients taking Coumadin. Use of this formula during pregnancy should be supervised by qualified practitioners.

Further Reading:

Bensky et al, p. 583
Chen & Chen, p. 928
Ellis, p. 121

SHAO FU ZHU YU TANG

Formula: *shào fŭ zhú yū tāng* (少腹逐瘀汤)
"Lower Abdomen Drive-Out Stasis Decoction"
Author: Wáng Qīng-Rèn (王清任)
Source: *Yī Lín Găi Cuò* (医林改错), 1830
Literal: "Physicians' Circle, Correction (of) Errors"

Availability:

Fennel Seed & Corydalis Combination (EG)
Cnidium & Bulrush Combination (EG)
Shao Fu Zhu Yu Tang (BP, TZ)
Shao Fu Zhu Yu Wan (HT)
Stasis In The Lower Palace Teapills (PF)
* Lower Palace Tablets (SF)

Ingredients: (from the standardized *"Fennel Seed & Corydalis Combination"*)

dāng guī (当归), Radix Angelicae Sinensis	21.1 %	AB
pú huáng (蒲黄), Pollen Typhae	21.1	J
chì sháo (赤芍), Radix Paeoniae Rubra	14.1	K
wŭ líng zhī (五灵脂), Faeces Trogopterori	14.1	K
yán hú suŏ (延胡索), Rhizoma Corydalis	7.0	K
chuān xiōng (川芎), Rhizoma Ligustici Chuanxiong	7.0	K
mò yào (没药), Myrrha	7.0	K
ròu guì (肉桂), Cortex Cinnamomi	7.0	E
gān jiāng (干姜), Rhizoma Zingiberis	1.4	E
xiăo huí xiāng (小茴香), Fructus Foeniculi	0.2	E

Ingredients: (from Herbal Times *"Shao Fu Zhu Yu Wan"*)

chì sháo (赤芍), Radix Paeoniae Rubra	13. %	K
dāng guī (当归), Radix Angelicae Sinensis	13	AB
pú huáng (蒲黄), Pollen Typhae	13	J
yán hú suŏ (延胡索), Rhizoma Corydalis	13	K
chuān xiōng (川芎), Rhizoma Ligustici Chuanxiong	8	K
gān jiāng (干姜), Rhizoma Zingiberis	8	E
hóng huā (红花), Flos Carthami	8	K
mò yào (没药), Myrrha	8	K
ròu guì (肉桂), Cortex Cinnamomi	8	E
xiăo huí xiāng (小茴香), Fructus Foeniculi	8	E

Invigorates blood, breaks blood stasis, dissipates masses, warms the uterus, relieves pain. Use for blood stagnation due to accumulation of cold causing menstrual cramps, postpartum cramping, uterine fibroids or ovarian cysts. Also for uterine blood stagnation causing amenorrhea, irregular menses or infertility. Appropriate for small uterine fibroids (>5cm). Can also be used for hepatomegaly, splenomegaly, and scrotal swelling due to blood stasis and cold.

Pulse: Choppy, slippery or wiry
Tongue: Normal or dark

Comments: In the early 19th century, Wang Qing-Ren developed numerous formulas to address blood stasis, including *Ge Xia Zhu Yu Tang* (Chapter 7A), *Shen Tong Zhu Yu Tang* (Chapter 4B), *Xue Fu Zhu Yu* Tang (Chapter 10) and *Tong Qiao Huo Xue Tang* (Chapter 10).

Shao Fu Zhu Yu Tang is Wang's formula for dysmenorrhea with pain, clots, and heavy bleeding due to cold in the uterus, and is also used for uterine masses. The uterus becomes cold because of exposure to cold and damp during the menstrual period or following childbirth. In some cases, cold is due to an underlying deficiency of kidney *yang*. *Ròu guì*, *xiǎo huí xiāng* and *gān jiāng* warm the uterus, while the remainder of the formula consists of strong blood invigorators (*pú huáng*, *chì sháo*, *wǔ líng zhī*, *yán hú suǒ*, *chuān xiōng*, and *mò yào*).

The original formula combines *wǔ líng zhī* with *pú huáng,* which dissolves clots without aggravating heavy bleeding. Herbal Times substitutes *hóng huā* for *wǔ líng zhī,* and in the Plum Flower version, *rǔ xiāng* (乳香, Olibanum/Boswelliae) is substituted. Both Herbal Times and Plum Flower increase the amount of *xiǎo huí xiāng* to enhance warming of the uterus.

The formula can also be used for hepatomegaly, splenomegaly, and scrotal swelling due to blood stasis and cold.

Caution: All of these formulas contain herbs that are prohibited during pregnancy, and with patients taking blood thinners such as Coumadin. Discontinue during the period once cramping and the discharge of clots is complete, to avoid excessing bleeding.

Further Reading:

Bensky et al, p. 567
Chen & Chen, p. 889
Ellis, p. 257

TAO HONG SI WU TANG

Formula: *táo hóng sì wù tāng* (桃红四物汤)
"Persica, Carthamus Four Substance Decoction"
Author: Wú Qiān (吴谦)
Source: *Yī Zōng Jīn Jiàn* (医宗金鉴), 1742
Literal: "Medical Tradition Golden Mirror"
Also attributed to:
Author: Wáng Hào-Gû (王好古)
Source: *Yī Lêi Yuán Róng* (医垒元戎), 1291
Literal: "Medical Ramparts Supreme Commanders"

Availability:

Augmented Four Substances (K)
Tangkuei Four, Persica, & Carthamus Combination (EG)
Tao Hong Si Wu Tang (BP, TZ)
Tao Hong Si Wu Tang Teapills (PF)
Tao Hong Si Wu Tang Wan (TL)
*Invigorate Blood & Stem Flow (TT)
* Jade Moon Flow (JW)
* Jade Moon Phase 1 (JW)

Ingredients: (from the standardized *"Tangkuei Four, Persica, & Carthamus Combination"* and from Plum Flower "*Tao Hong Si Wu Teapills*")

dāng guī (当归), Radix Angelicae Sinensis	20. %	AB
táo rén (桃仁), Semen Persicae	20	K
bái sháo (白芍), Radix Paeoniae Alba	20	AB
shú dì huáng (熟地黄), Radix Rehmanniae Praep.	20	AB
hóng huā (红花), Flos Carthami	10	K
chuān xiōng (川芎), Rhizoma Ligustici Chuanxiong	10	K

Tonifies blood, invigorates blood in the liver and uterus, regulates menses. Use for blood stagnation with blood deficiency, causing menstrual cramps with dark blood or clots. Also applicable for shortened periods with heavy bleeding, amenorrhea, irregular menses or infertility due to blood deficiency with blood stasis. Can be used for hepatomegaly and splenomegaly with anemia.

Pulse: Thin, choppy or wiry
Tongue: Pale or dark

Comments: *Tao Hong Si Wu Tang* is an enhancement of the 9th century blood-building prescription *Si Wu Tang* (Chapter 16B), adding two blood-moving and stasis-breaking herbs, *táo rén* and *hóng huā.* It is appropriate for mild cramping accompanying blood deficiency during the period. Experienced Chinese doctors prefer this formula to *Si Wu Tang* for blood tonification, anticipating blood stagnation as a common gynecological presentation.

Caution, Both *táo rén* and *hóng huā* are contraindicated in the second and third trimesters of pregnancy, and for patients taking Coumadin. Use of this formula during pregnancy should be supervised by qualified practitioners. Also, discontinue once cramps cease so as not to aggravate menstrual bleeding.

Further Reading:

Bensky et al, p. 337
Chen & Chen, p. 571
Ellis, p. 303

Modern Formulas:

TONG JING WAN

Formula: *tòng jīng wán* (痛经丸), "Painful Menstruation Pills"
Source: Modern patent medicine

Availability:

Calm In The Sea of Life Teapills (PF)
Tojing Wan (PM)
Tong Jing Wan (HT, PM, TL)
* Cramp Bark Plus (HC)

Ingredients: (from China National Chemicals; Hangzhou *"To Jing Wan"*)

é zhú (莪术), Rhizoma Curcumae	20. %	K
sān léng (三棱), Rhizoma Sparganii	20	K
chì sháo (赤芍), Radix Paeoniae Rubra	20	K
dāng guī (当归), Radix Angelicae Sinensis	10	AB
chuān xiōng (川芎), Rhizoma Ligustici Chuanxiong	10	K
dān shen (丹参), Radix/Rhiz. Salviae Miltiorrhizae	10	K
hóng huā (红花), Flos Carthami	10	K

Ingredients: (from Kingsway *"Menstrual Support/Tong Jing Wan"*)

táo rén (桃仁), Semen Persicae	17.3 %	K
dāng guī (当归), Radix Angelicae Sinensis	17.3	AB
hóng huā (红花), Flos Carthami	17.3	K
huái niú xī (怀牛膝), Radix Achyranthis Bidentatae	17.3	K
mŭ dān pí (牡丹皮), Cortex Moutan	17.3	DC
chuān xiōng (川芎), Rhizoma Ligustici Chuanxiong	8.1	K
é zhú (莪术), Rhizoma Curcumae	3.5	K
sān léng (三棱), Rhizoma Sparganii	1.7	K

Ingredients: (from Plum Flower *"Calm in the Sea of Life"*)

táo rén (桃仁), Semen Persicae	12.7 %	K
bái sháo (白芍), Radix Paeoniae Alba	12.7	AB
dān shen (丹参), Radix/Rhiz. Salviae Miltiorrhizae	10.6	K
pú huáng (蒲黄), Pollen Typhae	10.6	J
wū yào (乌药), Radix Linderae	10.6	G
yán hú suǒ (延胡索), Rhizoma Corydalis	10.6	K
dāng guī (当归), Radix Angelicae Sinensis	8.5	AB
xiāng fù (香附), Rhizoma Cyperi	8.4	G
hóng huā (红花), Flos Carthami	6.3	K
tián qī (田七), Radix/Rhizoma Notoginseng	5.3	J
chuān xiōng (川芎), Rhizoma Ligustici Chuanxiong	3.7	K

Ingredients: (from Herbal Times *"Tong Jing Wan"*)

yì mǔ cǎo (益母草), Herba Leonuri	25.7 %	K
shú dì huáng (熟地黄), Radix Rehmanniae Praep.	10.3	AB
dān shen (丹参), Radix/Rhiz. Salviae Miltiorrhizae	7.7	K
dāng guī (当归), Radix Angelicae Sinensis	7.7	AB
shān zhā (山楂), Fructus Crataegi	7.7	H
xiāng fù (香附), Rhizoma Cyperi	7.7	G
bái sháo (白芍), Radix Paeoniae Alba	5.1	AB
mù xiāng (木香), Radix Aucklandiae	5.1	G
tù sī zǐ (菟丝子), Semen Cuscutae	5.1	AC
yán hú suǒ (延胡索), Rhizoma Corydalis	5.1	K
chuān xiōng (川芎), Rhizoma Ligustici Chuanxiong	3.8	K
chōng wèi zǐ (茺蔚子), Fructus Leonuri	2.6	K
hóng huā (红花), Flos Carthami	2.6	K
páo jiāng (炮姜), Rhizoma Zingiberis Praeparatum	1.3	E
qīng pí (青皮), Pericarpium Citri Reticulatae Viride	1.3	G
ròu guì (肉桂), Cortex Cinnamomi	1.3	E

Invigorates blood, breaks blood stasis, regulates menses, relieves pain. Use for blood stagnation causing menstrual cramps with accompanying signs of amenorrhea, irregular menses or infertility. Symptoms include abdominal pain preceding and during menses, as well as the discharge of blood clots. May also be used for hepatomegaly and splenomegaly associated with trauma, cirrhosis, hepatitis or AIDS.

Pulse: Wiry, choppy
Tongue: Dark or with dark spots

Comments: The *Tong Jing Wan* formulas are effective for menstrual cramping with or without clots. There are many versions of formulas using this name. The original is the patent medicine from Hangzhou, while Plum Flower, Herbal Times, Tanglong and others have made their own formulas.

The ability of the formula to stop menstrual pain can be gauged by how many herbs are included that break blood stasis (Category K), especially *é zhú, sān léng, hóng huā* or *táo rén.* The original Hangzhou formula is the strongest, containing 90% K herbs, while the Kingsway version ("Menstrual Support"), which is packaged almost identically, only contains 48% break-stasis herbs.

The other formulas that are listed move blood and break stasis, but also address underlying conditions that lead to dysmenorrhea. For the Plum Flower version, 60% of the formula moves blood and breaks stasis, while 21% builds blood and 19% moves liver *qi*. For the Herbal Times and Tanglong versions, 47.5% moves blood and break stasis, while 23% tonifies blood and 14% moves liver *qi*. These formulas should be considered equally effective.

Caution: All of these formulas contain herbs that are prohibited during pregnancy, and for patients taking blood thinners such as Coumadin. Discontinue during the period once cramping and the discharge of clots is complete, to avoid excessing bleeding.

OTHER FORMULAS APPLICABLE TO THIS CATEGORY:

Classical Formulas:

Ge Xia Zhu Yu Tang

See Chapter 7A

Tian Tai Wu Yao San

See Chapter 7A

Modern Formulas:

Ji Sheng Ju He Wan

Ji Sheng Ju He Wan (MS, PM, TL)

Yan Hu Suo Zhi Tong Wan

See Chapter 5C

Other:

Blood Palace Formula (GF)
Butiao Tablets (PM)
Chong Release Formula (GF)
Mense-Ease (EV)
Moon Pearls (CP)
Stasis-Transforming Formula (GF)
Upbear Yang & Lift The Menses (BP)
Women's Rhythm (K)

Uterine Fibroid

Resolve-Lower (EV)
Sparganium 12 (SF)
Stasis-Transforming Formula (GF)

Ovarian Cysts

Cinnamon/Rehmannia (SF)
Phlegm-Transforming Formula (GF)
Stasis-Transforming Formula (GF)

Endometriosis

Jade Moon Cool (JW)
Resolve-EM (EV)
Stasis-Transforming Formula (GF)
Turtle Shell Tablets (SF)
Unlocking Formula (HC)

8. GYNECOLOGICAL DISORDERS

8D. VAGINAL DISCHARGE (LEUKORRHEA)

Classical Formulas:

Qian Jin Zhi Dai Wan (Chien Chin Chih Tai Wan) *qiān jīn zhǐ dài wán* (千金止带丸)

Modern Formulas:

Yu Dai Wan *yù dài wán* (瘉带丸)

Vaginal discharge, also known as leukorrhea, is marked by an increased volume of discharged liquid with changes in color, texture or odor. It can be due to exogenous pathogenic microbes such as Candida albicans or Trichomonas, or to endogenous causes, including an underlying deficiency of spleen *qi* complicated by liver stagnation, descent of damp-heat to the lower *jiao,* deficiency of the kidneys or blood stagnation.

Vaginal discharge can occur in numerous medical conditions, including chronic vaginitis, cervicitis, salpingitis (inflammation of the fallopian tube), or oophoritis (inflammation of the ovary). Other symptoms include vaginal irritation, slightly bloody discharge, localized pain, pain during intercourse, or symptoms aggravated during ovulation or menstruation.

Yellow discharge indicates heat and tends to have a thick creamy texture with a bad odor and itching. This is due to damp-heat descending into the lower jiao, or due to exogenous pathogenic factors. Chronic cases may indicate underlying candidiasis in the intestines. The two formulas in this chapter address this presentation.

Vaginal discharge due to deficiency of spleen or kidney has a clear or watery discharge without itching or odor. When complicated by cold, the discharge has a thicker whitish color, again without odor. Appropriate formulas include *Wen Jing Tang* (Chapter 8A).

Discharge with blood or pus may be due to chronic infection. In prolonged cases it may indicate cancer of the cervix, ovary, or uterus, and a gynecological medical evaluation is recommended.

Classical Formulas:

QIAN JIN ZHI DAI WAN
CHIEN CHIN CHIH TAI WAN

Formula: *qiān jīn zhǐ dài wán* (千金止带丸)
"Thousand Gold (Pieces), Stop Vaginal-Discharge Pill"
Author: Wǔ Zhī-Wàng (武之望)
Source: *Jì Yīn Gāng Mù* (济阴纲目), 1620
Literal: "Helping *Yin* (Women), Guiding Outline"

Availability:

Chien Chin Chih Tai Wan (PM)
Qian Jin Zhi Dai Wan (PIM, PM)

Ingredients: (From Great Wall Brand, Tianjin Lerongjin Pharmaceutical Factory, *"Chien Chin Chih Tai Wan"*)

xiāng fù (香附), Rhizoma Cyperi	15.4 %	G
chūn pí (椿皮), Cortex Ailanthi	15.4	L
jī guān huā (鸡冠花), Flos Celosiae Cristatae	15.4	DC
chuān xiōng (川芎), Rhizoma Ligustici Chuanxiong	7.7	K
dāng guī (当归), Radix Angelicae Sinensis	7.7	AB
bái sháo (白芍), Radix Paeoniae Alba	3.8	AB
shā rén (砂仁), Fructus Amomi	3.8	FB
xiǎo huí xiāng (小茴香), Fructus Foeniculi	3.8	E
bái zhú (白术), Rhizoma Atractylodis Macrocephalae	3.8	AA
dǎng shēn (党参), Radix Codonopsis	3.8	AA
bǔ gǔ zhī (补骨脂), Fructus Psoraleae	3.8	AC
xù duàn (续断), Radix Dipsaci	3.8	AC
yán hú suǒ (延胡索), Rhizoma Corydalis	3.8	K
dù zhòng (杜仲), Cortex Eucommiae	3.8	AC
mǔ lì (牡蛎), Concha Ostreae	3.8	N

Ingredients: (from Pine Mountain *"Qian Jin Zhi Dai Wan"*)

qīng dài (青黛), Indigo Naturalis	12. %	DD
hǎi piāo xiāo (海螵蛸), Endoconcha Sepiae	12	L
chūn pí (椿皮), Cortex Ailanthi	10	L
dǎng shēn (党参), Radix Codonopsis	10	AA
bái zhú (白术), Rhizoma Atractylodis Macrocephalae	10	AA
shān yào (山药), Rhizoma Dioscoreae	10	AA
xù duàn (续断), Radix Dipsaci	8	AC
mù xiāng (木香), Radix Aucklandiae	8	G
dāng guī (当归), Radix Angelicae Sinensis	8	AB
xiǎo huí xiāng (小茴香), Fructus Foeniculi	6	E
huáng bǎi (黄柏), Cortex Phellodendri	6	DB

Clears heat, resolves toxins, tonifies spleen qi, boosts yang, eliminates damp, relieves vaginal discharge, relieves itching. Use for vaginal discharge due to heat toxins with underlying deficiency of *qi* and *yang*. Symptoms include a watery or creamy vaginal discharge with or without itching. Clinical applications include chronic vaginitis, cervicitis, salpingitis (inflammation of the fallopian tube), or oophoritis (inflammation of the ovary) with symptoms of vaginal irritation, localized pain and pain during intercourse.

Pulses: Soft, wide, slippery, possibly rapid
Tongue: Normal, or wet with a yellow or white coat

Comments: This formula treats leukorrhea and vaginal discharge due to the presence of Trichomonas or Candida, with an underlying deficiency of *qi*, blood and *yang*. It can also be used for infections in the ovaries or uterus, including PID (pelvic inflammatory disease). It is preferred for more chronic presentations.

The Great Wall version is a popular patent medicine, with 45% of the formula consisting of *xiāng fù, chūn pí* and *jī guān huā. Xiāng fù* directs the formula along the liver channel into the vagina. *Chūn pí* and *jī guān huā,* two uncommonly used herbs, are effective for treating leukorrhea due to Trichomonas or Candida. Additional herbs tonify *qi*, blood and *yang*. It is a large formula, containing 15 herbs.

The Pine Mountain version, a smaller formula containing 11 herbs, substitutes *qīng dài* for *jī guān huā,* and also adds in 12% *hǎi piāo xiāo* (cuttlefish bone) to astringe dampness. It also boosts herbs that tonify *wei qi* to 30% of the formula, using *dǎng shen, bái zhú* and *shān yào*. It does not include *xiāng fù*.

Modern Formulas:

YU DAI WAN

Formula: *yù dài wán* (瘉带丸), "Heal Vaginal-Discharge Pill"
Source: Modern patent medicine

Availability:

Yu Dai Teapills (PF)
Yu Dai Wan (HT, MS, PM)

Ingredients: (from Herbal Times *"Yu Dai Wan"*)

chūn pí (椿皮), Cortex Ailanthi	47.0 %	L
bái sháo (白芍), Radix Paeoniae Alba	15.5	AB
shú dì huáng (熟地黄), Radix Rehmanniae Praep.	12.5	AB
dāng guī (当归), Radix Angelicae Sinensis	9.0	AB
gāo liáng jiāng (高良姜), Rhizoma Alpiniae Offic.	6.5	E
huáng bǎi (黄柏), Cortex Phellodendri	6.5	DB
chuān xiōng (川芎), Rhizoma Ligustici Chuanxiong	3.0	K

Clears heat, resolves toxins, eliminates damp, relieves vaginal discharge, relieves itching, nourishes blood. Use for vaginal discharge due to heat toxins. Symptoms include a creamy or thick yellow discharge, accompanied by itching, burning urination, or blood in the urine. Clinical applications include chronic vaginitis, cervicitis, salpingitis (inflammation of the fallopian tube), or oophoritis (inflammation of the ovary) with symptoms of vaginal irritation, localized pain and pain during intercourse.

Pulses: Soft, wide, slippery, possibly rapid
Tongue: Normal, or wet with a yellow or white coat

Comments: This is an effective formula for leukorrhea and vaginal discharge due to pathogenic heat toxins such as Trichomonas or Candida albicans, and can also be used for ovarian or uterine infection, including PID. It is preferred for acute presentations.

The Herbal Times, Minshan and Plum Flower versions are virtually identical, and contain 7 herbs. Here 47% of the formula is *chūn pí,* the main ingredient to stop discharge and attack pathogenic microbes. *Huáng bǎi* reinforces the effecting of clearing damp-heat, and *gāo liáng jiāng* mitigates the coldness of *chūn pí* and *huáng bǎi*. The rest of the formula consists of the blood-tonifying *Si Wu Tang* (see Chapter 16B), which makes up 40% of the formula.

OTHER FORMULAS APPROPRIATE FOR THIS CATEGORY:

Classical Formulas:

Bi Xie Fen Qing Yin
See Chapter 11A

Bi Xie Sheng Shi Wan
See Chapter 11B

Jie Jie Wan –1 (Kai Kit Pill)
See Chapter 11A

Long Dan Xie Gan Tang
See Chapter 7C

Wen Jing Tang
See Chapter 8A

Modern Formulas:

Butiao Tablets (PM)
Clearing (HC)
Clear the Lower Palace (K)
Immortal Valley Formula (GF)
Isatis Cooling (HC)
Ocean Pearls (CP)
Vagistatin (HC)
V-Statin (EV)
Yin Valley Formula (GF)

8E. MENOPAUSAL DISORDER AND DEFICIENCY FIRE

Classical Formulas:

Da Bu Yin Wan	*dà bǔ yīn wán* (大补阴丸)
Qing Gu San	*qīng gǔ sǎn* (清骨散)
Zhi Bai Di Huang Wan	*zhī bǎi dì huáng wán* (知柏地黄丸)

Modern Formulas:

Er Xian Tang	*èr xiān tāng* (二仙汤)
Geng Nian An Wan	*gēng nián ān wán* (更年安丸)

MENOPAUSAL DISORDER is marked by periodic hot flashes with flushed complexion and perspiration. Other symptoms may include dizziness, blurred vision, tinnitus, palpitations, insomnia, emotional sensitivity or irritability. It can also involve menstrual disturbances (irregularity, cramping, excessive bleeding), occasional edema of the face and lower limbs, loss of appetite, loose stools, depression or pronounced anxiety. In many ways, the symptoms can resemble those associated with premenstrual syndrome.

In Chinese medicine, the root cause is deficiency of kidney *yin*, *yang*, or *qi* (deficiency of both kidney *yin* and *yang*), although the liver, heart, and spleen can also be involved. In all of these cases, aspects of kidney *qi* have become depleted, affecting production and distribution of *qi* and blood. This may be aggravated by a history of weak constitution, exhaustion from childbirth, excessive menstrual bleeding, or long-standing deficiencies of the heart or spleen.

Deficiency of kidney *yin* is the most common pattern, with symptoms of heat, dryness and hot flashing being most noticeable. When kidney *yin* is exhausted, heart fire can blaze out of control. In extreme cases of *yin* deficiency, sweating may occur, especially at nighttime. Stagnation of liver *qi* also follows, allowing liver fire to flame upwards, or to overact on spleen *qi*, causing premenstrual-like symptoms of irritability and anxiety. Estrogen is the most *yin* substance in the body, and its levels are reduced during menopause, leading to *yin-deficiency* signs of heat and dryness.

Formulas listed in this chapter can be of significant benefit, especially in mild and moderate presentations. In severe cases unresponsive to Chinese herbs, bio-identical hormone replacement is recommended, at least for the duration of menopausal symptoms. When symptoms include those due to stagnation of liver *qi*, you can combine with formulas from *7A. Liver Stagnation* or *Chapter 8B. Pre-menstrual Tension.*

DEFICIENCY FIRE SYNDROMES have symptoms that overlap those found in menopausal disorders, and the formulas can be interchanged in both conditions. Deficiency-fire syndromes manifest during chronic fevers, excessive exposure to heat and dryness, or loss of blood, and are found in tuberculosis, AIDS, dengue fever and malaria, as well as acute hyperthyroidism. Fire presentation due to *yin* or blood deficiency produces symptoms of systemic internal heat, heat along the *yin* channels, and heat in the palms, soles and sternum ("the five hearts"). There can be heat-flashes with day or night sweating. Night sweats in particular are considered a serious sign of exhaustion of *yin,* and may be accompanied by spermatorrhea in men - involuntary loss of semen with or without an erection, as well as "wet dream".

Deficiency fire should be distinguished from excess heat or fire. In deficiency fire, the red tongue is a little more dull or glossy, versus the bright red tongue of excess heat. The tongue in deficiency fire is often geographic with sores or patches. The pulse, while rapid, is weaker or thinner.

Classical Formulas:

DA BU YIN WAN

Formula: *dà bŭ yīn wán* (大补阴丸), "Great Tonify *Yin* Pill"
Author: Zhū Zhèn-Hēng (朱震亨) *aka* Zhū Dān-Xī (朱丹溪)
Source: *Dān Xī Xīn Fă* (丹溪心法), 1481
Literal: "Dan-Xi's Heart Method (eg, Personal Insights)"

Availability:

Abundant Yin Teapills (PF)
Da Bu Yin Wan (BP, HT, MS, PM)
Great Yin (HC)
Rehmannia & Testudinis Combination (EG)

Ingredients: (from the standardized *"Rehmannia & Testudinis Combination"*)

shú dì huáng (熟地黄), Radix Rehmanniae Praep.	30. %	AB
guī băn (龟板), Plastrum Testudinis/Chinemys	30	AD
huáng băi (黄柏), Cortex Phellodendri	20	DB
zhī mŭ (知母), Rhizoma Anemarrhenae	20	DA

Ingredients: (from Herbal Times *"Da Bu Yin Wan"*)

guī băn (龟板), Plastrum Testudinis/Chinemys	20. %	AD
huáng băi (黄柏), Cortex Phellodendri	20	DB
zhī mŭ (知母), Rhizoma Anemarrhenae	20	DA
shēng dì huáng (生地黄), Radix Rehmanniae	20	DC
zhū suĭ (猪髓), Medulla Porci	20	

Nourishes kidney yin, clears heat, subdues deficiency fire, stops sweating. Use for *yin* deficiency fire flaming upwards, causing hot flashes, day or night sweating, feverish palms and soles, palpitations, insomnia, and anxiety. Can also be used for low-grade tidal fevers, spermatorrhea (nocturnal ejaculation), and weak lower back. Also for deficiency-heat bleeding, including bleeding from nose, lung, stomach, rectum, vagina and urethra. Used in menopausal disorder, hyperthyroidism, tuberculosis, malaria and AIDS.

Pulse: Thin, rapid
Tongue: Glossy red, no coat or geographic coat

Comments: This is an effective formula for deficiency *yin* fire conditions with sweating, and is often used for menopausal hot flashing. *Guī bǎn* uses turtle bones from the plastron, the more *yin* underside (as opposed to the carapace bones on the back). They astringe *jing* and *yin*, and stop sweating due to *yin* deficiency. These turtles are bred in captivity for food and medicine, and not taken from the wild. *Huáng bǎi* clears heat in the lower burner, while *shēng dì huáng* and *zhī mǔ* cool while promoting *yin*.

The Herbal Times version adds 20% *zhū suǐ*, the marrow of pig bone, which helps replenish *yin* and draw it back into the interior. It also counters "bone steaming", characterized by deep internal heat with day or night sweating. This addition was mentioned in original source books on preparation.

Versions from Minshan and Plum Flower follow the same formula as the standardized Taiwan extract granules.

Caution: *Guī bǎn* is contraindicated during pregnancy.

Further Reading:

Bensky et al, p. 372
Chen & Chen, p. 649
Ellis, p. 56

QING GU WAN

Formula: *qīng gŭ săn* (清骨散), "Clear Bones Powder"
Author: Wáng Kĕn-Tāng (王肯堂)
Source: *Zhèng Zhì Zhŭn Shéng* (证治准绳), 1602
Literal: "Pattern Treatment Standards"

Availability:

Cool Bones Teapills (PF)

Ingredients: (from Plum Flower *"Cool Bone Teapills"*)

yín chái hú (银柴胡), Radix Stellariae	18.4 %	DE
zhī mŭ (知母), Rhizoma Anemarrhenae	12.6	DA
hú huáng lián (胡黄连), Rhizoma Picrorhizae	12.6	DB
dì gŭ pí (地骨皮), Cortex Lycii	12.5	DE
qīng hāo (青蒿), Herba Artemisiae Annuae	12.5	DE
qín jiāo (秦艽), Radix Gentianae Macrophyllae	12.5	FA
biē jiă (鳖甲), Carapax Trionycis/Amydae	12.5	AD
gān căo (甘草), Radix Glycyrrhizae	6.4	AA

Clears deficiency heat, nourishes yin, stops sweating. Use for deficiency of *yin* with heat causing "steaming bone disorder". Symptoms include afternoon tidal fever or chronic low-grade fever, heat in the palms and soles, irritability and restlessness, lethargy, palpitations, insomnia, and night sweating. Useful in chronic tuberculosis, AIDS, chronic hepatitis, malaria, hyperthyroid, and certain stages of menopausal disorder.

Pulse: Thin, rapid
Tongue: Glossy red, no coat or geographic coat

Comments: This formula is useful for menopausal heat and flushing. It's original application was for "steaming bone disorder", a prolonged fever with bone pain associated with tuberculosis. In this regard, it is being used for fevers due to advanced AIDS and chronic hepatitis, fevers of unknown origin, and tidal fevers found in malaria. In "steaming bone disorder", the patient feels heat or burning deep in the body, although the flesh seems cool or normal to the touch.

In this formula, the *yin* is nourished, astringed and cooled with *yín chái hú, zhī mǔ, dì gǔ pí, qīng hāo* and *biē jiǎ*. The herb *hú huáng lián* clears heat. In cases accompanied by night sweating, combine with astringent formulas such as *Da Bu Yin Wan* (above).

Note: *Biē jiǎ* are bones from the carapace (dorsal aspect) of the Chinese soft shell turtle, Amyda sinensis. It is bred in captivity for food and medicine.

Caution: *Biē jiǎ* is contraindicated during pregnancy.

Further Reading:

Bensky et al, p. 214

ZHI BAI DI HUANG WAN

Formula: *zhī bǎi dì huáng wán* (知柏地黄丸)
"Anemarrhena, Phellodendron Rehmannia Pill"
Author: Wú Qiān (吴谦)
Source: *Yī Zōng Jīn Jiàn* (医宗金鉴), 1742
Literal: "Medical Tradition Golden Mirror"
also attributed to:
Author: Wú Kūn (吴昆)
Source: *Yī Fāng Kǎo* (医方考), 1584
Literal: "Medical Formulas Investigations"

Availability:

Anemarrhena, Phellodendron & Rehmannia Formula (EG)
Anem-Phello & Rehmannia (CC)
Eight Flavor Rehmannia Teapills (PF)
Menopause/Kidney Yin (JD)
Nourish (EV)
Temper Fire (K)
Zhi Bai Di Huang Wan (BP, HT, MS, PIM, PM, TL, TZ)
* Rehmannia And Scrophularia Formula (GF)
* Water Passages (TT)

Ingredients: (from the standardized *"Anemarrhena, Phellodendron & Rehmannia Formula"*)

shú dì huáng (熟地黄), Radix Rehmanniae Praep.	27.7 %	AB
shān zhū yú (山茱萸), Fructus Corni	13.8	L
shān yào (山药), Rhizoma Dioscoreae	13.8	AA
mǔ dān pí (牡丹皮), Cortex Mouta	10.3	DC
zé xiè (泽泻), Rhizoma Alismatis	10.3	FC
fú líng (茯苓), Poria	10.3	FC
zhī mǔ (知母), Rhizoma Anemarrhenae	6.9	DA
huáng bǎi (黄柏), Cortex Phellodendri	6.9	DB

Nourishes kidney yin, clears heat, subdues deficiency fire flourishing upwards. Use for *yin* deficiency fire flourishing upwards causing low grade tidal fever, feverish palms and soles, dry mouth, hot flashes, palpitations, insomnia and anxiety. Applicable for deficiency heat associated with menopausal disorder, hypertension, hyperthyroid and rheumatoid arthritis. It is also used for urinary difficulty and back pain due to kidney deficiency.

Pulse: Thin, rapid, may be flooding in the proximal position
Tongue: Glossy red, no coat or geographic coat

Comments: This formula is a variation of *Liu Wei Di Huang Wan* (Chapter 17A), the foundation formula for kidney *yin* deficiency. It has been modified by adding *zhī mŭ* and *huáng băi* to address deficiency *yin* fire flourishing upwards. Chronic kidney *yin* deficiencies easily turn to heat or fire, and the herbal additions cool deficiency heat while the foundation formula boosts *yin*.

The formula is frequently used for menopausal disorder, prolonged deficiency fever, or following episodes of involuntary night ejaculation (wet dream). If extreme sweating or night-sweats are involved, consider combining with *Da Bu Yin Wan* (above).

Further Reading:

Bensky et al, p. 369
Chen & Chen, p. 636
Ellis, p. 407

Modern Formulas:

ER XIAN TANG

Formula: *èr xiān tāng* (二仙汤), "Two Immortals Decoction"
Author: Zhāng Bó-Nè (张伯讷)
Source: *Zhōng Yī Fāng Jì Lín Chuáng Shǒu Cè* (中医方剂临床手册), 1950s
Literal: "Chinese Medicine Formulas Dosing Clinical Manual"

Availability:

Curculigo & Epimedium Combination (EG)
Er Xian Tang (BP, TZ)
Er Xian Wan (HT, TL)
Two Immortals (K)
Two Immortals Teapills (PF)
Two-Immortals Formula (CC)
* Dr. Shen's Two Immortals (DS)
* Supplement Yin (BP)
* Two Immortals Formula (GF)

Ingredients: (from Herbal Times *"Er Xian Wan"*)

xiān máo (仙茅), Rhizoma Curculiginis	23. %	AC
yín yáng huò (淫羊藿), Herba Epimedii	23	AC
bā jǐ tiān (巴戟天), Radix Morindae Officinalis	14	AC
dāng guī (当归), Radix Angelicae Sinensis	14	AB
huáng bǎi (黄柏), Cortex Phellodendri	13	DB
zhī mǔ (知母), Rhizoma Anemarrhenae	13	DA

Warms kidney yang, tonifies jing, clears kidney fire, tonifies blood. Use for kidney deficiency leading to high blood pressure with signs of heat . Also useful during menopause with symptoms of hot flashing, facial flushing, headache, anxiety, irritability, fatigue, insomnia or palpitation. May be useful in pituitary dysfunction causing polycystic ovarian disorder, and in hyperthyroid,

Pulse: Thin, deep, may be wiry or rapid
Tongue: Normal, or red

Comments: This modern formula was developed by Dr. Zhang Bo-Ne, Shanghai College of TCM, to address episodes of hypertension during menopause. This is seen as kidney *yang* deficiency but with excessive signs of heat. Most menopausal formulas nourish kidney *yin;* this formula takes a unique approach by tonifying kidney *yang* (*xiān máo, yín yáng huò* and *bā jǐ tiān*) while clearing kidney fire (*huáng bǎi* and *zhī mǔ*).

Kidney *yang* corresponds to adrenal cortisol, whose deficiency can affect hormone production, particularly cortisol, receptivity to ACTH, or overproduction of testosterone. It is useful during the early stage of perimenopause to nourish the kidney so as to prevent more severe menopausal symptoms. The formula is also being used clinically to regulate the pituitary in polycystic ovarian disorder, in glomerulonephritis, and in hyperthyroid.

Further Reading:

Bensky et al, p. 410
Chen & Chen, p. 684
Ellis, p. 90

GENG NIAN AN WAN

Formula: *gēng nián ān wán* (更年安丸), "Menopause Peaceful Pills"
Source: Modern patent medicine

Availability:

Geng Nian An - Menopause Comfort Pills (TZ)
Geng Nian An Wan (HT, PM)
Geng Nian An Wan - Menopause Comfort Pill (TL)

Ingredients: (from TCM Zone *"Geng Nian An - Menopause Comfort"*)

zhēn zhū mǔ (珍珠母), Concha Margaritiferae Usta	15.6 %	N
cí shí (磁石), Magnetitum	15.6	N
yè jiāo téng (夜交藤), Caulis Polygoni Multiflori	7.8	N
fú xiǎo mài (浮小麦), Fructus Tritici Levis	7.8	L
shēng dì huáng (生地黄), Radix Rehmanniae	5.2	DC
hé shǒu wū (何首乌), Radix Polygoni Multiflori	5.2	AB
mài mén dōng (麦门冬), Radix Ophiopogonis	5.2	AD
zé xiè (泽泻), Rhizoma Alismatis	5.2	FC
xuán shēn (玄参), Radix Scrophulariae	5.2	DC
shú dì huáng (熟地黄), Radix Rehmanniae Praep.	5.2	AB
xiān máo (仙茅), Rhizoma Curculiginis	5.2	AC
gōu téng (钩藤), Ramulus Uncariae cum Uncis	5.2	O
fú líng (茯苓), Poria	5.2	FC
wǔ wèi zǐ (五味子), Fructus Schisandrae	3.2	L
mǔ dān pí (牡丹皮), Cortex Moutan	3.2	DC

Ingredients: (from Herbal Times *"Geng Nian An Wan"*)

fú líng (茯苓), Poria	9.2 %	FC
fú xiǎo mài (浮小麦), Fructus Tritici Levis	9.2	L
shān yào (山药), Rhizoma Dioscoreae	9.2	AA
hé shǒu wū (何首乌), Radix Polygoni Multiflori	9.2	N
yè jiāo téng (夜交藤), Caulis Polygoni Multiflori	9.2	N
xiān máo (仙茅), Rhizoma Curculiginis	9.2	AC
zhēn zhū mǔ (珍珠母), Concha Margaritiferae Usta	9.2	N
shēng dì huáng (生地黄), Radix Rehmanniae	4.6	DC
shú dì huáng (熟地黄), Radix Rehmanniae Praep.	4.6	AB
zhì gān cǎo (炙甘草), Radix Glycyrrhizae Praep.	4.6	AA
shān zhū yú (山茱萸), Fructus Corni	4.6	L

wǔ wèi zǐ (五味子), Fructus Schisandrae	4.6	L
xuán shēn (玄参), Radix Scrophulariae	4.6	DC
zé xiè (泽泻), Rhizoma Alismatis	4.6	FC
mǔ dān pí (牡丹皮), Cortex Mouta	3.1	DC

Ingredients: (from Tanglong *"Geng Nian An Wan - Menopause Comfort"*)

zhēn zhū mǔ (珍珠母), Concha Margaritiferae Usta	19.9 %	N
fú xiǎo mài (浮小麦), Fructus Tritici Levis	19.9	L
fú líng (茯苓), Poria	9.9	FC
wǔ wèi zǐ (五味子), Fructus Schisandrae	9.9	L
hé shǒu wū (何首乌), Radix Polygoni Multiflori	9.9	AB
xuán shēn (玄参), Radix Scrophulariae	6.6	DC
shú dì huáng (熟地黄), Radix Rehmanniae Praep.	6.6	AB
dāng guī (当归), Radix Angelicae Sinensis	6.6	AB
zé xiè (泽泻), Rhizoma Alismatis	6.6	FC
lú huì (芦荟), Aloe	4.0	PA

Tonifies kidney qi, tonifies blood, stops sweating. Use for depletion of *yin* and blood causing day or night sweating. Other symptoms may include heat-flushing, fatigue, poor memory, dizziness, tinnitus, anxiety and restless sleep. Use for menopausal disorder and other cases of deficiency fire where sweating is the predominant symptom, including tuberculosis, AIDS, spermatorrhea and deficiency fever. Can be useful in menopausal hypertension.

Pulse: Rapid, thin
Tongue: Red, thin, glossy, no coat or geographic coat

Comments: There are several variations of *Geng Nian An Wan*, all of which address sweating as the predominant symptom. Towards this end, the combination of *zhēn zhū mǔ* (mother-of-pearl) and *fú xiǎo mài* (wheat berries) astringe sweating. Of the three versions shown here, the Tanglong formula uses 40% of this two-herb combination, the TCM Zone/Honso version has 23% and the Herbal Times version has 18%. The remaining herbs in each formula tonify blood and *yin* and calm *shen*. These formulas are not particularly cooling, and for hot flashing, they can be combined with other formulas, such as *Da Bu Yin Wan* or *Zhi Bai Di Huang Wan* (above).

Caution: *Lú huì*, found in the Tanglong version, is contraindicated during pregnancy. *Fú xiǎo mài*, the wheat berry, is contraindicated for patients with celiac disease or gluten sensitivity.

OTHER PRODUCTS APPROPRIATE TO THIS CATEGORY:

Modern Formulas:

Anemarrhena Tablets (SF)
Balance-Heat (EV)
Change and Enrich (BP)
Female Comfort (K)
Graceful Transition (K)
Guanyin Pearls (CP)
Haliotis 10 (SF)
Nulignan (HC)
Rehmannia Cool Blood Formula (GF)
Restorative Tablets (SF)
Supplement Yin (BP)
Three Immortals (HC)
Ultimate Immortals (BP)
Yin Valley Formula (GF)

9. DISTURBED SHEN
(Insomnia, Anxiety, Palpitation)

Classical formulas:

Bai Zi Yang Xin Tang	*bǎi zǐ yǎng xīn tāng* (柏子养心汤)
Gan Mai Da Zao Tang	*gān mài dà zǎo tāng* (甘麦大枣汤)
Gui Pi Tang	*guī pí tāng* (归脾汤)
Suan Zao Ren Tang	*suān zǎo rén tāng* (酸枣仁汤)
Tian Wang Bu Xin Dan	*tiān wáng bǔ xīn dān* (天王补心丹)

Modern Formulas:

An Mian Pian	*ān mián piàn* (安眠片)
An Mian Wan	*ān mián wán* (安眠丸)
An Shen Bu XIn Wan	*ān shén bǔ xīn wán* (安神补心丸)
An Shui Wan	*ān shuì wán* (安睡丸)
Bu Nao Wan	*bǔ nǎo wán* (补脑丸)
/Jian Nao Wan	*/ jiàn nǎo wán* (健脑丸)

The word *shén* (神) is often translated as "spirit", and disturbed *shen* implies that the spirit is agitated, especially as it affects the mind and emotional stability. Symptoms and disorders include insomnia or restless sleep, anxiety, palpitation, tachycardia and heart arrhythmias, and in some cases manic behavior. Other symptoms include poor concentration, memory or forgetfulness.

Disturbed *shen* disorders are divided between those of deficiency and those of excess. Deficiency syndromes are more common and are of two types: deficiency of both *yin* and blood, and deficiency of both *qi* and *yang*. In deficiency of *yin* and blood, deficiency-heat may lead to redness in the tip of the tongue, or the tongue may be pale. The pulse is thin and may be slightly rapid. The condition is due to over mental activity, exhaustion of *jing*, or deficiency of kidney *yin*. Symptoms include irregular heartbeat, disturbed dream-filled sleep and poor memory. In extreme cases of heart *yin* deficiency, there may be night sweats, "five heart fever" (heat in the palms, soles and sternum) and nocturnal emission.

In deficiency of heart *yang* or *qi*, the tongue can be dark or pale with a white coat, and the pulse is weak, thin or sunken. Dark facial discoloration on the nose and cheeks may also appear, although this is concurrent with heart blood stagnation. Symptoms of *qi* and *yang* deficiency are aggravated by fatigue or excessive mental activity. Palpitations or arrhythmias are not uncommon, triggered by overactivity. Breathing can be labored. These conditions are also addressed with *qi* tonics (*Chapter 16A*) or *yang* tonics (*Chapter 17B*).

Excess disorders are less common, and are due to phlegm-fire or stagnation of *qi* and blood. Phlegm-fire conditions can be due to acute infections affecting the heart, or may have an endogenous etiology such as liver fire. Signs include a very red tongue with a strong, bounding, rapid pulse. If phlegm is present, the tongue has a yellow greasy coat and the pulse is also slippery. Symptoms include insomnia with anxiety, and in severe cases, fever with delirium, or manic behavior. Most of the formulas in this chapter do not address this condition, with the exception of *An Mian Pian*.

Disturbed *shen* due to stagnation of *qi* and blood are addressed with formulas found in *Chapter 10: Heart Blood Stasis*.

These formulas are not sedatives in the pharmaceutical sense. They do not cause drowsiness or impair mental or physical function and can be taken throughout the day. In cases of insomnia, however, it is often beneficial to take one of the doses before bed, and, if necessary, another dose in the middle of the night. Chronic insomnia due to deficiency is stubborn and requires prolonged treatment before noticeable effects are achieved.

The formulas are also useful for sharpening the mind - to improve memory and concentration. This can be done on an ongoing basis, or short term such as preparing for exams.

QUICK REFERENCE:

Disturbed shen due to deficiency of heart yin and blood:

Bai Zi Yang Xin Tang
Gan Mai Da Zao Tang
Tian Wang Bu Xin Dan

Due to deficiency of yang and blood with accumulation of phlegm:

Bu Nao Wan

Due to deficiency of qi and blood:

Gui Pi Tang
Jian Nao Wan

Due to deficiency of qi, blood and yin:

An Mian Wan
An Shui Wan

Due deficiency heat:

Gan Mai Da Zao Tang
Suan Zao Ren Tang

Due to phlegm-fire:

An Mian Pian

Due to ascendant yang:

An Shen Bu Xin Wan

Due to blood stasis:

See formulas in *Chapter 10*

Classical Formulas:

BAI ZI YANG XIN TANG

Formula: *bǎi zǐ yǎng xīn tāng* (柏子养心汤)
"Biota Seed Nourish Heart Decoction"
Author: Péng Yòng-Guāng (彭用光)
Source: *Tǐ Rén Huì Biān* (体仁汇编), 1549
Literal: "Body Benevolent Collection-Compilation"

Availability:

Bai Zi Yang Xin Wan (MS, PM)
Bai Zi Zi Xin Wan (TL)
Heavenly Heart Teapills (PF)

Ingredients: (from Minshan *"Bai Zi Yang Xin Wan"*; also, Plum Flower "Heavenly Heart Teapills")

bǎi zǐ rén (柏子仁), Semen Platycladi/Biotae	25.8 %	N
gǒu qǐ zǐ (枸杞子), Fructus Lycii	19.4	AB
xuán shēn (玄参), Radix Scrophulariae	12.9	DC
shú dì huáng (熟地黄), Radix Rehmanniae Praep.	12.9	DC
mài mén dōng (麦门冬), Radix Ophiopogonis	6.5	AD
dāng guī (当归), Radix Angelicae Sinensis	6.5	AB
fú líng (茯苓), Poria	6.4	FC
shí chāng pú (石菖蒲), Rhizoma Acori Tatarinowii	6.4	M
gān cǎo (甘草), Radix Glycyrrhizae	3.2	AA

Nourishes heart blood, nourishes heart yin, cools blood heat, calms shen. Use for disturbed *shen* due to deficiency of heart blood and *yin* causing insomnia, restlessness, palpitation, anxiety, or uncomfortable dreaming. Also useful for poor concentration, clouded mind, and mental fatigue. Use in deficiency of *yin* and blood presentations.

Pulse: Thin, weak, rapid
Tongue: Pale with red tip, or dry or geographic

Comments: *Bai Zi Yang Xin Tang* is a good formula for disturbed *shen* patterns due to deficiency of blood and *yin*. The first three herbs (*bǎi zǐ rén, gǒu qǐ zǐ,* and *shú dì huáng*) comprise 58% of the formula, working together to tonify *yin* and blood. *Xuán shēn*, at 13% of the formula, cools the heart. The formula is effective for insomnia, anxiety and chronic palpitation. It does not contain any heavy minerals and can be used for long periods of time. *Bǎi zǐ rén*, the lead herb at 26%, moistens heart *yin* and blood and is valued for promoting sleep and calming anxiety.

Further Reading:

Bensky et al, p. 462
Chen & Chen, p. 729

GAN MAI DA ZAO TANG

Formula: *gān mài dà zǎo tāng* (甘麦大枣汤)
"Glycyrrhiza, Triticum, Jujube Decoction"
Author: Zhāng Zhòng-Jǐng (张仲景)
Source: *Jīn Guì Yào Lüè* (金匮要略), 220
Literal: "Golden Cabinet Essential Summary"

Availability:

Calm Spirit Teapills (PF)
Gan Mai Da Zao Tang (TZ)
Gan Mai Da Zao Wan (GC, HT, TL)
Licorice & Jujube Combination (EG)
Rescue Formula (K)

Ingredients: (from the standardized *"Licorice & Jujube Combination"*)

fú xiǎo mài (浮小麦), Fructus Tritici Levis	64.5 %	L
dà zǎo (大枣), Fructus Jujubae	19.4	AA
gān cǎo (甘草), Radix Glycyrrhizae	16.1	AA

Ingredients: (from Herbal Times *"Gan Mai Da Zao Wan"*)

fú xiǎo mài (浮小麦), Fructus Tritici Levis	25.0 %	L
dà zǎo (大枣), Fructus Jujubae	16.6	AA
gān cǎo (甘草), Radix Glycyrrhizae	12.5	AA
bǎi zǐ rén (柏子仁), Semen Platycladi/Biotae	12.5	N
suān zǎo rén (酸枣仁), Semen Ziziphi Spinosae	12.5	N
fú líng (茯苓), Poria	12.5	FC
hé huān pí (合欢皮), Cortex Albiziae	8.4	N

Ingredients: (from Plum Flower *"Calm Spirit Teapills"*)

yè jiāo téng (夜交藤), Caulis Polygoni Multiflori	18.1 %	N
fú xiǎo mài (浮小麦), Fructus Tritici Levis	15.0	L
dà zǎo (大枣), Fructus Jujubae	14.9	AA
fú líng (茯苓), Poria	14.9	FC
bǎi hé (百合), Bulbus Lilii	14.9	AD
gān cǎo (甘草), Radix Glycyrrhizae	12.0	AA
hé huān pí (合欢皮), Cortex Albiziae	10.2	N

Nourishes heart yin, boosts heart qi, soothes the liver, calms shen. Use for disturbed *shen* due to *yin* deficiency, causing emotional volatility including depression, anxiety, excessive worrying, or unprovoked crying. Also for restless sleep, clouded mind, or uncomfortable dreaming. Can be used for uncomfortable emotional states due to premenstrual tension and menopausal disorder.

Pulse: Thin
Tongue: Normal, or reddish with dry coat

Comments: We have two different formulas here; they both address restlessness due to disturbed *shen*, with emotional volatility and poor sleep. Modern applications include mental agitation with menopausal syndrome, and night-crying and terror among children.

The original formula recorded by Zhang Zhong-Jing consisted of three herbs (*fú xiǎo mài, gān cǎo* and *dà zǎo*), and was basically prescribed for hysteria. The original formula is used by the Taiwan granule companies, Kan and TCM Zone. In the standardized formula, *fú xiǎo mài* comprises 64.5% of the formula. This herb, an astringent, traditionally is used to bring *yin* back to the interior and stop sweating. In Zhang's time, it was thought to bring one's escaping soul back into the body during acute mental disturbance. Because the herb has the properties of moistening *yin* and cooling blood, it is used for deficiency heat in the heart disturbing the shen. *Gān cǎo* and *dà zǎo* boost *qi*, and in this case, heart *qi*.

The formulas offered by Herbal Times, Plum Flower, Guang Ci Tang and Tanglong reduce the quantity of *fú xiǎo mài* and add herbs to enhance tonification of *yin* and blood. Herbal Times adds *bǎi zǐ rén* and *suān zǎo rén* for another 25% of the formula, plus 8% *hé huān pí* to settle the liver and enhance treatment of anxiety. Taking a different track, the Plum Flower version adds 18% *yè jiāo téng* to tonify heart blood and 15% *bǎi hé* to nourish heart *yin*, and also adds 10% *hé huān pí*. The adjustments in both of these formulas boost heart *yin* and blood.

Caution: *Fú xiǎo mài* is the wheat seed, and is contraindicated for those with celiac disease or gluten sensitivities.

Further Reading:

Bensky et al, p. 471
Chen & Chen, 731
Ellis, p. 105

GUI PI WAN

Formula: *guī pí tāng* (归脾汤), "Restore Spleen Pill"
Author: Yán Yòng-Hé (严用和)
Source: *Jì Shēng Fāng* (济生方), 1253
Literal: "Aid (the) Living Formulas"

Availability:

Gather Vitality (K)
Ginseng & Longan Combination (EG)
Ginseng and Longan Formula (CC, GF)
Gui Pi Tang (BP, TZ)
Gui Pi Teapills (PF)
Gui Pi Wan (GC, HT, MS, PIM, TL)
Tonify Spleen (JD)
* Calm the Shen (TT)
* Shen-Gem (HC)

Ingredients: (from the standardized *"Ginseng & Longan Combination"*)

rén shēn (人参), Radix Ginseng	9.7 %	AA
bái zhú (白术), Rhizoma Atractylodis Macrocephalae	9.7	AA
fú líng (茯苓), Poria	9.7	FC
suān zǎo rén (酸枣仁), Semen Ziziphi Spinosae	9.7	N
lóng yǎn ròu (龙眼肉), Arillus Longan	9.7	AB
huáng qí (黄芪), Radix Astragali	9.7	AA
dāng guī (当归), Radix Angelicae Sinensis	9.7	AB
yuǎn zhì (远志), Radix Polygalae	9.7	N
shēng jiāng (生姜), Rhizoma Zingiberis Recens	6.5	BA
dà zǎo (大枣), Fructus Jujubae	6.5	AA
mù xiāng (木香), Radix Aucklandiae	4.7	G
zhì gān cǎo (炙甘草), Radix Glycyrrhizae Praep	4.7	AA

Ingredients: (from Herbal Times *"Gui Pi Wan"*)

bái zhú (白术), Rhizoma Atractylodis Macrocephalae	14. %	AA
dāng guī (当归), Radix Angelicae Sinensis	14	AB
fú líng (茯苓), Poria	14	FC
lóng yǎn ròu (龙眼肉), Arillus Longan	14	N
yuǎn zhì (远志), Radix Polygalae	14	N
dǎng shēn (党参), Radix Codonopsis	7	AA

huáng qí (黄芪), Radix Astragali	7	AA
suān zǎo rén (酸枣仁), Semen Ziziphi Spinosae	7	N
dà zǎo (大枣), Fructus Jujubae	3	AA
gān cǎo (甘草), Radix Glycyrrhizae	3	AA
mù xiāng (木香), Radix Aucklandiae	3	G

Calms shen, tonifies spleen and heart qi, nourishes heart blood. Use for heart *shen* disorders due to deficiency of *qi* and blood, characterized by insomnia or restless sleep, poor memory, excessive dreaming, dizziness, palpitations or anxiety. Also for fatigue or poor appetite, and deficiency ulcer. Can be used as a general *qi* and blood tonic for the aged or those recovering from illness or childbirth, and for gynecological conditions including amenorrhea and infertility. The formula is also used for spleen failing to control the blood, and is used for internal bleeding, thrombocytopenic purpura, and prolonged menstrual spotting.

Pulse: Normal, or thin, weak
Tongue: Normal, or pale

Comments: *Gui Pi Wan* is a famous formula for deficiency of heart blood and spleen *qi*. The underlying cause is taken to be obsessive thinking or over-use of the mind. It has a wide variety of applications, and is most often used for insomnia due to deficiency of *qi* and blood, as well as deficiency gynecological bleeding disorders. The formula uses *Si Jun Zi Tang* (Chapter 6A) as its foundation for promoting *qi,* with the addition of *huáng qí* and *dà zǎo*. *Huáng qí* and *rén shēn* are the principal herbs to promote *qi*, while *dāng guī* is the principal herb to promote blood. The herbs *yuǎn zhì*, *lóng yǎn ròu* and *suān zǎo rén* moisten *yin* and blood and direct the formula to the heart.

The ingredient percentages represented by Herbal Times are similar to those offered by Minshan, Plum Flower, and others.

Gui Pi Tang is particularly useful for disturbed sleep, anxiety, or palpitations in the elderly, constitutionally weak patients, or following illness, surgery or childbirth.

Further Reading:

Bensky et al, p. 353
Chen & Chen, p. 583
Ellis, p. 118

SUAN ZAO REN TANG

Formula: *suān zǎo rén tāng* (酸枣仁汤), "Zizyphus Decoction"
Author: Zhāng Zhòng-Jǐng (张仲景)
Source: *Jīn Guì Yào Lüè* (金匮要略), 220
Literal: "Golden Cabinet Essential Summary"

Availability:

Suan Zao Ren Tang (BP, PF)
Suan Zao Ren Wan (HT, PM, TL)
Zizyphus Combination (EG)
Zizyphus Formula (CC, GF)
Zizyphus Sleep Formula (K)
* Nourish The Soul (TT)
* Te Xiao Zao Ren An Mian Pian (GC)

Ingredients: (from the standardized "*Zizyphus Combination*")

suān zǎo rén (酸枣仁), Semen Ziziphi Spinosae	45.5 %	N
fú líng (茯苓), Poria	18.2	FC
chuān xiōng (川芎), Rhizoma Ligustici Chuanxiong	18.2	K
gān cǎo (甘草), Radix Glycyrrhizae	9.1	AA
zhī mǔ (知母), Rhizoma Anemarrhenae	9.1	DA

Ingredients: (from Herbal Times "*Suan Zao Ren Wan*")

suān zǎo rén (酸枣仁), Semen Ziziphi Spinosae	38.5 %	N
fú líng (茯苓), Poria	23.0	FC
chuān xiōng (川芎), Rhizoma Ligustici Chuanxiong	15.2	K
zhī mǔ (知母), Rhizoma Anemarrhenae	15.2	DA
gān cǎo (甘草), Radix Glycyrrhizae	8.0	AA

Ingredients: (from Plum Flower *"Suan Zao Ren Tang"*)

suān zǎo rén (酸枣仁), Semen Ziziphi Spinosae	78.5 %	N
chuān xiōng (川芎), Rhizoma Ligustici Chuanxiong	6.1	K
fú líng (茯苓), Poria	6.1	FC
zhī mǔ (知母), Rhizoma Anemarrhenae	6.1	DA
gān cǎo (甘草), Radix Glycyrrhizae	3.1	AA

Calms shen, nourishes heart and liver blood and yin, clears deficiency heat, invigorates blood. Use for deficiency presentations of disturbed *shen* causing insomnia, restlessness, palpitation, anxiety, irritability, or uncomfortable dreaming. Also useful for poor concentration or mental fatigue. Useful for agitation, insomnia and night-sweats during menopause, and for agitation, palpitation and insomnia the elderly.

Pulse: Thin, wiry or rapid
Tongue: Normal, may be dry

Comments: *Suan Zao Ren Tang* is well tolerated for long periods of time, and acts as a heart, *shen* and liver tonic. The principal herb is *suān zăo rén*, an oily seed that moistens blood and *yin* of both the heart and the liver. It is supported with herbs to cool deficiency heat (*zhī mŭ*), tonify *qi* (*gān căo*) and move blood (*chuān xiōng*). The amount of *suān zăo rén* is important, and Chinese doctors often prefer large amounts to achieve the desired effect. In that regard, the Plum Flower formula can be considered the strongest.

Further Reading:

Bensky et al, p. 462
Chen & Chen, p. 722
Ellis, p. 301

TIAN WANG BU XIN DAN

Formula: *tiān wáng bŭ xīn dān* (天王补心丹)
"Heavenly Emperor Tonify Heart Elixir"
Author: Hóng Jī (洪基) *aka* Hóng Jiŭ-Yŏu (洪九有)
Source: *Shè Shēng Mì Pōu* (摄生秘剖), 1638
Literal: "Sustaining Life Secrets, Explanation"
also attributed to:
Author: *Xuē Jĭ* (薛己) *aka* Xuē Xīn-Fŭ (薛新甫) *aka* Xuē Lì-Zhāi (薛立斋)
Source: *Jiào Zhù Fù Rén Liáng Fāng* (校注妇人良方), mid-16th c.
Literal: "Corrections (and) Annotations (to) Women's Fine Formulas"

Availability:

Celestial Emperor's Blend (K)
Emperor's Teapills (PF)
Emperor's Heart Yin Formula (JD)
Ginseng & Zizyphus Formula (CC, EG)
Heavenly Emperor's Formula (GF)
Tian Wang Bu Xin Dan (BP, PIM, TZ)
Tian Wang Bu Xin Wan (GC, HT, JD, MS, TL)

Ingredients: (from Minshan *"Tian Wang Bu Xin Wan"*)

shú dì huáng (熟地黄), Radix Rehmanniae Praeparata	29.7 %	AB
dāng guī (当归), Radix Angelicae Sinensis	7.4	AB
wŭ wèi zĭ (五味子), Fructus Schisandrae	7.4	L
suān zăo rén (酸枣仁), Semen Ziziphi Spinosae	7.4	N
băi zĭ rén (柏子仁), Semen Platycladi	7.4	N
tiān mén dōng (天门冬), Radix Asparagi	7.4	AD
mài mén dōng (麦门冬), Radix Ophiopogonis	7.4	AD
xuán shēn (玄参), Radix Scrophulariae	7.4	DC
dān shēn (丹参), Radix/Rhizoma Salviae Miltiorrhizae	3.7	K
dăng shēn (党参), Radix Codonopsis	3.7	AA
fú ling (茯苓), Poria	3.7	FC
jié gĕng (桔梗), Radix Platycodonis	3.7	CA
yuăn zhì (远志), Radix Polygalae	3.7	N

Calms shen, cools blood heat, nourishes heart blood, yin and qi, clears heart heat. Use for disturbed *shen* causing insomnia, restlessness, palpitation, anxiety or uncomfortable dreaming. Also for poor memory or concentration, or mental fatigue. Can be used for hyperthyroid, menopausal disorder and chronic myocarditis. Can also be used for chronic mouth ulcers and nocturnal emissions. Use in presentations with deficiency heat rather than real fire.

Pulse: Thin, rapid
Tongue: Red in tip, dry

Comments: *Tian Wang Bu Xin Dan* is commonly used for disturbed *shen* due to deficiency of *yin* and blood with signs of insomnia, irritability and anxiety. *Shú dì huáng* makes up 28-29% of most of the formulas, with the exception of the standardized Taiwan formula, where it is kept at 5.6%. This herb moistens heart *yin* and blood, and is reinforced with *suān zǎo rén* and *bǎi zǐ rén* for another 15% of the formula. *Tiān mén dōng* and *mài mén dōng* further moisten heart *yin*, while *xuán shēn* clears heat in the heart.

This formula contains no heavy minerals to subdue *yang*, and is intended for heart and *shen* conditions marked by blood and *yin* deficiency. (The original formula contained *zhū shā* (朱砂, Cinnabaris), which is no longer used.). The efficacy for insomnia and anxiety is gradual, and is used in chronic cases.

Further Reading:

Bensky et al, p. 459
Chen & Chen, p. 725
Ellis, p. 308

Modern Formulas:

AN MIAN PIAN

Formula: *ān mián piàn* (安眠片), "Calm Sleep Tablets"
Source: Modern patent medicine

Availability:

An Mian Pian (BP)
An Mien Pian (PF)
An Mien Pien (PM)

Ingredients: (from Plum Flower *"An Mien Pian"*)

suān zǎo rén (酸枣仁), Semen Ziziphi Spinosae	30. %	N
yuǎn zhì (远志), Radix Polygalae	20	N
fú líng (茯苓), Poria	15	FC
zhī zǐ (栀子), Fructus Gardeniae	15	DA
shén qū (神曲), Massa Medicata Fermentata	15	H
gān cǎo (甘草), Radix Glycyrrhizae	5	AA

Calms shen, clears heart heat, resolves phlegm-fire, moistens heart yin and blood, resolves food stasis. Use for disturbed *shen* causing insomnia, restlessness, agitation, and vivid or uncomfortable dreaming. Can be used in mild cases of disturbed *shen* due to phlegm-fire with signs of mania or panic. Also useful for inability to sleep following overeating. Useful for chronic anxiety or panic disorders, and depression.

Pulse: Wiry, rapid; may be slippery and bounding
Tongue: Normal, or reddish with a greasy coat

Comments: *An Mian Pian* represents one of the few available products that address insomnia and disturbed mind due to phlegm-fire. 50% of the formula combines *suān zăo rén, yuăn zhì* and *fú líng* to nourish heart *shen, yin* and blood, while 30% combines *zhī zĭ* and *shén qū* to clear phlegm-fire. Although serious cases of manic behavior require experienced practitioners, this formula is useful for mild cases of mania or agitated mind, as well as insomnia.

The formula can also be used for inability to sleep or disturbed sleep due to over-eating, as well as chronic deficiency-heat in the heart.

Caution: *Shén qū* contains a wheat binder and is contraindicated for people with celiac disease or gluten allergy.

AN MIAN WAN

Formula: *ān mián wán* (安眠丸), "Calm Sleep Pills"
Source: Modern patent medicine

Availability:

An Mian Wan (HT)

Ingredients: (from Herbal Times *"An Mian Wan"*)

bǎi zǐ rén (柏子仁), Semen Platycladi/Biotae	10.0 %	N
shú dì huáng (熟地黄), Radix Rehmanniae Praep.	10.0	AB
yuǎn zhì (远志), Radix Polygalae	10.0	N
jié gěng (桔梗), Radix Platycodonis	9.7	CA
suān zǎo rén (酸枣仁), Semen Ziziphi Spinosae	8.0	N
chén pí (陈皮), Pericarpium Citri Reticulatae	7.4	G
dāng guī (当归), Radix Angelicae Sinensis	5.5	AB
dǎng shēn (党参), Radix Codonopsis	5.5	AA
gān cǎo (甘草), Radix Glycyrrhizae	5.5	AA
shān yào (山药), Rhizoma Dioscoreae	5.5	AA
mài mén dōng (麦门冬), Radix Ophiopogonis	5.5	AD
xuán shēn (玄参), Radix Scrophulariae	5.5	DC
bái zhǐ (白芷), Radix Angelicae Dahuricae	4.5	BB
jiǔ jié chāng pú (九节菖蒲), Rhizoma Anemones Altaicae	4.5	M
wǔ wèi zǐ (五味子), Fructus Schisandrae	2.9	L

Calms shen, tonifies qi, nourishes blood, nourishes yin, clears heat. Use for disturbed *shen* due to deficiency of *qi* and blood, with symptoms of insomnia, restlessness, palpitation, anxiety, and vivid uncomfortable dreaming. Also useful for poor memory or concentration, clouded mind, headache, dizziness, or mental fatigue. Can be useful for chronic low-level anxiety disorders and depression. Useful for insomnia following childbirth or surgery.

Pulse: Weak or thin
Tongue: Normal, or slightly swollen and moist

Comments: Although having the same name as *An Mian Pian* (above), this is a very different formula. While both formulas nourish heart *yin* and blood, the former clears phlegm-fire, while this formula boosts heart *yin*, blood and *qi*. In this product offered by Herbal Times, 32% nourishes heart *shen*, *yin* and blood (*suān zǎo rén, bǎi zǐ rén, yuǎn zhì, jiǔ jié chāng pú*), while another 32% boosts *qi* and blood (*dǎng shēn, gān cǎo, shān yào, shú dì huáng, dāng guī*). It is particularly useful for disturbed sleep, anxiety, or palpitations in the elderly, constitutionally weak patients, or following illness, surgery or childbirth.

The formula is similar to *An Shui Wan* (below), sharing 14 of the same ingredients. Both formulas are for disturbed *shen* due to deficiency of *qi*, blood and *yin*.

AN SHEN BU XIN WAN

Formula: *ān shén bŭ xīn wán* (安神补心丸), "Calm *Shen* Tonify Heart Pill"
Source: Modern patent medicine

Availability:

An Shen Bu Xin Teapills (PF)
An Shen Bu Xin Wan (GC, HT, MS, PM)
Soothwell (PM)

Ingredients: (from Minshan *"An Shen Bu Xin Wan"* and Plum Flower *"An Shen Bu Shen Teapills"*)

zhēn zhū mŭ (珍珠母), Concha Margaritiferae Usta	44.0 %	N
yè jiāo téng (夜交藤), Caulis Polygoni Multiflori	11.0	N
nǚ zhēn zĭ (女贞子), Fructus Ligustri Lucidi	8.8	AD
dān shēn (丹参), Radix/Rhizoma Salviae Miltiorrhizae	6.6	K
hàn lián căo (旱莲草), Herba Ecliptae	6.6	AD
tù sī zĭ (菟丝子), Semen Cuscutae	6.6	AC
hé huān pí (合欢皮), Cortex Albiziae	6.6	N
shēng dì huáng (生地黄), Radix Rehmanniae	4.4	AB
wŭ wèi zĭ (五味子), Fructus Schisandrae	3.3	L
shí chāng pú (石菖蒲), Rhizoma Acori Tatarinowii	2.2	M

Ingredients: (from Herbal Times *"An Shen Bu Xin Wan"*)

dān shēn (丹参), Radix/Rhizoma Salviae Miltiorrhizae	20. %	K
tù sī zĭ (菟丝子), Semen Cuscutae	20	AC
hàn lián căo (旱莲草), Herba Ecliptae	15	AD
shí chāng pú (石菖蒲), Rhizoma Acori Tatarinowii	15	M
wŭ wèi zĭ (五味子), Fructus Schisandrae	15	L
zhēn zhū (珍珠), Margarita	15	N

Ingredients: (Shanghai Chinese Medicine Works *"Soothwell"*)

dān shēn (丹参), Radix/Rhizoma Salviae Miltiorrhizae	25. %	K
wŭ wèi zĭ (五味子), Fructus Schisandrae	20	L
nǚ zhēn zĭ (女贞子), Fructus Ligustri Lucidi	15	AD
hàn lián căo (旱莲草), Herba Ecliptae	15	AD
hé huān pí (合欢皮), Cortex Albiziae	10	N
yè jiāo téng (夜交藤), Caulis Polygoni Multiflori	10	N
shēng dì huáng (生地黄), Radix Rehmanniae	5	AB

Calms shen, subdues ascendant yang, invigorates blood, settles the liver, secures the kidney. Use for disturbed *shen* due to ascendant *yang* with symptoms of insomnia with active mental dialogue, vivid or uncomfortable dreaming, palpitation, dizziness, restlessness or anxiety.

Pulse: Normal, or thin, wiry or rapid
Tongue: Normal, or reddish with a dry coat

Comments: The original *An Shen Bu Xin Wan* formula is the patent medicine from Minshan, which is also duplicated by Plum Flower. In this version, 44% of the formula uses *zhēn zhū mǔ* (mother-of-pearl shell), a heavy mineral substance that settles ascendant *yang* causing overactive mind and an inability to sleep. The *yang* ascends due to the kidney losing its rooting strength, and the formula uses herbs that strengthen kidney *qi* (combining *tù sī zǐ, nǚ zhēn zǐ* and *hàn lián cǎo*) to pull *yang* downwards. Other herbs reinforce the effect to settle or calm *shen* and ascendant liver *yang* (*yè jiāo téng, hé huān pí* and *shí chāng pú*). Due to the large amount of *zhēn zhū mǔ*, the original ten herb formula offers a strong and effective medicine for insomnia with excessive mental chatter.

Two other products exist with the same name, each a smaller version of the original formula. They both boost the amount of *dān shēn* to move heart blood and *wǔ wèi zǐ* to astringe the formula into the heart, while also boosting kidney *qi* to attract ascendant *yang*. The Herbal Times formula uses 6 herbs of the original formula, with *zhēn zhū* (the whole pearl) as 15% of the formula. *Soothwell*, a product from Shanghai Medicine Works, uses 7 herbs from the original formula, but does not include *zhēn zhū* or *zhēn zhū mǔ*.

Caution: Overuse of *zhēn zhū mǔ* may injure spleen *qi*, leading to indigestion or gastric pain. Limit use if necessary.

AN SHUI WAN

Formula: *ān shuì wán* (安睡丸), "Peaceful Sleep Pills"
Source: Modern patent medicine

Availability:

An Shui Teapills (PF)

Ingredients: (from Plum Flower *"An Shui Teapills"*)

yè jiāo téng (夜交藤), Caulis Polygoni Multiflori	10.0 %	N
fú xiǎo mài (浮小麦), Fructus Tritici Levis	10.0	L
yuǎn zhì (远志), Radix Polygalae	8.0	N
shú dì huáng (熟地黄), Radix Rehmanniae Praep.	8.0	AB
bǎi zǐ rén (柏子仁), Semen Platycladi/Biotae	8.0	N
suān zǎo rén (酸枣仁), Semen Ziziphi Spinosae	6.0	N
chén pí (陈皮), Pericarpium Citri Reticulatae	6.0	G
fú líng (茯苓), Poria	4.5	FC
dāng guī (当归), Radix Angelicae Sinensis	4.5	AB
shān yào (山药), Rhizoma Dioscoreae	4.5	AA
dǎng shēn (党参), Radix Codonopsis	4.5	AA
xuán shēn (玄参), Radix Scrophulariae	4.5	DC
mài mén dōng (麦门冬), Radix Ophiopogonis	4.5	AD
jié gěng (桔梗), Radix Platycodonis	4.5	CA
bái zhú (白术), Rhizoma Atractylodis Macrocephalae	3.5	AA
shí chāng pú (石菖蒲), Rhizoma Acori Tatarinowii	3.5	M
gān cǎo (甘草), Radix Glycyrrhizae	3.5	AA
wǔ wèi zǐ (五味子), Fructus Schisandrae	2.0	L

Calms shen, tonifies qi, nourishes blood, moistens heart yin, clears heat. Use for disturbed *shen* due to deficiency of *qi* and blood, with symptoms of insomnia, restlessness, palpitation, anxiety, and vivid uncomfortable dreaming. Also useful for poor memory or concentration, clouded mind, deficiency headache, dizziness, or mental fatigue. Can be useful for chronic low-level anxiety disorders and depression. Useful for insomnia following childbirth or surgery, or during menopause.

Pulse: Weak or thin
Tongue: Normal, or slightly swollen and moist

Comments: This large 18-herb formula is similar to Herbal Times' *An Mian Wan* (above), sharing 14 of the same ingredients. Plum Flower's *An Shui Wan*, however, uses *yè jiāo téng* and *fú xiǎo mài* for 20% of the formula, two herbs that are not included in the Herbal Times product. *Yè jiāo téng* settles ascendant *yang*, while *fú xiǎo mài* clears heart heat and astringes *yin* back into the heart.

35% of the formula nourishes heart *shen* (*fú xiǎo mài, yè jiāo téng, yuǎn zhì, bǎi zǐ rén, suān zǎo rén*), and 28% tonifies *qi* and blood (*dǎng shēn, shān yào, gān cǎo, shú dì huáng, dāng guī*). It is particularly useful for disturbed sleep, anxiety, or palpitations in the elderly, constitutionally weak patients, or following illness, surgery or childbirth. Because *fú xiǎo mài* has properties for astringing sweating, the formula is also useful for menopausal insomnia with night sweats.

Caution: *Fú xiǎo mài* is the wheat seed, and is contraindicated for those with celiac disease or gluten sensitivity.

BU NAO WAN / JIAN NAO WAN

Formula: *bŭ nǎo wán* (补脑丸), "Tonify Brain Pill"
Source: Modern patent medicine

Availability:

Bu Nao Wan (HT, PIM, TL)
Bu Nao Pian (PF)
Cerebral Tonic Pill (PM)
Clear Mind (K)
Polygala Combo (PM)

Formula: *jiàn nǎo wán* (健脑丸), "Healthy Brain Pills"
Source: Modern patent medicine

Availability:

Healthy Brain Pills (PM)

Ingredients: (from Xian TCM Factory *"Cerebral Tonic Pill / Polygala Combo"*)

wŭ wèi zǐ (五味子), Fructus Schisandrae	20. %	L
suān zǎo rén (酸枣仁), Semen Ziziphi Spinosae	16	N
dāng guī (当归), Radix Angelicae Sinensis	10	AB
suǒ yáng (锁阳), Herba Cynomorii	8	AC
hú táo rén (胡桃仁), Semen Juglans Regiae	8	AC
gǒu qǐ zǐ (枸杞子), Fructus Lycii	8	AB
bǎi zǐ rén (柏子仁), Semen Platycladi/Biotae	6	N
gōu téng (钩藤), Ramulus Uncariae cum Uncis	4	O
yuǎn zhì (远志), Radix Polygalae	4	N
tiān nán xīng (天南星), Rhizoma Arisaematis	4	CA
shí chāng pú (石菖蒲), Rhizoma Acori Tatarinowii	4	M
hǔ pò (琥珀), Succinum	4	N
lóng chǐ (龙齿), Dens Draconis	4	N

The Plum Flower formula *"Bu Nao Pian"* follows the same formula, but substitutes *hé huān pí* (合欢皮, Cortex Albiziae) for *hŭ pò*, and *zhēn zhū* (珍珠, Margarita) for *lóng chǐ*.

Ingredients: (from Herbal Times *"Bu Nao Wan"*)

suān zǎo rén (酸枣仁), Semen Ziziphi Spinosae	18.0 %	N
dāng guī (当归), Radix Angelicae Sinensis	12.0	AB
hú táo rén (胡桃仁), Semen Juglans Regiae	10.0	AC
wǔ wèi zǐ (五味子), Fructus Schisandrae	10.0	L
gǒu qǐ zǐ (枸杞子), Fructus Lycii	7.0	AB
shí chāng pú (石菖蒲), Rhizoma Acori Tatarinowii	7.0	M
yì zhì rén (益智仁), Fructus Alpiniae Oxyphyllae	7.0	AC
tiān má (天麻), Rhizoma Gastrodiae	5.0	O
tiān zhú huáng (天竹黄), Concretio Silicea Bambusae	5.0	CB
yuǎn zhì (远志), Radix Polygalae	5.0	N
bái zhǐ (白芷), Radix Angelicae Dahuricae	3.5	BA
chuān xiōng (川芎), Rhizoma Ligustici Chuanxiong	3.5	K

Ingredients: (from Qingdao Traditional Chinese Medicine Factory *"Healthy Brain Pills"*)

suān zǎo rén (酸枣仁), Semen Ziziphi Spinosae	22.5 %	N
dāng guī (当归), Radix Angelicae Sinensis	15.0	AB
shān yào (山药), Rhizoma Dioscoreae	12.5	AA
gǒu qǐ zǐ (枸杞子), Fructus Lycii	9.0	AB
wǔ wèi zǐ (五味子), Fructus Schisandrae	7.5	L
yì zhì rén (益智仁), Fructus Alpiniae Oxyphyllae	7.5	AC
tiān zhú huáng (天竹黄), Concretio Silicea Bambusae	5.2	CB
jiǔ jié chāng pú (九节菖蒲), Rhizoma Anemones Altaicae	5.2	M
dān shēn (丹参), Radix/Rhiz. Salviae Miltiorrhizae	5.2	K
rén shēn (人参), Radix Ginseng	5.2	AA
bǎi zǐ rén (柏子仁), Semen Platycladi/Biotae	5.2	N

Calms shen, nourishes heart blood, tonifies heart qi and yang, moves blood, subdues ascendant yang. Use for *shen* disturbance due to deficiency of heart blood and *yin* and deficiency of heart *qi* and *yang*. Indicated for insomnia, restlessness, palpitation, anxiety, uncomfortable dreaming, poor memory or concentration.

Pulse: Weak or thin
Tongue: Normal, or slightly swollen and moist

Comments: The *Bu Nao* and *Jian Nao* formulas are used to treat deficiencies affecting heart *shen*, causing muddled thinking and poor concentration. These *shen* disturbances are thought to be due to overuse of the mind including over concentration or over-studying, and also from the affects of aging. It is recommended for students preparing for exams, and to boost mental abilities in the aged or following illness or childbirth.

The three formulas listed here are similar in composition, with certain variations. Plum Flower's *Bu Nao Pian* and Xian's *Cerebral Tonic Pills/Polygala Combo* are virtually the same formula, with 38% treating disturbed *shen,* 18% tonifying blood, and 16% boosting *yang.* The Herbal Times version uses 37% of the formula to treat disturbed *shen,* 19% to tonify blood, and 17% to boost *yang.* The *yang* boosting herbs include *suŏ yang, hú táo rén* (walnut) and *yì zhì rén.*

The formula *Healthy Brain Pills,* from Qingdao TCM Factory, is a bit different. It uses 33% to treat disturbed *shen* and 24% to tonify blood, with an additional 18% to tonify *qi,* but only 7.5% to boost *yang.* It is preferred for deficiency of *qi* and blood, versus deficiency of *yang* and blood.

All three formulas include herbs that dispel phlegm blocking the heart orifices (*tiān nán xīng, shí chāng pú, jiŭ jié chāng pú,* or *tiān zhú huáng*). Heart phlegm leads to muddled or confused thinking, poor concentration and poor memory. The inclusion of these herbs boosts the ability to clear the mind.

OTHER FORMULAS APPROPRIATE FOR THIS CATEGORY:

Classical Formulas:

shen qi wu wei zi wan

See Chapter 14A.

zhi gan cao tang

See Chapter 16A.

Modern Formulas:

Acorus Tablets (SF)
An Shen Ding Zhi Wan (TL)
Bu Nao Yang Shen Pian (GC)
Calm Spirit (HC)
Calm-Jr. (EV)
Clear & Calm (BP)
Comfort Shen (CMS)
Compassionate Sage (K)
Dr. Shen's Good Sleep & Worry Free Pill (DS)
Enhance Memory (EV)
Fu-Shen 16 (SF)
Ginkgo Formula (GF)
Harmonize Kidney & Heart (CMS)
Kavaseng (HC)
Peace Pearls (CP)
Peaceful Spirit Formula (GF)
Resolve Depression & Stabilize Sleep (BP)
Restful Sleep Formula (GF)
Salvia/Amber Tablets (SF)
Schisandra ZZZ (EV)
Schizandra Dreams (HC)
Settle the Will Decoction (AL)
Shen Jing Shuai Ruo Wan (PM)
Shui De An (PM)
St. John's Seng (HC)
Strengthen Heart (CMS)
Te Xiao Zao Ren An Mian Pian/Wan (GC)
Zizyphus 18 (SF)

10. HEART BLOOD STASIS AND ACCUMULATION OF HEART PHLEGM
(Chest Pain, Headache, Arterial Plaque, Hypercholesteremia)

Classical Formulas:

Dan Shen Yin	*dān shēn yǐn* (丹参饮)
Tong Qiao Huo Xue Tang	*tōng qiào huó xuè tāng* (通窍活血汤)
Xue Fu Zhu Yu Tang	*xuè fŭ zhú yū tāng* (血府逐瘀汤)

Modern Formulas:

Cholisma (EV)	
Shan Zha Jiang Zhi Wan	*shān zhā jiàng zhī wán* (山楂降脂丸)

Formulas for heart blood stagnation are used to treat or prevent chest *bi* syndrome (*xiōng bì*, 胸痹); they also address headache due to blood stasis and trauma. Chest *bi* includes the modern diseases of angina pectoris and coronary heart disease, and symptoms include chest pain, shortness of breath or shallow breathing when lying down, dizziness, poor concentration and fatigue. Mild cases may show discomfort in the chest, while severe cases can have a sense of twisting pain in the chest with short breath and difficult respiration. With continued development, chest *bi* syndrome can result in intense, prolonged chest pain with sweating, cold limbs, pale complexion, cyanotic lips, hands and feet.

In modern medicine, coronary heart disease is due a thickening of coronary heart vessels due to atherosclerosis, a plaque build-up of cholesterol and fatty deposits. When it causes heart pain, it is called angina. With sustained blockage, the heart muscles become damaged, resulting in a heart attack. If soft plaque breaks off and lodges in blood vessels of the brain, the result is a stroke or heart attack.

The formulas in this chapter use herbs that move blood and break blood stasis, as well as herbs that open the coronary blood vessels (referred to in Chinese medicine as the heart orifices). Besides treating pain and constriction due to blood stasis in the coronary vessels, the formulas can be used preventatively to reduce accumulation of arterial plaque, both soft and hard. This makes them a valuable adjunct in the management of heart disease and the prevention of stroke. Many patients in China self-prescribe these formula to reduce blood vessel plaque.

The formulas are also used for blood stasis patterns causing palpitation, anxiety, insomnia, and hypertension; they are specific for stabbing headaches due to old or new trauma; and and also used to repair and treat stomach ulcers. The formulas are also given for diminished blood flow to the brain, affecting memory and concentration, and following a stroke.

As people age, heart blood stasis may be due to the gradual diminishing of kidney *mingmen* fire. In these cases, the heart actually becomes cold, and some of the formulas will incorporate warming herbs. In other cases, it can be beneficial to combine with kidney *yang* formulas (see *Chapter 17B. Kidney and Jing Tonics*).

Formulas for heart phlegm reduce accumulated fats in the blood, and are indicated for elevated cholesterol and triglycerides. Elevated blood fats are due to diets rich in sugars (including refined carbohydrates and alcohol), saturated fats or poor quality cooking oils. In persons with healthy diets, genetic factors can be an underlying cause.

In Chinese medicine, heart phlegm may be a result of chronic food stagnation. It exhibits signs of a greasy tongue coating and a wide or slippery pulse. Other symptoms include dizziness, feelings of heavy headedness, dull mind, poor digestion, loose or erratic stools, oily skin or hair, and excess weight.

In modern functional medicine, elevated cholesterol is not necessarily a risk to health unless it is also coupled with inflammation to the walls of the arterial blood vessels. In inflammation, cholesterol binds during repair, leading to plaque and arteriosclerosis. Inflammation is triggered by free radical damage (due to bad oils, environmental chemicals, and a diet lacking fruits and vegetables) or bacteria found in red meat. Another risk is chronically elevated serum insulin, which irritates and inflames the epithelia of blood vessels. Insulin should clear the blood within and hour or so of eating, but "insulin resistance" develops from chronic consumption of sugars, refined carbohydrates and alcohol. In both Chinese and functional medicine, diet is both the cause and cure for elevated blood lipids.

The formulas discussed in this chapter offer an alternative to modern pharmaceuticals for reducing cholesterol, especially when combined with diet and nutritional medicines such as nicotinic acid, Nattokinase, red rice yeast and so on. Pharmaceutical statins that reduce cholesterol reduce levels of coenzyme Q10, which is important for scavenging free radicals and supporting cellular mitochondria. The Chinese herbal approach is not only effective, but is non-toxic and can be taken for long periods of time.

Classical Formulas:

DAN SHEN YIN

Formula: *dān shēn yǐn* (丹参饮), "Salvia Cool-Decoction"
Author: Chén Niàn-Zǔ *aka* Chén Xiū-Yuán (陈念祖 / 陈修园)
Source: *Shí Fāng Gē Kuò* (时方歌括), 1801
Literal: "Contemporary Formulas (as a) Song Collection"
also attributed to:
Author: Wú Qiān (吴谦)
Source: *Yī Zōng Jīn Jiàn* (医宗金鉴), 1742
Literal: "Medical Tradition Golden Mirror"

Availability:

Compound Dan Shen Pill (PM)
Cool Salvia Formula (K)
Dan Shen Pian (PIM, PM)
Dan Shen Tablet (PM)
Dan Shen Wan (HT)
Dan Shen Yin (BP)
Dan Shen Yin Wan (TL)
Fu Fang Dan Shen Pian/Wan (GC, PM)
Salvia & Pseudoginseng (KP)
Salvia Plus Formula (CC)
Salvia Root Formula (KP)
Salvia Teapills (PF)

Ingredients: (From Herbal Times *"Dan Shen Wan"*)

dān shēn (丹参), Radix/Rhiz. Salviae Miltiorrhizae	72. %	K
tán xiāng (檀香), Lignum Santali Albi	14	G
shā rén (砂仁), Fructus Amomi	14	FB

Ingredients: (from Plum Flower *"Salvia Teapills"*)

dān shēn (丹参), Radix/Rhiz. Salviae Miltiorrhizae	69.8 %	K
tán xiāng (檀香), Lignum Santali Albi	13.9	G
shā rén (砂仁), Fructus Amomi	13.9	FB
gān cǎo (甘草), Radix Glycyrrhizae	2.4	AA

Invigorates blood, breaks blood stasis, calms shen, resolves chest oppression, opens the heart orifices. Use for upper *jiao* blood stasis causing chest pain, shortness of breath, palpitations, tachycardia, arrhythmia and restless sleep. Can also be used for blood stasis headache or dizziness, or to treat head trauma, or to increase blood flow to the brain. Also for blood stasis involved in stomach ulcer, hepatomegaly, splenomegaly, and dysmenorrhea. Recommended following stroke, or as a preventative against thrombus formation.

Pulses: Wiry or choppy
Tongue: Dark or red, may have yellow coat

Comments: *Dan Shen Wan* follows a basic formula of *dān shēn* 70%, *tán xiāng* 14%, and *shā rén* 14%. *Dān shēn* is highly regarded for treating chest and gastric pain. In Chinese hospitals, it is given to reduce blood emboli and soft plaque affecting the heart or brain, and as a treatment following heart attack or stroke. The herb *dān shēn* also treats disturbed *shen* disorders causing palpitations, arrhythmias and insomnia. The aromatic herbs *tán xiāng* (sandlewood) and *shā rén* open the blood vessels and invigorate blood flow. Together, the herbs can break down soft and hard blood plaque, reduce serum cholesterol, and stop chest pain.

Caution: *Dān shēn* is contraindicated for patients taking blood thinners such as Coumadin. *Dān shēn* and *tán xiāng* are used with caution during pregnancy.

Further Reading:

Bensky et al, p. 594
Chen & Chen, p. 917

TONG QIAO HUO XUE TANG

Formula: *tōng qiào huó xuè tāng* (通窍活血汤)
"Open Orifices Invigorate Blood Decoction"
Author: Wáng Qīng-Rèn (王清任)
Source: *Yī Lín Gǎi Cuò* (医林改错), 1830
Literal: "Physicians' Circle, Correction (of) Errors"

Availability:

Persica & Cnidum Combination (EG)
Persica & Ligusticum Combination (KP)
Tong Qiao Huo Xue Tang (BP)
Tong Qiao Huo Xue Teapills (PF)

Ingredients: (from the standardized *"Persica & Ligusticum/Cnidium Combination"*)

táo rén (桃仁), Semen Persicae	20.7 %	K
gān jiāng (干姜), Rhizoma Zingiberis	20.7	BA
hóng huā (红花), Flos Carthami	20.7	K
dà zǎo (大枣), Fructus Jujubae	17.2	AA
chuān xiōng (川芎), Rhizoma Ligustici Chuanxiong	6.9	K
chì sháo (赤芍), Radix Paeoniae Rubra	6.9	K
cōng bái (葱白), Bulbus Allii Fistulosi	6.9	BA

Ingredients: (from Plum Flower *"Tong Qiao Huo Xue Teapills"*)

táo rén (桃仁), Semen Persicae	19.8 %	K
hóng huā (红花), Flos Carthami	19.8	K
chì sháo (赤芍), Radix Paeoniae Rubra	10.1	K
chuān xiōng (川芎), Rhizoma Ligustici Chuanxiong	10.1	K
bái zhǐ (白芷), Radix Angelicae Dahuricae	10.1	BA
dà zǎo (大枣), Fructus Jujubae	10.1	AA
gān jiāng (干姜), Rhizoma Zingiberis	10.0	BA
shí chāng pú (石菖蒲), Rhizoma Acori Tatarinowii	10.0	BA

Invigorates blood, breaks blood stasis, opens heart orifices, opens channels and collaterals, boosts heart yang and qi, relieves chest oppression. Use for blood stagnation in the upper *jiao* affecting the heart and causing chest oppression, costal distension, angina, and numbness and tingling in the chest and arms. Also for blood stasis or trauma affecting the head, causing stabbing headache, dizziness, tinnitus, and darkness to the face and nose. Can be used for general stasis in the blood vessels and capillaries, and as a formula for hepatomegaly, splenomegaly, or uterine blood stasis. Can also be used for skin disorders such as vitiligo, varicosities, and spider veins It is also used as a preventative against stroke.

Pulses: Wiry or choppy
Tongue: Dark

Comments: In the early 19th century, Wang Qing-Ren developed numerous formulas to address blood stasis, including *Shen Tong Zhu Yu Tang* for blood stasis *bi* syndrome (Chapter 4B), *Ge Xia Zhu Yu Tang* for hepatomegaly (Chapter 7A), *Shao Fu Zhu Yu Tang* for dysmenorrhea (Chapter 8C), and *Xue Fu Zhu Yu Tang* (below).

Tong Qiao Huo Xue Tang addresses blood stasis in the upper *jiao* causing chest pain, difficulty breathing, or headache due to trauma. *Táo rén, hóng huā, chuān xiōng* and *chì sháo* are the principal herbs to move blood and break stasis. The formula also addresses an underlying diminishing of *mingmen* fire, causing the heart to go cold. Herbs such as *gān jiāng* and *dà zǎo* boost heart *yang* and *qi*. *Cōng bái*, the warming and aromatic wild onion, opens the channels allowing the formula to better get to the vessels.

In heart blood stasis with cold, typically, there is dark discoloration on the face, affecting the nose and cheeks. The formula can also be used for stabbing headaches or sudden deafness due to trauma. Also, it can be taken prophylactically to minimize the risk of stroke, and is used to treat skin conditions such as vitiligo and rosacea.

The Plum Flower version substitutes *shí chāng pú* and *bái zhǐ* for *cōng bái*; it is also stronger in percentages of blood moving and breaking herbs. Wang Qing-Ren's original formula contained musk gland *shè xiāng* (麝香, Moschus) to open the heart orifices. This expensive animal-source medicinal is omitted in the available products.

Caution: *Táo rén* and *hóng huā* are prohibited during pregnancy, and for patients on blood thinners such as Coumadin.

Further Reading:

Bensky et al, p. 567
Chen & Chen, 877
Ellis, p. 312

XUE FU ZHU YU TANG

Formula: *xuè fǔ zhú yū tāng* (血府逐瘀汤)
"Blood Mansion Drive-Out Stasis Decoction"
Author: Wáng Qīng-Rèn (王清任)
Source: *Yī Lín Gǎi Cuò* (医林改错), 1830
Literal: "Physicians' Circle, Correction (of) Errors"

Availability:

Blood Palace Formula (GF)
Drive Out Stasis in the Mansion of Blood Formula (HS)
Persica & Carthamus Combination (EG)
Stasis in the Mansion Of Blood (PF)
Xue Fu Zhu Yu Tang (BP)
Xue Fu Zhu Yu Wan (HT, TL)
Blood's Mansion (AL)
Red Stirring (TT)
Upper Palace Tablets (SF)

Ingredients: (from the standardized "Persica & Carthamus Combination")

táo rén (桃仁), Semen Persicae	16. %	K
dāng guī (当归), Radix Angelicae Sinensis	12	AB
shēng dì huáng (生地黄), Radix Rehmanniae	12	DC
hóng huā (红花), Flos Carthami	12	K
chuān niú xī (川牛膝), Radix Cyathulae	12	K
zhǐ ké (枳壳), Fructus Aurantii	8	G
chì sháo (赤芍), Radix Paeoniae Rubra	8	K
jié gěng (桔梗), Radix Platycodonis	6	CA
chuān xiōng (川芎), Rhizoma Ligustici Chuanxiong	6	K
chái hú (柴胡), Radix Bupleuri	4	BB
gān cǎo (甘草), Radix Glycyrrhizae	4	AA

Invigorates blood, breaks blood stasis, soothes the liver, opens heart orifices, relieves chest oppression and pain. Use for stagnation of *qi* and blood in the upper burner, including the chest, epigastrium, or head. Symptoms include chest or costal pain accompanied by restless sleep, palpitation, dizziness, irritability or depression. Also for chronic stabbing headache due to trauma; also for oppression in the epigastrium causing belching, prolonged hiccoughs or a choking sensation. Use in coronary heart disease, angina, arrhythmia and head trauma, and hypertension due to blood stagnation. Can be used as a preventative before or following stroke.

Pulses: Wiry or choppy
Tongue: Dark or with purple spots

Comments: In chronic blood stagnation in the upper burner (*jiao*), there will be a dark or reddened face, dark tongue, and choppy, wiry pulse. It is aggravated by stagnation of liver *qi* and may be seen in aging patients, patients with a history of alcohol abuse. It can also appear following head trauma. This formula has three distinct clinical applications: chest pain including angina, stabbing headache, and epigastric oppression with belching. It is commonly used for chest pain, and for headache due to trauma or concussion.

Xue Fu Zhu Yu Tang can be considered an elaboration of the 13th century formula *Tao Hong Si Wu Tang* (Chapter 6C), which comprises 66% of the formula. Like *Tong Qiao Huo Xue Tang*, above, this formula contains the blood movers *táo rén, chì sháo, hóng huā* and *chuān xiōng*. *Tong Qiao Huo Xue Tang* is preferred for blood stasis with deficiency of *yang* and *qi*, while *Xue Fu Zhu Yu Tang* is preferred for deficiency of blood with a bit of liver stasis.

The author Wang Qing-Ren developed three *Zhu Yu* formulas to address blood stasis. *Xue Fu Zhu Yu Tang* addresses stasis in the upper jiao affecting the heart and head; *Ge Xia Zhu Yu Tang* addresses blood stasis in the middle and lower *jiao* affecting the liver and lower abdomen (*Chapter 7A*); and *Shao Fu Zhu Yu Tang* addresses lower jiao blood stagnation causing dysmenorrhea (*Chapter 6C*).

Caution: *Táo rén, chuān niú xī* and *hóng huā* are prohibited during pregnancy, and for patients on blood thinners such as Coumadin.

Further Reading:

Bensky et al, p. 564
Chen & Chen, 879
Ellis, p. 372

Modern Formulas:

CHOLISMA

Source: Evergreen Herbs
Author: John Chen

Ingredients: (Ingredient percentages are not given)

cāng zhú (苍术), Rhizoma Atractylodis	FB
dān shēn (丹参), Radix/Rhiz. Salviae Miltiorrhizae	K
gé gēn (葛根), Radix Puerariae Lobatae	BB
hé shǒu wū (何首乌), Radix Polygoni Multiflori	AB
hé yè (荷叶), Folium Nelumbinis	DF
hǔ zhàng (虎杖), Rhizoma Polygoni Cuspidati	K
jiǎo gǔ lán (绞股蓝), Herba Gynostemmatis Pentaphylli	AA
jú huā (菊花), Flos Chrysanthemi	BB
jué míng zǐ (决明子), Semen Cassiae	DA
shān zhā (山楂), Fructus Crataegi	H
yì yǐ rén (薏苡仁), Semen Coicis	FB
zé xiè (泽泻), Rhizoma Alismatis	FB
zǐ mù sù (紫苜蓿), Herba Medicago Sativa (alfalfa)	

Dispels phlegm and dampness, transforms turbidity, tonifies blood. Use to reduce elevated blood lipids including cholesterol and triglycerides.

Pulses: Normal, or wide and slippery
Tongue: Normal, or yellow coat

Comments: The Evergreen formula is a newer prescription for addressing elevated blood lipids, and is based on modern clinical research from China and Japan. It combines *shān zhā*, which addresses phlegm and food stasis, with herbs that dispel dampness (*cāng zhú, yì yǐ rén* and *zé xiè*) and herbs that move or tonify blood (*dān shēn, hé shǒu wū*). Herbs are included that have been shown in modern research to lower cholesterol, including *jué míng zǐ, hé yè, jú huā, jiǎo gǔ lán,* and *zǐ mù sù*. *Hǔ zhàng* reduces arterial wall inflammation.

Caution: *Dān shēn* is contraindicated in patients taking blood thinners such as Coumadin.

SHAN ZHA JIANG ZHI WAN

Formula: *shān zhā jiàng zhī wán* (山楂降脂丸)
"Crataegus Lower Lipids Pill"
Source: Modern patent medicine

Availability:

Shan Zha Jiang Zhi Wan (GC, HT, PM, TL)

Ingredients: (from Herbal Times *"Shan Zha Jiang Zhi Wan"*)

shān zhā (山楂), Fructus Crataegi	70.0 %	H
shén qū (神曲), Massa Medicata Fermentata	11.5	H
mài yá (麦芽), Fructus Hordei Germinatus	11.5	H
tián qī (田七), Radix/Rhizoma Notoginseng	7.0	J

Ingredients: (from Tanglong *"Shan Zha Jiang Zhi Wan"*)

shān zhā (山楂), Fructus Crataegi	23.1 %	H
dān shēn (丹参), Radix/Rhiz. Salviae Miltiorrhizae	23.1	K
hé shǒu wū (何首乌), Radix Polygoni Multiflori	23.0	AB
dà huáng (大黄), Radix/Rhizoma Rhei	15.4	PA
tiān kuí zǐ (天葵子), Radix Semiaquilegiae	15.4	DD

Dispels phlegm and dampness, transforms turbidity, tonifies blood. Use to reduce elevated blood lipids. Also useful in weight loss. Can be used for chronic food stagnation leading to fullness, belching and discomfort.

Pulses: Normal, or wide and slippery
Tongue: Normal, or yellow coat

Comments: The *Shan Zha Jiang Zhi Wan* formulas are based on recent Chinese research validating the effects of *shān zhā* in the lowering of blood lipids and triglycerides; they are quite popular in China for reducing cholesterol. In Herbal Times and most of the other versions, *shān zhā* accounts for 70% of the formula, and is reinforced with herbs to break food stasis and reduce blood fats (*shén qū* and *mài yá*). *Tián qī* takes the formula to the blood, and has it own beneficial effects in reducing cholesterol. This formula is also used to treat obesity, when combined with appropriate diet and exercise.

The Tanglong version, a different formula, uses 28% *shān zhā*, reinforced with 23% *dān shēn* to move blood and break stasis, and 23% *hé shǒu wū* to benefit the blood. *Dà huáng* and *tiān kuí zǐ* reduce inflammation in the blood vessels. Blood vessel inflammation aggravates atherosclerosis by allowing excess fats to be trapped during arterial repair and are transformed into plaque.

Caution: *Shén qū* contains a wheat binder and is contraindicated for people with celiac disease or gluten allergy.

OTHER FORMULAS APPROPRIATE FOR THIS CATEGORY:

Modern Formulas for heart blood stasis:

Zhong Guo Tong Xue Wan (China Tung Hsueh Pills)

See Chapter 4B

Other:

Cardioshen (HS)
Circulation (EV)
Cir-Q (HC)
Dry Ginger Tablets (SF)
Flavonex (HC)
Heart Clear (DR.KA)
Heart Pearls (CP)
Huo Xue Tong Mai Wan (TL)
Pomexcellent (HC)
Red Stirring (TT)
Rhodiola 8 (SF)
Salvia Shou Wu (SF)
Vitality Tablets (SF)

Modern Formulas for heart phlegm and blood lipids:

Astra Garlic (HC)
Jiang Dan Gu Chun Pian/Wan (GC)
Polilipid (HC)
Rhubarb Teapills (PF)

11. UROGENITAL DISORDERS

11A. URINARY DIFFICULTY AND PROSTATE SWELLING

Classical Formulas:

Bi Xie Fen Qing Yin — *bì xiè fēn qīng yǐn* (萆薢分清饮)

Modern Formulas:

Jie Jie Wan –1 (Kai Kit Pill) — *jiě jiē wán* (解结丸)

Urinary difficulty includes frequent, urgent, scanty or dribbling urination, as well as difficulty maintaining a stream. It incorporates the TCM disorders Urinary Disturbance (*lìn zhèng*, 淋证) and Retention of Urine (*lóng bì*, 癃闭). Urinary disturbance (*lìn zhèng*), sometimes called stranguria, basically means straining to urinate. Retention of urine (*lóng bì*) is characterized by diminished volume of urine, dribbling urination, and, in its extreme, inability to pass urine without accompanying pain.

In Chinese medicine, urinary difficulty is most often due to a deficiency of kidney *yang*, and the formulas in this chapter tonify kidney *yang* while restraining urine with astringent herbs. Symptoms may also be due to swollen prostate. In the elderly, failure to control urine may accompany a depletion of *jing* and *yang*. Supportive formulas can be found in *Chapter 17B.*

Urinary disturbance also includes bladder infections and stone blockage; these are discussed separately in *Chapter 11B. Bladder or Prostate Infection* and *Chapter 11D. Kidney Stone*. Other formulas for frequent urination are included in *Chapter 11C. Spermatorrhea and Urinary Incontinence.*

Chinese medicine distinguishes two types of **prostate swelling**, one due to excess and the other due to deficiency. The excess type is seen in acute prostatitis, and is discussed in Chapter *11B.* The deficiency type, discussed here, involves a benign, noncancerous, swollen prostate. Symptoms include a downward-bearing sensation or pain in the inguinal groin area, and frequency of urination with difficulty stopping the flow. In chronic cases of prostate swelling, laboratory values may show an elevated PSA (prostate specific antigen). Formulas presented here are effective for regulating urine, reducing swelling, and lowering the PSA value.

Classical Formulas:

BI XIE FEN QING YIN

Formula: *bì xiè fēn qīng yǐn* (萆薢分清饮)
"Dioscorea *Bi Xie* Separate (the) Clear Cool-Decoction"
Author: Wāng Áng (汪昂)
Source: *Yī Fāng Jí Jiě* (医方集解), 1682
Literal: "Medical Formulas Collected, Explained"

The formula is based on:

Formula: *bì xiè fēn qīng yǐn* (萆薢分清饮)
"Dioscorea *Bi Xie* Separate (the) Clear Cool-Decoction"
Author: Zhū Zhèn-Hěng (朱震亨) *aka* Zhū Dān-Xī (朱丹溪)
Source: *Dān Xī Xīn Fǎ* (丹溪心法), 1481
Literal: "Dan-Xi's Heart Method" (eg, "Personal Insights")

Availability:

Bi Xie Fen Qing Teapills (PF)
Bi Xie Fen Qing Wan (HT)
Bi Xie Fen Qing Yin (BP, PM)
Separate Clear and Turbid (TT)
Tokoro Combination (EG)

Ingredients: (from Herbal Times *"Bi Xie Fen Qing Wan"*)

bì xiè (萆薢), Rhizoma Dioscoreae Hypoglaucae	48.5 %	FC
gān cǎo (甘草), Radix Glycyrrhizae	24.2	AA
wū yào (乌药), Radix Linderae	12.1	G
shí chāng pú (石菖蒲), Rhizoma Acori Tatarinowii	9.1	M
yì zhì rén (益智仁), Fructus Alpiniae Oxyphyllae	6.1	AC

Ingredients: (from Plum Flower *"Bi Xie Fen Qing Teapills"*)

yì zhì rén (益智仁), Fructus Alpiniae Oxyphyllae	18.2 %	AC
fú líng (茯苓), Poria	18.2	FC
bì xiè (萆薢), Rhizoma Dioscoreae Hypoglaucae	18.1	FC
jīn qián cǎo (金钱草), Herba Lysimachiae	18.1	FC
wū yào (乌药), Radix Linderae	18.1	G
gān cǎo (甘草), Radix Glycyrrhizae	9.3	AA

Warms and benefits the kidney, dispels damp, dispels turbidity, stops pain. Use for urinary difficulty with cloudy urine (chyluria), frequent urination, difficulty starting or stopping the stream, urinary dribbling, and a distended sensation in the lower abdomen. Effective for chronic prostatitis or chronic cystitis. May be applied in leukorrhea (vaginal discharge) due to cold.

Pulse: Deep; may be soft or slippery
Tongue: Normal with thin white coat

Comments: This remedy treats urinary disorders due to deficiency-cold kidney patterns causing cloudy urine. It can be found in chronic prostatitis without infection or cold-damp leukorrhea. Zhu Dan-Xi (1481), commenting on the foundation formula, said that the urine of the patient would be "white as rice soup and thick as dilute paste", what is currently referred to as cloudy urine, chyluria or galacturia. *Bì xiè* resolves turbid dampness, and is the principal herb to resolve cloudy urine. *Wū yào* and *yì zhì rén* warm the bladder and kidney; *shí chāng pú* helps to transform turbid to clear, and to warm the bladder.

The original formula used four herbs in equal doses*: bì xiè, yì zhì rén, wū yào,* and *shí chāng pú*. The later formula from Wang Ang added *gān cǎo* and *fú líng*. The two versions represented here have been further adjusted. The version from Herbal Times increases *bì xiè* to 48.5% of the formula and *gān cǎo* at 24%, but removes *fú ling*. This enrichment of *bì xiè* addresses the primary symptom of cloudy urine. The version from Plum Flower retains equal dosing of the original ingredients, but uncharacteristically adds *jīn qián cǎo*, a cold herb normally used to treat urinary calculi.

Bi Xie Fen Qing Yin should not be confused with *Bi Xie Sheng Shi Wan*, found in *Chapter 11B*. The latter is used for prostate or urinary tract infection.

Further Reading:

Bensky et al, p. 751
Chen & Chen, p. 1140
Ellis, p. 30

Modern Formulas:

JIE JIE WAN (1)
KAI KIT PILL

Formula: *jiě jiē wán* (解结丸), "Relieve Knotty-Swelling Pill"
Origin: Modern patent medicine

Availability:

Kai Kit Pill (PM)
Kai Kit Wan (PF)
Prostate Gland Pills (PM)

Ingredients: (from Plum Flower "*Kai Kit Wan*". The current formula is proprietary. The ingredient percentages listed are from an earlier version, which may be the same. It is similar to Guangzhou First Chinese Medicine Factory "Prostate Gland Pills")

wáng bù liú xíng (王不留行), Semen Vaccariae	16. %	K
bài jiàng cǎo (败酱草), Herba Patriniae	16	DD
chì sháo (赤芍), Radix Paeoniae Rubra	12	K
huáng qí (黄芪), Radix Astragali	12	AA
mǔ dān pí (牡丹皮), Cortex Moutan	10	DC
mù tōng (木通), Caulis Akebiae	10	FC
tǔ mù xiāng (土木香), Radix Inulae	8	G
yán hú suǒ (延胡索), Rhizoma Corydalis	8	K
gān cǎo (甘草), Radix Glycyrrhizae	8	AA

Ingredients: (from Hanyang Pharmaceutical Works, Hubei *"Kai Kit Pill"*)

shú dì huáng (熟地黄), Radix Rehmanniae Praep.	20. %	AB
huáng qí (黄芪), Radix Astragali	20	AA
dǎng shēn (党参), Radix Codonopsis	20	AA
nǚ zhēn zǐ (女贞子), Fructus Ligustri Lucidi	10	AD
huái niú xī (怀牛膝), Radix Achyranthis Bidentatae	5	K
dān shēn (丹参), Radix/Rhiz. Salviae Miltiorrhizae	5	K
zé xiè (泽泻), Rhizoma Alismatis	5	FC
tù sī zǐ (菟丝子), Semen Cuscutae	5	AC
sāng piāo xiāo (桑螵蛸), Oötheca Mantidis	5	L
chē qián cǎo (车前草), Herba Plantaginis	5	FC

Tonifies qi, invigorates blood, benefits the movement of urine, resolves swelling and dissipates masses, clears heat and resolves toxins. Use for chronic swollen prostate due to deficiency, with symptoms of downward inguinal sensation, and difficult or painful urination with urinary dribbling or urinary retention. Also applicable in chronic prostatitis, and leukorrhea due to both cold-damp or heat-toxins.

Pulse: Normal, or wide and slippery
Tongue: Normal, or pale or dark

Comments: The "*Kai Kit*" products are popular in the Chinatown herb stores for treating swollen prostate. (*Kai kit* is the Cantonese pronunciation/spelling of *jiě jiē,* 解结). Each *Kai Kit* product, however, has a different formula, with slightly different applications. The two versions presented here are more applicable for chronic swollen prostate without acute infection.

The first is manufactured by Plum Flower, which copies the original formula from Guangzhou's *Prostate Gland Pills.* In the main, the formula is directed towards treating enlarged prostate affecting urination. *Wáng bù liú xíng, chì sháo* and *yán hú suǒ* are the primary ingredients to reduce swelling by moving blood, with *mù tōng* promoting normal urination. *Huáng qí* and *gān cǎo* boost spleen *qi* to raise clear fluid, while *mù tōng* directs the turbid fluid downwards. *Bái jiāng cán* is used to clear residual infectious toxins, and in this regard this product could be used for chronic prostate infection or damp-heat leukorrhea.

The second formula, Hanyang's *Kai Kit Pill,* is a very different formula, and does not contain any herbs to treat infection. This product is indicated for chronic swollen prostate due to deficiency of spleen *qi* and kidney *qi. Dǎng shēn* and *huáng qí* raise spleen *qi, shú dì huáng* benefits blood and *yin, tù sī zǐ* and *nǚ zhēn zǐ* tonify kidney *qi, huái niú xī* and *dān shēn* move blood, and *zé xiè* with *chē qián cǎo* benefit the movement of urine. *Sāng piāo xiāo,* the egg case of the praying mantis, inhibits urinary frequency and helps lead the formula to the prostate area.

Although having the same name, *Jie Jie Wan* (2) from Herbal Times (see *Chapter 11B*), is a different formula; it is indicated for acute prostatitis.

Caution 1: *Dān shēn* is used with caution with patients on blood thinners such as Coumadin. At 5% of the formula, this formula should not pose a risk.

Caution 2: *Wáng bù liú xíng* is contraindicated during pregnancy.

OTHER FORMULAS IN THIS CATEGORY:

Modern Formulas:

Consolidate Moisture (CMS)
Cuscuta 15 (SF)
Essence Chamber (HC)
Jade Chamber (BP)
P-Statin (EV)
Prostate Formula (DJ, GF)
Restore Integrity (K)
Saw Palmetto Complex (EV)
Unlocking the Gate (CMS)
Water Pearls (CP)

For hernia and testicular swelling:

Ji Sheng Ju He Wan

Ji Sheng Ju He Wan (MS, PM, TL)

11B. BLADDER OR PROSTATE INFECTION

Classical Formulas:

Ba Zheng San	*bā zhèng sǎn* (八正散)

Modern Formulas:

Bi Xie Sheng Shi Wan	*bì xiè shèng shī wán* (萆薢胜湿丸)
Jie Jie Wan (2)	*jiě jiē wán* (解结丸)
Qian Lie Xian Wan	*qián liè xiàn wán* (前列腺丸)

Infections of the urinary bladder or prostate are included under the TCM category Urinary Disturbance (*lìn zhèng*, 淋证) with the differentiation of damp-heat in the lower *jiao*. In both bladder infection and acute prostatitis, there is burning urination that may include pus or blood, and the urine tends to be dark and odorous. Symptoms include frequent, scanty or dribbling urination. There may be pain in the inguinal, pubic or lumbar regions.

Kidney-bladder damp-heat is usually triggered by exogenous pathogens, but may have a root in internal heat generated from over-indulgence in spicy food, sugar or alcohol. Diagnosis of an infection can be confirmed with a urinary dipstick showing elevated leukocytes. While bladder and prostate infections are treated with antibiotics in modern medicine, the Chinese have created herbal formulas that are equally effective, with relief often obtained within twenty-four hours. The herbs used in the Chinese formulas clear heat and resolve toxin, and are effective at treating bacterial infection. For cases unresponsive to herbs after several days, or if migration into the kidney occurs, marked by fever and pain in the kidney region, pharmaceutical antibiotics are recommended.

Classical Formulas:

BA ZHENG SAN

Formula: *bā zhèng sǎn* (八正散), "Eight Corrections Powder"
Author: Imperial Medical Bureau (*tài yī jú*, 太医局);
revised by Chén Shī-Wén (陈师文)
Source: *Tài Píng Huì Mín Hé Jì Jú Fāng* (太平惠民和剂局方), 1078
Literal: "(Era of) Great Peace, Benefit People Harmonious Medicines, Office (of) Formulas"

Availability:

Ba Zheng San (BP, PM, TZ)
Ba Zheng Wan (HT, TL)
Dianthus Formula (EG)
Eight Righteous Teapills (PF)
Relieving Formula (K)
Urinary Health (JD)
* Akebia Moist Heat (HC)
* Polyporus & Dianthus Formula (GF)
* Pyrrosia 14 (SF)

Ingredients: (from the standardized *"Dianthus Formula"*)

qú mài (瞿麦), Herba Dianthi	11.5 %	FC
biǎn xù (萹蓄), Herba Polygoni Avicularis	11.5	FC
chē qián cǎo (车前草), Herba Plantaginis	11.5	FC
gān cǎo (甘草), Radix Glycyrrhizae	11.5	AA
zhī zǐ (栀子), Fructus Gardeniae	11.5	DA
mù tōng (木通), Caulis Akebiae	11.5	FC
dà huáng (大黄), Radix/Rhizoma Rhei	11.5	PA
huá shí (滑石), Talcum	11.5	FC
dēng xīn cǎo (灯心草), Medulla Junci	8.0	FC

Clears heat, dispels damp, benefits the movement of urine, relieves pain. Use for acute urinary tract infections due to exogenous or endogenous factors, with symptoms of dark, turbid or bloody urine, pain during urination, scanty or frequent urination, and lower back pain. Also for strangury (frequent, difficult or painful urination) due to damp-heat. Also used in acute kidney and bladder infections, glomerulonephritis, cystitis and acute prostatitis.

Pulse: Slippery, rapid
Tongue: Yellow, greasy coat

Comments: This is the formula of choice for the treatment of acute bladder infection. It is also effective for early stage kidney infection, as a formula to prevent bladder infections from reaching the kidney, and can also treat acute prostatitis. The herbs in this formula go directly to the kidney and bladder, and have strong properties against heat, damp-heat and bacterial heat toxins. These herbs include *qú mài, biǎn xù, zhī zǐ, dà huáng and huá shí.* The herbs *chē qián cǎo, dēng xīn cǎo* and *mù tōng* benefit the movement of water.

Caution 1: Not recommended for long-term use; the cold nature of the herbs can injure *yang* and *qi*. If the symptoms are not relieved in 36 hours, consider pharmaceutical antibiotics.

Caution 2: *Dà huáng* is prohibited during pregnancy.

Further Reading:

Bensky et al, p. 713
Chen & Chen, p. 1103
Ellis, p. 11

Modern Formulas:

BI XIE SHENG SHI WAN

Formula: *bì xiè shèng shī wán* (萆薢胜湿丸)
"Dioscorea *Bi Xie* Victory (Over) Dampness Pill"
Source: Modern patent medicine

Availability:

Bi Xie Sheng Shi Wan (PM)
Subdue The Dampness Teapills (PF)

Ingredients: (from Plum Flower *"Subdue the Dampness Teapills"*)

yì yǐ rén (薏苡仁), Semen Coicis	16.2 %	AC
fú líng (茯苓), Poria	12.8	FC
bì xiè (萆薢), Rhizoma Dioscoreae Hypoglaucae	10.9	FC
bái xiān pí (白鲜皮), Cortex Dictamni	10.9	DD
tōng cǎo (通草), Medulla Tetrapanacis	10.9	FC
huáng bǎi (黄柏), Cortex Phellodendri	10.9	DB
zé xiè (泽泻), Rhizoma Alismatis	9.8	FC
mǔ dān pí (牡丹皮), Cortex Moutan	8.8	DC
zhī zǐ (栀子), Fructus Gardeniae	8.8	DA

Dispels damp-heat, disperses swelling, clears heat, resolves toxin, cools blood. Use for painful, burning or difficult urination, or vaginal or penile discharge. Use for acute or chronic urinary tract infection, prostatitis, vaginitis, and discharge due to venereal disease. Can also be used for acute skin inflammations marked by raised wheals, weeping or greasy exudate, redness and itching, particularly rashes in the groin or anus.

Pulse: Wiry or slippery, rapid
Tongue: Swollen, red with yellow coat

Comments: This formula treats damp-heat discharge from the penis or vagina due to local infection, including bacterial or fungal infection, and is useful for irritation or infection following catheterization of the penis. It is appropriate for acute prostatitis or urinary tract infection. The formula can also be used for rashes found in the groin due to venereal disease.

61% of the herbs dispel damp (*yì yǐ rén, fú líng, bì xiè, tōng cǎo, zé xiè*), while the remaining 39% clear heat (*bái xiān pí, huáng bǎi, mǔ dān pí, zhī zǐ*).

JIE JIE WAN (2)

Formula: *jiě jiē wán* (解结丸), "Relieve Knotty-Swelling Pill"
Origin: Modern patent medicine

Availability:

Jie Jie Wan (HT)

Ingredients: (from Herbal Times *"Jie Jie Wan"*)

shí wéi (石韦), Folium Pyrrosiae	27. %	FC
jīn qián cǎo (金钱草), Herba Lysimachiae	23	FC
huáng qí (黄芪), Radix Astragali	7	AA
é zhú (莪术), Rhizoma Curcumae	7	K
sān léng (三棱), Rhizoma Sparganii	7	K
tōng cǎo (通草), Medulla Tetrapanacis	7	FC
dà huáng (大黄), Radix/Rhizoma Rhei	4	PA
tǔ xiāng rú (土香薷), Herba Origanum vulgare	4	DE
chē qián cǎo (车前草), Herba Plantaginis	4	FC
yán hú suǒ (延胡索), Rhizoma Corydalis	4	K
hǎi jīn shā (海金沙), Spora Lygodii	4	DD
gān cǎo (甘草), Radix Glycyrrhizae	2	AA

Clears heat, resolves toxins, frees and benefits the movement of urine, invigorates blood, tonifies qi, stops pain. Use for acute or chronic prostatitis or bladder infection with symptoms of swelling, painful urination, urinary pus, urinary dribbling or retention, distended sensation in the lower abdomen or testicular pain.

Pulse: Thin, wiry, rapid
Tongue: Normal, or red with a yellow coat in the back of the tongue

Comments: This formula addresses acute and chronic prostate infection, although it can also be used to treat a bladder infection. The lead herbs, *shí wéi* and *jīn qián cǎo*, make up 50% of the formula, and they aggressively clear damp-heat while regulating urination. The formula is reinforced with herbs to move blood and break blood stasis, including *é zhú* and *sān léng*, which helps reduce swelling. *Tǔ xiāng rú*, the leaf of the oregano plant, plus *dà huáng*, are used to clear heat-toxin. *Hǎi jīn shā* is specific for treating painful urination due to damp-heat. *Tōng cǎo* and *chē qián cǎo* promote the free flow of urine. *Huáng qí* boosts the *wei qi* to help support the immune system, and also, with *gān cǎo* raises spleen *qi* in order to separate the clear from the turbid.

Although having the same name, *Jie Jie Wan* (1) (Kai Kit Pills), offered by Plum Flower and described in Chapter 11A, is a different formula; it is indicated for chronic swollen prostate without infection.

Caution: *É zhú, sān léng* and *dà huáng* are contraindicated during pregnancy, and for patients taking blood thinners such as Coumadin.

QIAN LIE XIAN WAN

Formula: *qián liè xiàn wán* (前列腺丸), "Prostate Pill"
Source: Modern patent medicine

Availability:

Prostate Gland Care (PM)
Qian Lie Xian Wan (HT, PM, TL)

Ingredients: (from Herbal Times' *"Qian Lie Xin Wan"* and Tanglong *"Qian Lie Xian Pian"*)

huáng qí (黄芪), Radix Astragali	17. %	AA
bì lì (薜荔), Fructus Ficus Pumilae	15	AC
huáng băi (黄柏), Cortex Phellodendri	13	DB
liăng tóu jiān (两头尖), Rhizoma Anemones Raddeanae	13	FA
pú gōng yīng (蒲公英), Herba Taraxaci	13	DD
zé lán (泽兰), Herba Lycopi	13	K
chē qián căo (车前草), Herba Plantaginis	10	FC
hŭ pò (琥珀), Succinum	6	N

Clears heat, resolves toxins, frees and benefits the movement of urine, invigorates blood, raises spleen qi, stops pain. Use for acute or chronic prostatitis with symptoms of swelling, painful urination, urinary pus, urinary dribbling or retention, distended sensation in the lower abdomen or testicular pain. Can also be used for acute bladder infection or testicular infection.

Pulse: Thin, wiry, rapid
Tongue: Normal, or red with a yellow coat in the back of the tongue

Comments: This formula is indicated for chronic prostate infection with swelling and pain, and can also be used for chronic urinary tract infections. It includes herbs to dispel dampness and swelling, combined with herbs to clear heat and resolve toxin. One of the main herbs is *bì lì*, not well known medicinally, but commonly used in China for a fruit jelly. It is used to tonify the kidney, astringe discharge, and reduce swelling. *Zé lán* helps promote urination, and it is also useful for reducing painful swelling. It is reinforced by *chē qián cǎo* to drain dampness, and *hǔ pò* to relieve swelling. *Huáng bǎi* and *pú gōng yīng* are used to clear heat and resolve toxin. *Liǎng tóu jiān,* another uncommon herb, reduces swelling by addressing phlegm and infectious abscesses. *Huáng qí* boosts the *wei qi* to help support the immune system, and also raises spleen *qi* in order to separate the clear from the turbid.

OTHER FORMULAS IN THIS CATEGORY:

Classical Formulas:

zhu ling tang

Polyporus Combination (EG)
Polyporus Formula (HS)

Modern Formulas:

Kidney DTX (EV)
Qian Lie Shu Pian (GC)
Rabdosia Prostate Formula (GF)
San Jin Pian/Wan (GC)

11C. SPERMATORRHEA AND URINARY INCONTINENCE

Classical Formulas:

Jin Suo Gu Jing Wan	*jīn suǒ gù jīng wán* (金锁固精丸)
Sang Piao Xiao San	*sāng piāo xiāo sǎn* (桑螵蛸散)

Spermatorrhea includes spontaneous erection with ejaculation of semen, spontaneous le*aka*ge of semen without erection, and nocturnal emission (wet dream). One or two instances of spermatorrhea per month are considered normal in young adult males. It is considered pathological with episodes occurring more than twice per week, or when spontaneous seminal discharge is accompanied by dizziness, listlessness, poor concentration, weak lower back and legs, palpitations or insomnia. **Urinary incontinence**, usually seen in the elderly, responds to the formulas described in this section. It indicates an urgency to urinate, or an inability to terminate the urine stream.

In Chinese medicine, spermatorrhea or urinary incontinence, in the absence of prostate or testicular disease, is due to a weakness of kidney *qi* and its failure to astringe and secure *jing*. Both disorders can result from emotional stress, overindulgent sexual activity, or weakened kidney energy with adrenal fatigue. In most cases, a heart and kidney imbalance ensues, with kidney deficiency precipitating heart excess. The disorders may be due to lowered *mingmen* and kidney *yang* function alone, without heart involvement.

The formulas in this chapter astringe and consolidate *jing* by using astringent herbs, and addresses heart-kidney imbalance. They may not correct other underlying imbalances, including deficiency of kidney *yin*, deficiency of kidney *yin* with fire, deficiency of kidney *yang,* exhaustion of *jing* and *yang,* or descent of damp-heat into the lower *jiao.* Refer to the appropriate chapters for treating the root cause:

- 7C. Liver-Gallbladder Damp-Heat and Fire.
- 8E. Menopausal Disorder and Deficiency Fire
- 17A. Kidney *Yin* Tonics
- 17B. Kidney *Yang* and *Jing* Tonics

Classical Formulas:

JIN SUO GU JING WAN

Formula: *jīn suǒ gù jīng wán* (金锁固精丸), "Golden Lock Consolidate *Jing* Pill"
Author: Wāng Áng (汪昂)
Source: *Yī Fāng Jí Jiě* (医方集解), 1682
Literal: "Medical Formulas Collected, Explained"

Availability:

Golden Lock Teapills (PF)
Jin Suo Gu Jing Tang (TZ)
Jin Suo Gu Jing Wan (MS, PM, TL)
Lotus Stamen Formula (EG)

Ingredients: (from the standardized *"Lotus Stamen Formula"*)

lián zǐ (莲子), Semen Nelumbinis	20. %	L
qiàn shí (芡实), Semen Euryales	20	L
lián xū (莲须), Stamen Nelumbinis	20	L
mǔ lì (牡蛎), Concha Ostreae	20	N
shā yuàn zǐ (沙苑子), Semen Astragali Complanati	10	AC
lóng gǔ (龙骨), Os Draconis	10	N

Ingredients: (from Minshan *"Jin Suo Gu Jing Wan"* and Plum Flower "*Golden Lock Teapills*")

lián zǐ (莲子), Semen Nelumbinis	33.3 %	L
qiàn shí (芡实), Semen Euryales	16.7	L
lián xū (莲须), Stamen Nelumbinis	16.7	L
shā yuàn zǐ (沙苑子), Semen Astragali Complanati	16.7	AC
duàn mǔ lì (煅牡蛎), Concha Ostreae Praeparatum	8.3	N
duàn lóng gǔ (煅龙骨), Os Draconis Praeparatum	8.3	N

Consolidates jing, benefits and consolidates the kidneys, astringes urine. Use for male sexual dysfunction causing nocturnal emission, spermatorrhea, or premature ejaculation due to deficiency of kidney *qi*. Accompanying symptoms may include lower back pain, fatigue, tinnitus or palpitation. Can be used as an astringent for urinary dribbling or frequency, leukorrhea (vaginal discharge), excessive sweating, diarrhea and pediatric enuresis. Also useful for treating swollen prostate.

Pulses: Normal, or thready and feeble
Tongue: Pale with white coat

Comments: This formula is intended for nocturnal emission (wet dream) and spermatorrhea (unintentional le*aka*ge of semen); it can also used for urinary dribbling or frequency. It is somewhat helpful for ejaculation control recommended in Daoist sexual practices. It can be taken alone, or combined with a root treatment for nocturnal emission, which includes deficiency of kidney *yang*, deficiency of *jing* or deficiency of kidney *yin*. (See the appropriate chapters.)

The original formula used baked or calcined *mŭ lì* and *lóng gŭ*, which is followed in the Minshan and Plum Flower versions (but not the standardized Taiwan formulas). This allows those substances to act as astringents, adding to the other astringent herbs *lián zĭ*, *qiàn shí*, and *lián xū*.

In cases of nocturnal emission accompanied by night sweats, combine with *Zhi Bai Di Huang Wan* or *Da Bu Yin Wan* (Chapter 8E).

Further Reading:

Bensky et al, p. 435
Chen & Chen, p. 789
Ellis, p. 168

SANG PIAO XIAO SAN

Formula: *sāng piāo xiāo sǎn* (桑螵蛸散), "Mantidis Powder Pills"
Author: Kòu Zōng-Shì (寇宗奭)
Source: *Běn Cǎo Yǎn Yì* (本草衍义), 1116
Literal: "Materia Medica Extended Meanings"

Availability:

Mantis Cocoon Formula (EG)
Mantis Cradle Teapills (PF)
* Restore Integrity (K)

Ingredients: (from the standardized *"Mantis Cocoon Formula"*)

rén shēn (人参), Radix Ginseng	12.5 %	AA
rén shēn (茯神), Sclerotium Poriae Pararadicis	12.5	N
yuǎn zhì (远志), Radix Polygalae	12.5	N
sāng piāo xiāo (桑螵蛸), Oötheca Mantidis	12.5	L
lóng gǔ (龙骨), Os Draconis	12.5	N
zhì guī bǎn (炙龟板), Plastrum Testudinis/Chinemys	12.5	AD
dāng guī (当归), Radix Angelicae Sinensis	12.5	AB
shí chāng pú (石菖蒲), Rhizoma Acori Tatarinowii	12.5	M

Ingredients: (from Plum Flower *"Mantis Cradle Teapills"*)

lóng gǔ (龙骨), Os Draconis	28.5 %	N
zhì guī bǎn (炙龟板), Plastrum Testudinis/Chinemys	14.0	AD
sāng piāo xiāo (桑螵蛸), Oötheca Mantidis	11.5	L
rén shēn (人参), Radix Ginseng	11.5	AA
fú shēn (茯神), Sclerotium Poriae Pararadicis	11.5	N
shí chāng pú (石菖蒲), Rhizoma Acori Tatarinowii	8.5	M
dāng guī (当归), Radix Angelicae Sinensis	8.5	AB
yuǎn zhì (远志), Radix Polygalae	6.0	N

Settles the heart, calms shen, harmonizes heart and kidney, consolidates jing, astringes urine. Use for or nocturnal emission or spermatorrhea (le*aka*ge of sperm) due to poor interaction between heart and kidney. The formula can also be used for frequent urination, urinary incontinence, and pediatric enuresis (bed-wetting). Other symptoms may include insomnia, poor memory, fatigue and palpitation, weak limbs, and tinnitus.

Pulse: Thin or weak pulse
Tongue: Pale

Comments: This formula is indicated for heart and kidney failing to interact, causing spermatorrhea, nocturnal emission, frequent urination or incontinence. *Lóng gǔ, zhì guī bǎn,* and *sāng piāo xiāo* are astringent herbs and make up half of the formula, while the remaining herbs (*rén shēn, dāng guī, shí chāng pú* and *yuǎn zhì*) tonify heart *qi* and blood. *Sāng piāo xiāo*, the egg case of the praying mantis, is the principal herb. It tonifies kidney, while *lóng gǔ* calms and settles disturbed *shen*.

The formula was originally used for excessive sexual activity leading to le*aka*ge of sperm, premature ejaculation, disorientation, and fatigue. It is now commonly used in pediatric enuresis, and urinary incontinence in the elderly.

Further Reading:

Bensky et al, p. 436
Chen & Chen, p. 792
Ellis, p. 254

OTHER FORMULAS APPROPRIATE FOR THIS CATEGORY:

Classical Formulas:

Huan Shao Dan
See Chapter 18A

Jin Gui Shen Qi Wan
See Chapter 17B

Wu Zi Yan Zong Wan
See Chapter 17B

You Gui Wan
See Chapter 17B

Modern Formulas:

Cong Rong Bu Shen Wan
See Chapter 17B

Ge Jie Bu Shen Wan
See Chapter 17B

Ge Jie Da Bu Wan
See Chapter 17B

Gui Ling Ji (*Kwei Ling Chi*)
See Chapter 17B

Gui Zhi Jia Long Gu Mu Li Tang
Cinnamon & Dragon Bone Combination (EG)
Cinnamon D Formula (GF)
Cinnamon Twig Decoction Plus Dragon Bone and Oyster Shell (AL)
Gui Zhi Jia Long Gu Mu Li Tang (TZ)

Ren Shen Bu Wan (Ginseng Tonic Capsules)
See Chapter 18A

Ren Shen Lu Rong (Ginseng Deer Horn)
See Chapter 18A

Other:
Lotus Nourishing Formula (K)

For spermatorrhea:

He Shou Wu (*hé shǒu wū,* 何首乌*,* Radix Polygoni Multiflori)
See Chapter 16B

11D. KIDNEY STONE

Modern Formulas:

Pai Shi Wan (Passwan) *pái shí wán* (排石丸)

In TCM, chronic damp-heat in the kidney or bladder causes the formation of stones (calculi). Modern medicine attributes it to an oxalate-rich diet, reduced fluid intake, and genetic proclivity. Stones have sharp fin-like protrusions, which damage tissue and cause bleeding. When stones are large enough (>3mm), they can block vessels draining the kidney, causing the kidney to enlarge. This causes acute and unrelenting pain, which does not dissipate until the stone can pass from the kidney into the urinary bladder. Occasionally, a bladder stone can block the urethra, causing distending pain of the bladder. Symptoms usually begin as occasional pains over the kidney region in the back. As the kidney swells, pain may radiate to the costal or abdominal areas, or in the inguinal area. In cases where kidney stone is suspected, a urine dipstick will reveal blood. Medical confirmation includes a CT scan or MRI.

Chinese medicine does not distinguish calcium oxalate from uric acid or struvite stones; all are treated the same. The synergistic combination of *jīn qián cǎo* (金钱草, Herba Lysimachiae) and *hǎi jīn shā* (海金沙, Spora Lygodii) can dissolve stones; the formulas include herbs to fight inflammation and stop bleeding. In cases of acute stone impaction, taking the herbal formula every 2-3 hours helps smooth and reduce the size of the stone, allowing it to pass.

An acupuncture protocol using micro-amp or milli-amp electric-stim can help dilate and vibrate the ureter, allowing the stone to pass. The points used are BL 23 (*shèn shū*, 肾俞) and BL 52 (*zhì shì*, 志室) (using the closest *ā shì* point), plus SP 6 (*sān yīn jiāo*, 三阴交) and KI 5 (*shuǐ quán*, 水泉), all on the affected side. Cable pairs connect an upper and lower point, with treatments 20-40 minutes long, twice daily. Often one treatment will allow passage of the stone. Some large stones may require 3 days of treatment.

Patients with a tendency towards urinary stones are advised to take a stone formula 5-7 days per month as a preventative, or at least 2-3 times a year. Chinese *tui na* therapy also recommends pounding the upper back with closed fists every day to keep casts and debris from accumulating in the renal tubes.

Modern Formulas:

PAI SHI WAN
PASSWAN

Formula: *pái shí wán* (排石丸), "Discharge Stone Pill"
Origin: Modern patent medicine

Availability:

Amber Stone Formula (GF)
Specific Passwan (PM)
Specific Drug Passwan (PM)

Ingredients: (from Guang Xing Tang Pharmaceutical, Guangzhou *"Specific Passwan"*)

jīn qián cǎo (金钱草), Herba Lysimachiae	25.0 %	FC
hǎi jīn shā (海金沙), Spora Lygodii	20.0	DD
bái zhǐ (白芷), Radix Angelicae Dahuricae	10.0	BA
chuān xīn lián (穿心莲), Herba Andrographis	10.0	DD
huái niú xī (牛膝), Radix Achyranthis Bidentatae	7.5	K
dà huáng (大黄), Radix/Rhizoma Rhei	5.0	PA
wǔ zhǐ máo táo (五指毛桃), Radix Ficus Simplicissima	5.5	FA
niú dà lì (牛大力), Radix Millettia Speciosae	5.0	DD
hǔ pò (琥珀), Succinum	5.0	N
tián qī (田七), Radix/Rhizoma Notoginseng	3.0	J
Other	4.0	

Ingredients: (from Golden Flower *"Amber Stone-Transforming Formula"*)

jīn qián cǎo (金钱草), Herba Lysimachiae	15 %	FC
hǎi jīn shā (海金沙), Spora Lygodii	15	DD
bái máo gēn (白茅根), Rhizoma Imperatae	12	J
shí wéi (石韦), Folium Pyrrosiae	12	FC
jin yín huā (金银花), Flos Lonicerae Japonicae	9	DD
jī xuè téng (鸡血藤), Caulis Spatholobi/Millettiae	8	K
qú mài (瞿麦), Herba Dianthi	7	FC
hǔ pò (琥珀), Succinum	7	N
huá shí (滑石), Talcum	7	FC

Expels stones, dispels damp heat, moves qi, clears heat and resolves toxins, invigorates blood, stops bleeding, frees the stool, relieves pain. Use for acute and chronic kidney and bladder stone attacks, with symptoms of lower back pain and pressure which may radiate through or around to the naval area, and hematuria.

Pulse: Forceful
Tongue: Normal, possible coating in back

Comments: These formulas dissolve stones, reduce bleeding, and reduce inflammation. In acute blockage, it is necessary to take frequently and in larger amounts, but it can actually dissolve the stone enough to allow passage. For patients with a history of repeat kidney stones, doing a course for three or four days once a month, or one week courses 3 times per year, can prevent stone formation.

The synergistic combination of *jin qián cǎo* and *hǎi jīn shā* is effective for dissolving stones. The first formula, the original *Passwan*, lists *jin qián cǎo* at 25% of the formula and *hǎi jīn shā* at 20%. The Golden Flower version has a combined percentage of 30% for these two herbs. Supportive herbs in both formulas stop bleeding, move blood, dispel damp-heat and clear inflammation.

Both formulas are also useful following shock wave lithotripsy, which breaks stones into smaller particles. This procedure can injure the kidney and ureter, and the *Pai Shi* formulas can help repair the tissues, and stop bleeding and inflammation.

Caution: *Huái niú xī, dà huáng* and *ji xuè téng* are contraindicated during pregnancy. *Jī xuè téng* is contraindicated for patients of blood thinners including Coumadin.

OTHER FORMULAS APPROPRIATE FOR THIS CATEGORY:

Modern Formulas:

- Dissolve KS (EV)
- Jin Qian Cao Stone Formula (HC)
- Li Niao Pai Shi Pian/Wan (GC)
- Lysimachia 3 (SF)
- San Jin Pian/Wan (GC)
- Stone Formula (PF)

12. WATER RETENTION AND EDEMA

Classical Formulas:

Fang Ji Huang Qi Tang	*fáng jǐ huáng qí tāng* (防己黄芪汤)
Wu Ling San	*wǔ líng sǎn* (五苓散)
Wu Pi Yin	*wǔ pí yǐn* (五皮饮)
Zhen Wu Tang	*zhēn wǔ tāng* (真武汤)

Water retention and edema (*shuī zhǒng* 水肿 or *zhèng shuǐ* 正水) indicates accumulation of fluid in the body causing swelling of the eyelids, face, limbs, trunk, or the entire body. It can be due to exogenous pathogenic factors including exposure to wind and damp, or involve internal disorders of the lung, spleen or kidney, particularly the kidney. In some cases, there may be an obstruction of the water passages of the *san jiao* by stagnant blood.

The formulas in this category act as diuretics. The Chinese use the expression *lǐ shuǐ xiāo zhǒng* (理水消肿): "benefit (the movement of) water, reduce swelling". They do not act harshly on the kidney like pharmaceutical diuretics, yet can be as effective with the correct dosage.

Edema is a common symptom of many diseases of modern medicine including congestive heart failure, kidney disease, endocrine disease and ascites due to liver disease. Swelling can be found in trauma and arthritis-rheumatism, as well as post-surgery, particularly the removal of lymph glands in breast cancer procedures. These formulas may be used alone, or adjunctively with other prescriptions for the underlying cause in order to reinforce a diuretic effect. For edema in the limbs, combining with appropriate formulas for treating wind-damp *bi* syndrome is beneficial (see *Chapter 4A*).

All four formulas in this chapter date back to the second century CE, indicative perhaps of the prevalence of wind-damp swelling due to exposure to the elements with underlying deficiencies of *zong* and *wei qi.* Their continued usage is a testament to their efficacy.

Quick Comparison:

Fang Ji Huang Qi Tang	Mild, chronic edema
Wu Ling San	Acute or stubborn edema
Wu Pi Yin	Mild, chronic edema
Zhen Wu Tang	Mild, chronic edema

Classical Formulas:

FANG JI HUANG QI TANG

Formula: *fáng jǐ huáng qí tāng* (防己黄芪汤), "Stephania, Astragalus Decoction"
Author: Zhāng Zhòng-Jǐng (张仲景)
Source: *Jīn Guì Yào Lüè* (金匮要略), 220
Literal: "Golden Cabinet Essential Summary"

Availability:

Fang Ji Huang Qi Tang (TZ)
Stephania & Astragalus Combination (EG)
Stephania & Astragalus Teapills (PF)
Stephania and Astragalus (HS)

Ingredients: (from the standardized *"Stephania & Astragalus Combination"*)

hàn fáng jǐ (汉防己), Radix Stephaniae Tetrandrae	26.7 %	FC
huáng qí (黄芪), Radix Astragali	26.7	AA
bái zhú (白术), Rhizoma Atractylodis Macrocephalae	20.0	AA
zhì gān cǎo (炙甘草), Radix Glycyrrhizae Praep.	13.2	AA
shēng jiāng (生姜), Rhizoma Zingiberis Recens	6.7	BA
dà zǎo (大枣), Fructus Jujubae	6.7	AA

Ingredients: (from Plum Flower *"Stephania & Astragalus Teapills"*)

huáng qí (黄芪), Radix Astragali	38.2 %	AA
hàn fáng jǐ (汉防己), Radix Stephaniae Tetrandrae	19.9	FC
bái zhú (白术), Rhizoma Atractylodis Macrocephalae	13.2	BA
dà zǎo (大枣), Fructus Jujubae	10.1	AA
shēng jiāng (生姜), Rhizoma Zingiberis Recens	10.1	BA
gān cǎo (甘草), Radix Glycyrrhizae	8.5	AA

Dispels damp, tonifies spleen, benefits the movement of water, dispels wind and dampness, disperses swelling. Use to dispel dampness found in edema, ascites, watery diarrhea, and wind-damp *bi* syndromes. Symptoms include heaviness in the limbs and a superficial edema that comes and goes. Useful in chronic nephritic edema, arthritis with swelling, edema during pregnancy, congestive heart disease, and early ascites due to liver cirrhosis. Good for swelling of the knee or ankle.

Pulse: Floating, or wide
Tongue: Pale, may be swollen, with a white coat

Comments: This formula was originally developed for superficial edema due to deficiency of *wei qi* with susceptibility to wind. It is also used for edema associated with pregnancy and liver disease. It is particularly suited to edema in the ankles and knees.

Most of the formula is used to build genuine *qi* in order to dispel pathogenic *qi. Hàn fáng jǐ* drains dampness in the lower limbs and lower *jiao*. The formula can be used alone or to augment other formulas when treating swollen joints in arthritis and rheumatism. In systemic cases with edema, combine with *Wu Ling San*, below.

Further Reading:

Bensky et al, p. 735
Chen & Chen, p. 1118
Ellis, p. 95

WU LING SAN

Formula: *wŭ líng săn* (五苓散), "Five (ingredients) Poria Powder"
Author: Zhāng Zhòng-Jĭng (张仲景)
Source: *Shāng Hán Lùn* (伤寒论), 220
Literal: "Injury (by) Cold, Discussion"

Availability:

Drain Dampness (HC)
Poria/Hoelen Five Herb Formula (EG)
Poria Five Formula (GF)
Water's Way (K)
Wu Ling San (BP, PM, TL, TZ)
Wu Ling San Wan (PF)
Wu Ling Wan (HT)

Ingredients: (from the standardized *"Poria/Hoelen Five Herb Formula"*)

zé xiè (泽泻), Rhizoma Alismatis	26.7 %	FC
fú líng (茯苓), Poria	20.0	FC
zhū líng (猪苓), Polyporus	20.0	FC
bái zhú (白术), Rhizoma Atractylodis Macrocephalae	20.0	AA
guì zhī (桂枝), Ramulus Cinnamomi	13.3	BA

Dispels damp, dispels wind, benefits the movement of water, benefits kidney and spleen, warms yang, disperses swelling. Use to dispel damp found in edema, ascites, and watery diarrhea; also for wind-damp *bi* syndromes characterized by heaviness of the limbs. Symptoms may include headache, dizziness, shortness of breath, difficulty urinating, or watery stool. Applicable for water accumulation due to kidney or heart disease including congestive heart failure, nephritis, edema during pregnancy and abdominal ascites due to liver cirrhosis.

Pulse: Thin or wide, weak, floating or deep
Tongue: Normal, or pale or watery, with white coat

Comments: This *Shang Han Lun* prescription treats accumulation of water in the limbs, joints, organs and digestive tract. Zhang Zhong-Jing originally indicated it for wind invasions that had penetrated to the bladder, causing "water rebellion": water retention with vomiting of fluids. In the modern clinic, it is the most effective of the herbal diuretics, for both the abdominal cavity and limbs. The principal herbs, *zé xiè, fú líng*, and *zhū líng,* are strong diuretics, and make up 67% of the standardized formula. If spleen *qi* deficiency with damp is present, one might combine with *Fang Ji Huang Qi Tang,* above.

Besides edema of the limbs and abdomen, *Wu Ling San* is also being used for the treatment of headache in chronic fatigue syndrome, where the headache is due to slight swelling in the brain. In functional medicine terms, the formula also assists the kidney in drainage of accumulated toxins.

Further Reading:

Bensky et al, p. 724
Chen & Chen, p. 1109
Ellis, p. 325

WU PI YIN

Formula: *wǔ pí yǐn* (五皮饮), "Five Peel Cool-Decoction"
Author: Huà Tuó (华佗)
Source: *Zhōng Zàng Jīng* (中藏经), 2nd C.
Literal: "Central Depository Classic"

Availability:

Five Peel Teapills (PF)
Poria/Hoelen & Areca Combination (EG)
Wu Pi Wan (HT)
Wu Pi Yin Wan (TL)

Ingredients: (from Herbal Times *"Wu Pi Wan"*)

dà fù pí (大腹皮), Pericarpium Arecae	23. %	G
fú líng pí (茯苓皮), Pericarpium Poria	23	FC
sāng bái pí (桑白皮), Cortex Mori	23	CC
chén pí (陈皮), Pericarpium Citri Reticulatae	16	G
shēng jiāng pí (生姜皮), Pericarpium Zingiberis Recens	15	E

Ingredients: (from Plum Flower *"Five Peel Teapills"* and Tanglong "*Wu Pi Yin Wan*")

fú líng (茯苓), Poria	20. %	FC
zé xiè (泽泻), Rhizoma Alismatis	20	FC
sāng bái pí (桑白皮), Cortex Mori	20	CC
shēng jiāng (生姜), Rhizoma Zingiberis Recens	20	E
bǎi biǎn dòu (百扁豆), Semen Dolichos/Lablab Album	10	DF
chén pí (陈皮), Pericarpium Citri Reticulatae	10	G

Ingredients: (from KP *"Poria and Areca Combination"*)

wǔ jiā pí (五加皮), Cortex Acanthopanacis	20. %	FA
dì gǔ pí (地骨皮), Cortex Lycii	20	DE
fú líng (茯苓), Poria	20	FC
dà fù pí (大腹皮), Pericarpium Arecae	20	G
shēng jiāng (生姜), Rhizoma Zingiberis Recens	20	E

Dispels damp, benefits the movement of water, benefits kidney, warms and tonifies spleen, benefits (movement of) water and disperses swelling. Use to dispel wind-damp edema with heavy, swollen joints, or abdominal ascites. Also for labored breathing due to accumulation of fluid in the lungs. Useful in edema during pregnancy, liver cirrhosis and congestive heart failure.

Pulse: Thin or wide, weak, floating or deep
Tongue: Normal, or pale or watery, with white coat

Comments: This prescription, one of the earliest recorded herbal formulas, treats accumulation of water in the skin, limbs and joints, as well as the lungs. The original formula uses the skin (*pí, 皮*) of the medicinal plants, which better facilitates treating superficial edema in the limbs and over the abdomen. Herbal Times and the standardized versions from the Taiwan manufacturers (EG) follow the original formula.

Curiously, KP's version is a variation, containing only 3 herbs of the original formula, but then using *wǔ jiā pí* (五加皮, Cortex Acanthopanacis). The Plum Flower version includes 4 of the basic 5 herbs of the formula, and adds *zé xiè* and *bǎi biǎn dòu* to reinforce the effect. The applications of the formula are the same.

Further Reading:

Bensky et al, p. 732
Chen & Chen, p. 1121

ZHEN WU TANG

Formula: *zhēn wǔ tāng* (真武汤), "True Warrior Decoction"
Author: Zhāng Zhòng-Jǐng (张仲景)
Source: *Shāng Hán Lùn* (伤寒论), 220
Literal: "Injury (by) Cold, Discussion"

Availability:

Ginger, Aconite, Poria & Peony Combination (KP)
Ginger, Aconite, Hoelen & Peony Combination (EG)
True Warrior Formula (K)
True Warrior Teapills (PF)
Vitality Combination (EG)
Zhen Wu Tang (BP, HT)
* Vitality-GC Tablets (SF)

Ingredients: (from the standardized *"Ginger, Aconite, Poria/Hoelen & Peony Combination"*)

fú líng (茯苓), Poria	25.0 %	FC
bái sháo (白芍), Radix Paeoniae Alba	25.0	AB
shēng jiāng (生姜), Rhizoma Zingiberis Recens	25.0	BA
bái zhú (白术), Rhizoma Atractylodis Macrocephalae	16.7	AA
zhì fù zǐ (炙附子), Radix Aconiti Lateralis Praeparata	8.3	E

Ingredients: (from Herbal Times *"Zhen Wu Wan"*)

bái zhú (白术), Rhizoma Atractylodis Macrocephalae	25. %	BA
fú líng (茯苓), Poria	25	FC
zhì fù zǐ (炙), Radix Aconiti Lateralis Praeparata	20	E
bái sháo (白芍), Radix Paeoniae Alba	15	AB
shēng jiāng (生姜), Rhizoma Zingiberis Recens	15	BA

Warms spleen and kidney yang, dispels damp, benefits the movement of urine, invigorates blood and fluids. Use for deficiency of spleen and kidney *yang* leading to water retention, urinary difficulty, or watery diarrhea. Also for heavy limbs, swollen joints, or heavy abdominal distension with pain. Applicable in edema, congestive heart failure, chronic nephritis, liver cirrhosis, ascites, and wind-damp arthritis. Also for dizziness and vertigo due to retention of dampness.

Pulse: Deep, thin or wide, weak
Tongue: Pale or dark, may be wet or with a white coat

Comments: *Zhen Wu Tang* treats chronic accumulation of damp due to deficiency of *yang*. It is applicable in edema, swollen joints, ascites and congestive heart failure. In China it is commonly used for congestive heart failure, chronic kidney disease, and to aid in nutritional absorption when the intestines have water, indicated by loose stool. It had also been used to treat Meniere's disease. *Zhen Wu*, translated as "True Warrior", is the name of the legendary Chinese god of water.

The Herbal Times and Plum Flower versions, compared to the standardized Taiwan versions, have a significantly higher amount of *zhì fù zǐ*, an herb that strongly warms *yang* in order to dispel dampness.

Caution: *Zhì fù zǐ* is used with caution during pregnancy.

Further Reading:

Bensky et al, p. 744
Chen & Chen, p. 1135
Ellis, p. 404

OTHER PRODUCTS APPROPRIATE FOR THIS CATEGORY:

Classical Formulas:

Jin Gui Shen Qi Wan
See *Chapter 16B.*

Modern Formulas:

Alisma 16 (SF)
Lotus 9 (SF)
Purge Moisture (CMS)
Siler Tablets (SF)

13. DERMATOLOGICAL DISORDERS

13A. SKIN RASHES
(Acne, Eczema, Urticaria)

Classical Formulas:

Dang Gui Yin Zi	*dāng guī yǐn zǐ* (当归饮子)
Lian Qiao Bai Du Pian	*lián qiào bài dú piān* (连翘败独片)
Xiao Feng San	*xiāo fēng sǎn* (消风散)

Modern Formulas:

Hua She Jie Yang Wan (Kai Yeung Pill)	*huā shé jiě yǎng wán* (花蛇解痒丸)
Zhen Zhu An Zhuang Wan	*zhēn zhū ān chuāng wán* (珍珠暗疮丸)

For clinical purposes, we can divide common skin rashes into three categories: acne, eczema and urticaria.

Acne is characterized by raised red or white pimples, either in isolation or grouped along areas of the forehead, cheeks, chin, chest and upper back. The pimples form in hair follicle sebaceous glands. It is common among teenagers, although serious cases may persist well into the adult years. Modern medicine recognizes the role of hormonal changes as well as a diet rich in sweets and poor quality oils. Also, weak digestion can play a role in the incomplete digestion of foods, ultimately affecting the skin.

In Chinese, acne is is called *fěn cì* (粉刺), literally, "chalky thorns" based on the appearance of the white-head pustules. Differential diagnosis includes blood heat, liver heat, stomach heat, lung heat and damp-heat toxin with blood stasis. Usually, it is treated symptomatically with products that clear blood heat, but in stubborn cases attention should be given to the root pattern.

In acne, it is important to stay away from foods that aggravate heat and dampness; these include alcohol, oils, fats and sugars. For teenagers especially, care should be taken to avoid sugary soft drinks, processed cheeses, and oily or fried foods including French fries, cheeseburgers and pizza.

Eczema (*shī chuāng*, 湿疮) is a reddish inflammation of the skin, and can appear greasy or dry; heat is involved in all cases, which produces itching. Cases are differentiated as damp-heat or dry-heat, one with raised swellings and the other with flaking.

In functional and modern medicine, eczema is due to a combination of genetic and environmental factors. Environmental factors include a poor diversity of intestinal bacteria, and the presence of food triggers, particularly gluten grains, dairy, soybean products or eggs. Here, the reaction actually starts in the epithelia of the small intestine, and formulas that go to the skin also go to the "internal skin" of the small intestine. Ultimately, identification and avoidance of the food allergies is important for true control.

Some cases of eczema may be due to fungal infections of the skin, particularly Candida albicans. These present as a itching with dry skin, and include blood-dryness.

Urticaria, or acute hives, is due to damp-heat in the blood. The term *má zhěn* (麻疹) is applied to any skin condition showing raised wheals with itching, and is used for urticaria, but can also apply to pediatric heat-toxin illnesses such as chicken pox, measles or rubella. Itching hives can be due to contact with toxic plants such as poison ivy, or reactions to certain foods, particularly shellfish, or reactions to chemicals, including pharmaceutical drugs. The colder formulas can also be used for acute herpes zoster (shingles).

All skin rashes require herbs that dispel wind (in order to bring the formula to the surface), clear blood heat, and then mediate dampness or dryness. Chronic presentations also require tonification of *qi* and blood. In cases with hardenings, as found in chronic cystic acne, dispelling blood stasis is required. Skin rashes due to heat-toxins, such as impetigo, measles, chicken pox, etc, will include herbs that clear heat and resolve toxin.

The formulas of this chapter can be applied in psoriasis, an autoimmune condition, by addressing damp-heat and blood stasis. These cases are more stubborn then typical skin conditions.

Itching dry skin can be due to deficiency of *qi* and blood. Supportive formulas can be found in *Chapters 16B. Blood Tonics* and *16C. Qi and Blood Tonics.*

Quick Reference:

Dang Gui Yin Zi	Chronic dryness
Lian Qiao Bai Du Pian	Acute heat
Xiao Feng San	Acute wind-heat
Hua She Jie Yang Wan	Itching skin
Zhen Zhu An Zhuang Wan	Acne, or acute heat

Classical Formulas:

DANG GUI YIN ZI

Formula: *dāng guī yǐn zǐ* (当归饮子), "Angelica *Dang Gui* Drink"
Author: Yán Yòng-Hé (严用和)
Source: *Jì Shēng Fāng* (济生方), 1253
Literal: "Aid (the) Living Formulas"

Availability:

Dang Gui Yin Zi (BP)
Luminescence (K)
Nourish the Surface Teapills (PF)
Tangkuei & Tribulus Combination (EG)

Ingredients: (from Plum Flower *"Nourish the Surface"*)

dāng guī (当归), Radix Angelicae Sinensis	18.2 %	AB
shēng dì huáng (生地黄), Radix Rehmanniae	17.1	DC
chuān xiōng (川芎), Rhizoma Ligustici Chuanxiong	10.9	K
fáng fēng (防风), Radix Saposhnikov./Ledebouriellae	10.9	BA
bái sháo (白芍), Radix Paeoniae Alba	10.9	AB
bái jí lí (白蒺藜), Fructus Tribuli	10.9	O
hé shǒu wū (何首乌), Radix Polygoni Multiflori	6.9	AB
huáng qí (黄芪), Radix Astragali	5.1	AA
jīng jiè (荆芥), Herba Schizonepetae	5.1	BA
gān cǎo (甘草), Radix Glycyrrhizae	4.0	AA

Ingredients: (from the standardized *"Tangkuei & Tribulus Combination"*)

dāng guī (当归), Radix Angelicae Sinensis	11.1 %	AB
shēng dì huáng (生地黄), Radix Rehmanniae	11.1	DC
bái sháo (白芍), Radix Paeoniae Alba	11.1	AB
chuān xiōng (川芎), Rhizoma Ligustici Chuanxiong	11.1	K
hé shǒu wū (何首乌), Radix Polygoni Multiflori	11.1	AB
jīng jiè (荆芥), Herba Schizonepetae	11.1	BA
fáng fēng (防风), Radix Saposhnikov./Ledebouriellae	11.1	BA
bái jí lí (白蒺藜), Fructus Tribuli	11.1	O
huáng qí (黄芪), Radix Astragali	5.6	AA
gān cǎo (甘草), Radix Glycyrrhizae	5.6	AA

Tonifies blood, boosts qi, moistens dryness, invigorates blood, dispels wind, calms shen, relieves itching. Use for skin itching due to deficiency of *qi* and blood withs blood dryness. Symptoms include dry, scaly or thickened skin, dry hair and pale complexion. Can be used for neurodermatitis, dry eczema, alopecia, ichthyosis, and chronic psoriasis.

Pulse: Weak, floating
Tongue: Pale

Comments: This formula treats itching due to blood dryness. The foundation formula is *Si Wu Tang* (Chapter 16B), which boosts blood, and consists of *dāng guī, dì huáng, bái sháo* and *chuān xiōng*. *Shēng dì huáng* is preferred to *shú dì huáng* because it is more cooling and moistening to the *yin* aspect of the skin. In the Taiwan standardized products, *Si Wu Tang* accounts for 44% of the prescription. In the Plum Flower version, *Si Wu Tang* makes up 68% of the prescription. The addition of *jīng jiè* and *fáng fēng* takes the formula to the surface, namely the skin, while *bái jí lí* relieves itching.

The formula is appropriate for long-term usage, and is often used after heat stages have been cleared with other formulas.

Caution: *Bái jí lí* is contraindicated during pregnancy.

Further Reading:

Bensky, p. 639
Chen & Chen, p. 970
Ellis, p. 78

LIAN QIAO BAI DU PIAN

Formula: *lián qiào bài dú piān* (连翘敗毒片), "Forsythia Defeat Toxin Tablet"
Author: Anonymous, possibly Táo Huá, 陶华
Source: *Shāng Hán Quán Shēng Jí* (伤寒全生集), 1445
Literal: "Injury (by) Cold, Complete Health Collection"

Availability:

Lian Qiao Bai Du Pian (PM, PF)
Lienchiaopaitu Pien (PM)

Ingredients: (from Tianjin Drug Manufactory *"Lienchiaopaitu Pien"*)

lián qiào (连翘), Fructus Forsythiae	13.8 %	DD
dà huáng (大黄), Radix et Rhizoma Rhei	13.8	PA
bái jí lí (白蒺藜), Fructus Tribuli	13.8	DD
zhī zǐ (栀子), Fructus Gardeniae	10.4	DA
huáng qín (黄芩), Radix Scutellariae	10.4	DB
bái xiān pí (白鲜皮), Cortex Dictamni	10.4	DD
chì sháo (赤芍), Radix Paeoniae Rubra	10.4	K
fáng fēng (防风), Radix Saposhnikov./Ledebouriellae	10.4	BA
chán tuì (蝉蜕), Periostracum Cicadae	6.7	BB

Ingredients: (from Plum Flower *"Lian Qiao Bai Du Pian"*)

lián qiào (连翘), Fructus Forsythiae	7.8 %	DD
jīn yín huā (金银花), Flos Lonicerae Japonicae	7.8	DD
dà huáng (大黄), Radix et Rhizoma Rhei	7.8	PA
pú gōng yīng (蒲公英), Herba Taraxaci	5.9	DD
zǐ huā dì dīng (紫花地丁), Herba Violae	5.9	DD
bái xiān pí (白鲜皮), Cortex Dictamni	5.9	DD
huáng qín (黄芩), Radix Scutellariae	5.9	DB
chì sháo (赤芍), Radix Paeoniae Rubra	5.8	K
fáng fēng (防风), Radix Saposhnikov./Ledebouriellae	5.8	BA
zhè bèi mǔ (浙贝母), Bulbus Fritillariae Thunbergii	5.8	CB
jié gěng (桔梗), Radix Platycodonis	5.8	CA
bái zhǐ (白芷), Radix Angelicae Dahuricae	5.8	BA
xuán shēn (玄参), Radix Scrophulariae	4.1	DC
mù tōng (木通), Caulis Akebiae	4.1	G
gān cǎo (甘草), Radix Glycyrrhizae	4.1	AA
tiān huā fěn (天花粉), Radix Trichosanthis	3.9	CB
zhī zǐ (栀子), Fructus Gardeniae	3.9	DA
chán tuì (蝉蜕), Periostracum Cicadae	3.9	BB

Dispels wind, clears heat, resolves toxin, clears and discharges damp-heat, disperses swelling, cools blood. Use for acute skin inflammation marked by redness, heat and itching, including urticaria (allergic hives), boils, rash, hives, poison ivy, and carbuncles with pus. Can be used for herpes zoster, herpes simplex and impetigo. In the pediatric presentations of chicken pox, measles, roseola, rubella and mumps, the formula can be combined with *Yin Qiao San* (Chapter 1B).

Pulse: Floating, excess
Tongue: Red or red tip, yellow coat

Comments: This formula addresses skin itching due to heat in the blood, and is commonly used for acute eczema or urticaria. The use of cold anti-microbial herbs also makes it appropriate for the treatment of impetigo, measles, chicken pox, herpes zoster, rubella and roseola, as septicemia from infected wounds. All of the herbs in this formula are cool or cold, and act quickly to reduce itching and redness due to heat.

The original patent medicine, from Tianjin, contains 9 herbs, 7 of which are quite cold. The amount of *dà huáng* is high (almost 14%) and can lead to loose stools. The Plum Flower version is a larger formula with 18 herbs. It includes all of the original herbs (with the exception of *bái jí lí*), and a smaller amount of *dà huáng* (8%). Additions include herbs to enhance clearing of damp-heat, herbs to clear heat toxins, and others.

Caution: *Dà huáng, tiān huā fěn* and *bái jí lí* are prohibited during pregnancy. Also, reduce dosage if diarrhea or loose stool develops.

Further Reading:

Chen & Chen, p. 1331

XIAO FENG SAN

Formula: *xiāo fēng sǎn* (消风散), "Disperse Wind Powder"
Author: Chén Shí-Gōng (陈实功)
Source: *wài kē zhèng zōng* (外科正宗), 1617
Literal: "External Medicine True Lineage"

Availability:

Derma Wind Release (K)
Great Windkeeper Teapills (PF)
Tangkuei & Arctium Formula (EG)
Xiao Feng Pian (GC)
Xiao Feng San (BP, PM, TZ)
Xiao Feng San Wan (TL)
Xiao Feng Wan (HT)

Ingredients: (from the standardized "*Tangkuei & Arctium Formul*a")

jīng jiè (荆芥), Herba Schizonepetae	8.3 %	BA
fáng fēng (防风), Radix Saposhnikov./Ledebouriellae	8.3	BA
dāng guī (当归), Radix Angelicae Sinensis	8.3	AB
shēng dì huáng (生地黄), Radix Rehmanniae	8.3	DC
kǔ shēn (苦参), Radix Sophorae Flavescentis	8.3	DB
cāng zhú (苍术), Rhizoma Atractylodis	8.3	FB
chán tuì (蝉蜕), Periostracum Cicadae	8.3	BB
huǒ má rén (火麻仁), Fructus Cannabis	8.3	PB
niú bàng zǐ (牛蒡子), Fructus Arctii	8.3	BB
zhī mǔ (知母), Rhizoma Anemarrhenae	8.3	DA
shí gāo (石膏), Gypsum Fibrosum	8.3	DA
gān cǎo (甘草), Radix Glycyrrhizae	4.4	AA
mù tōng (木通), Caulis Akebiae	4.3	FC

Disperses wind, eliminates damp, clears heat, cools blood, relieves itching. Use for skin itching due to wind-dampness giving rise to wind toxins. Symptoms include red raised wheals, weepy skin lesions, or open sores with bleeding. Useful in weeping eczema, psoriasis, pruritus, dermatitis, allergic urticaria (hives), diaper rash and certain fungal infections. Also useful for rosacea and poison ivy.

Pulse: Floating, rapid, forceful
Tongue: White or yellow coat

Comments: This effective and popular formula addresses itching due to blood heat with wind-dampness. The formula is effective for allergic hives or eczema, and is also used for red rash, acne, and to a lesser extent, measles and chicken pox.

33% of the formula dispels wind (*jīng jiè, fáng fēng, chán tuì, niú bàng zǐ*), while 25% clears heat (*kǔ shēn, zhī mǔ, shí gāo*) and another 25% nourishes the blood and *yin* (*dāng guī, shēng dì huáng, huǒ má rén*).

Further Reading:

Bensky et al, p. 636
Chen & Chen, p. 967
Ellis, p. 348

Modern Formulas:

HUA SHI JIE YANG WAN
KAI YEUNG PILL

Formula *huā shé jiě yǎng wán* (花蛇解痒丸)
"Agkistrodon Relieve Itching Pill"
Source: Modern patent medicine

Availability:

Hua She Jie Yang Wan (PF, PM)
Jie Yang Wan (HT)
Kai Yeung Pill (PM)
* Dermatrol-Ps (EV)
* Zaocys Tablets (SF)

Ingredients: (from Hanyang Pharmaceutical *"Kai Yeung Pill"*)

bái huā shé (白花蛇), Agkistrodon bungarus	10. %	FA
rén shēn (人参), Radix Ginseng	10	AA
huáng qí (黄芪), Radix Astragali	10	AA
cāng zhú (苍术), Rhizoma Atractylodis	10	FB
chuān xiōng (川芎), Rhizoma Ligustici Chuanxiong	10	K
bái zhǐ (白芷), Radix Angelicae Dahuricae	10	BA
dāng guī (当归), Radix Angelicae Sinensis	10	AB
shé chuáng zǐ (蛇床子), Fructus Cnidii	10	R
fáng fēng (防风), Radix Saposhnikov./Ledebouriellae	5	BA
cāng ěr zǐ (苍耳子), Fructus Xanthii	5	FA
shēng dì huáng (生地黄), Radix Rehmanniae	5	DC
wū shāo shé (乌梢蛇), Zaocys dhumnades	5	FA

Ingredients: (from Herbal Times *"Jie Yang Wan"*)

wū shāo shé (乌梢蛇), Zaocys dhumnades	32. %	FA
bái xiān pí (白鲜皮), Cortex Dictamni	15	DD
huáng qín (黄芩), Radix Scutellariae	12	DB
fáng fēng (防风), Radix Saposhnikov./Ledebouriellae	10	BA
xuán shēn (玄参), Radix Scrophulariae	10	DC
chán tuì (蝉蜕), Periostracum Cicadae	8	BB
huáng bǎi (黄柏), Cortex Phellodendri	8	DB
dāng guī (当归), Radix Angelicae Sinensis	5	AB

Ingredients: (from Plum Flower *"Hua She Jie Yang Wan"*)

bái huā shé (白花蛇), Agkistrodon bungarus	10.0 %	FA
guī bǎn (龟板), Plastrum Testudinis/Chinemys *	10.0	AD
lù lù tong (路路通), Fructus Liquidambaris	9.5	K
cāng zhú (苍术), Rhizoma Atractylodis	7.0	FB
huáng qí (黄芪), Radix Astragali	6.0	AA
shé chuáng zǐ (蛇床子), Fructus Cnidii	6.0	R
wū shāo shé (乌梢蛇), Zaocys Dhumnades	6.0	FA
shēng dì huáng (生地黄), Radix Rehmanniae	6.0	DC
wū shāo shé (乌梢蛇), Zaocys dhumnades	6.0	FA
chuān xiōng (川芎), Rhizoma Ligustici Chuanxiong	5.0	K
rén shēn (人参), Radix Ginseng	5.0	AA
cāng ěr zǐ (苍耳子), Fructus Xanthii	5.0	FA
huáng bǎi (黄柏), Cortex Phellodendri	5.0	DB
dāng guī (当归), Radix Angelicae Sinensis	5.0	AB
bái zhǐ (白芷), Radix Angelicae Dahuricae	5.0	BA
rén gōng niú huáng (人工牛黄), Calculus Bovis Synth.	3.0	M
rén gōng shè xiāng (人工麝香), Moschus Syntheticum	0.5	M

* Plum Flower lists this as *Cao Gui*, Chinemys reevesii.

Dispels wind-damp, tonifies qi, nourishes blood, nourishes yin, invigorates blood, clears heat, dispels wind, generates tissue, relieves itching. Use for skin itching due to wind dryness damaging the blood, with symptoms of itching and dry flaky or red skin. Useful in eczema, allergic dermatitis, pruritus, allergic urticaria and certain fungal infections, including ringworm and scabies. Can be used for psoriasis and rosacea.

Pulse: Rapid, may be thin or slippery, floating
Tongue: Normal, or reddish with a yellow coat

Comments: The *Jie Yang* formulas (*kai yeung* in the Cantonese pronunciation/spelling) use various whole snakes as principal ingredients. The use of snake follows the "law of signatures": as a snake sheds its dry and old skin, use of these medicines can repair dry or damaged skin. Clinically, the medicinal use of snake is effective for treating itching with redness or dry scales.

Three versions of the formula are presented here. The original patent medicine *Kai Yeung Pills,* contains 12 herbs, with the snakes *bái huā shé* and *wū shāo shé* contributing 15% of the formula. Of the three formulas, it stands alone in devoting 20% of the formula to tonify *qi* (using *rén shēn* and *huáng qí*).

The version from Herbal Times, *Jie Yang Wan*, is the smallest of the formulas, having 8 herbs. The snake *wū shāo shé*, however, makes up 32% of the formula, with another 45% using heat-clearing herbs (*bái xiān pí, huáng qín, xuán shēn*, and *huáng bǎi*). *Chán tuì*, the sloughed shell of the cicada insect, also follows the law of signatures, by "sloughing off" old and impaired skin. It is the best of the three for heat presentations, but, lacking *shé chuáng zǐ*, is less effective for dry itching due to fungal infection.

The Plum Flower version, *Hua She Jie Yang Wan,* is a large formula, with 17 herbs. It contains three snakes - *bái huā shé, wǔ bù shé* and *wū shāo shé* (22%) - plus *guī bǎn,* the underbelly bones of the Chinese pond turtle, which nourishes *yin.* Including the snakes, 27% of the formula dispels wind-damp in order to relieve itching. Other herbs move blood (14%) and tonify *qi* (11%); only 5% clears heat (*huáng bǎi*).

Note: *Bái huā shé* (the poisonous Chinese krait snake), *wū shāo shé* (the non-poisonous Chinese rat snake) and *guī bǎn* (Chinemys reevesii, the Chinese pond turtle) are bred in captivity for food and medicinal purposes. Wild populations of Chinemys are listed as endangered.

Caution: Both *lù lù tong* and *guī bǎn*, ingredients in the Plum Flower version, are contraindicated during pregnancy. *Lù lù tong* is contraindicated for patients on blood thinners such as Coumadin.

ZHEN ZHU AN CHUANG WAN

Formula: *zhēn zhū ān chuāng wán* (珍珠暗疮丸), "Pearl Acne Pill"
Source: Modern patent medicine

Availability:

Clear Skin (JD)
Colorful Phoenix Pearl Combo (K)
Margarita Complexion Formula (GF)
Margarite Acne Pills (PF, PM)
Margarite Pills (PM)
Margarite Beauty Pills (HT)
Zhen Zhu An Chuang Wan (TL)

Ingredients: (from Herbal Times *"Margarite Beauty Pills"*)

zhēn zhū (珍珠), Margarita	8.5 %	N
bái xiān pí (白鲜皮), Cortex Dictamni	8.5	DD
bǎn lán gēn (板蓝根), Radix Isatidis	8.5	DD
shēng dì huáng (生地黄), Radix Rehmanniae	8.5	DC
huáng bǎi (黄柏), Cortex Phellodendri	8.5	DB
huáng qín (黄芩), Radix Scutellariae	8.5	DB
kǔ shēn (苦参), Radix Sophorae Flavescentis	8.5	DB
lián qiào (连翘), Fructus Forsythiae	8.5	DD
mǔ dān pí (牡丹皮), Cortex Moutan	8.5	DC
pú gōng yīng (蒲公英), Herba Taraxaci	8.5	DD
tǔ fú ling (土茯苓), Rhizoma Smilacis Glabrae	8.5	DD
lóng dǎn cǎo (龙胆草), Radix/Rhizoma Gentianae	6.5	DB

Ingredients: (from Plum Flower *"Margarite Acne Pills"*. The current formula is proprietary. The ingredient percentages listed have been previously published, and may be the same.)

jīn yín huā (金银花), Flos Lonicerae Japonicae	20. %	DD
shēng dì huáng (生地黄), Radix Rehmanniae	20	DC
hǎi dài cǎo (海带草), Herba Zosterae Marinae	20	CB
zhēn zhū (珍珠), Margarita	15	N
shuǐ niú jiao (水牛角), Cornu Bubali	15	DC
rén gōng niú huáng (人工牛黄), Calculus Bovis Synth.	10	M

Softens masses, clears heat, cools blood, resolves toxin, tonifies blood and yin. Use for blood heat with stasis causing acne, skin rash, or allergic hives. Can be applied to boils, hardened furuncles, and rosacea. Can also be used for eczema, psoriasis and hives. Can also be used in pediatric chicken pox, roseola and measles, as well as infected wounds. Use for skin conditions marked by heat and redness.

Pulse: Rapid, floating
Tongue: Red or reddish

Comments: There are numerous *Zhen Zhu An Chuang* formulas available, all of which feature *zhēn zhū* (powdered pearl) as a featured ingredient. *Zhēn zhū* is a heavy mineral substance that cools the blood, and is good for removing isolated red spots or pimples due to blood heat and inflammation. All versions contain herbs that clear heat, resolve toxins and cool blood heat.

Two versions are represented here, with somewhat different applications. The formula from Herbal Times, *Margarite Beauty Pills* (almost identical with the version from Tanglong, *Zhen Zhu An Chuang Wan*) contains herbs that clear heat and resolve toxin, or remove damp-heat. These account for 83% of the formula (the DD and DB herbs), making it a very cold formula. It is most appropriate for acne with pustular and inflamed heads, but the formula can also be used for eczema, psoriasis, acute hives, or infectious rash diseases like chicken pox or measles. It can also be used to treat infected wounds.

The second formula, from Plum Flower, addresses acne with hardened cysts (cystic acne). Several herbs clear heat in the surface: *jīn yín huā*, *shuǐ niú jiao* (water buffalo horn), *shēng dì huáng* and *rén gōng niú huáng*. *Hǎi dài cǎo* (kelp seaweed) breaks up cystic masses.

Caution: *Rén gōng niú huáng* is used with caution during pregnancy. Also, reduce dosage if diarrhea develops.

OTHER FORMULAS APPROPRIATE FOR THIS CATEGORY:

Classical Formulas:

Bi Xie Sheng Shi Wan
See *Chapter 11B*

Fang Feng Tong Shen San
See *Chapter 2B*

Shi Wei Bai Du Tang
Bupleurum & Schizonepeta Formula (EG)
Ten-Ingredient Detoxifying Formula (HS)

Modern Formulas:

Coix Tablets (SF)
Dr. Shen's Complexion Pills (DS)
Fire Fighter (GW)
Kochia 13 (SF)
Lonicera 13 (SF)
Plantago Seed Tablets (SF)
Quell the Surface Teapills (PF)
Red Peony Tablets (SF)
Siler & Coix Clearing Formula (K)
Silerex (EV)
Skin Balance (HC)
Ten-Ingredient Detoxifying Formula (HS)
Wind Pearls (CP)

Formulas for Topical Application:

Antifungal Ointment (BP)
Chapped Nipple Ointment (BP)
Ching Wan Hong (PM) (See *Chapter 5B*)
Clear Heat Ointment (BP)
Eczema Ointment (BP)
Jade Dew Ointment (BP)
Pearl Cream (PM)
Psoriaquell Ointment (BP)
Spring Wind Ointment (SE/GF)
Stop Itching Tincture (BP)
Tamu Oil (HC)

13. DERMATOLOGICAL DISORDERS

13B. HAIR LOSS
(Alopecia)

Classical Formulas:

Qi Bao Mei Ran Dan — *qī bǎo měi rán dān* (七宝美髯丹)

Modern Formulas:

Ban Tu Wan — *bān tū wán* (斑秃丸)

The formulas in this chapter are applicable for hair-loss disorders (alopecia). Alopecia can occur as patchy baldness on the scalp (alopecia areata), or involve all hair follicles on the body (alopecia universalis). The formulas are most commonly used for hair loss in women, which may be due to blood deficiency accompanying low thyroid or following childbirth; they are also appropriate for hair loss due to radiation or chemotherapy. The formulas are helpful in most cases, with the exception of alopecia universalis, which is an autoimmune disorder that has irreversibly destroyed hair follicles. The products may be helpful in male pattern baldness, although in this regard they are far less successful than in woman's hair loss.

In Chinese medicine, hair loss or patching is due to deficiency of blood, and the formulas are rich in blood tonics. The formulas also employ herbs to tonify kidney *qi*, acknowledging the Chinese medicine observation that kidney controls the hair of the head. It does this in its function of helping to create blood, as well as distribution of *qi* to the scalp via the Bladder channel. The formulas may include herbs that dispel wind-dryness, which affects both blood and scalp.

Other underlying causes may need to be addressed, including liver stagnation, blood stagnation, or deficiency of liver and kidney. Refer to the appropriate chapters. Additional formulas for treating blood deficiency can be found in *Chapters 16B. Blood Tonics,* and *16C. Qi and Blood Tonics.*

Classical Formulas:

QI BAO MEI RAN DAN

Formula: *qī bǎo měi rán dān* (七宝美髯丹)
"Seven Treasures Beautiful Hair Elixir"
Author: Wāng Áng (汪昂)
Source: *Yī Fāng Jí Jiě* (医方集解), 1682
Literal: "Medical Formulas Collected, Explained"
also attributed to:
Author: Lǐ Shí-Zhēn (李时珍) *aka* Lǐ Dōng-Bì (李东壁)
Source: *Běn Cǎo Gāng Mù* (本草纲目), 1578 or 1590
Literal: "Materia Medica Guiding Outline"

Availability:

He-Shou-Wu & Lycium Formula (EG)
Qi Bao Mei Ran Dan (GC, KP, PM)
Seven Treasures For Hair Teapills (PF)
Seven Treasures Formula (EG, GF)
Silken Tresses (K)

Ingredients: (from Plum Flower *"Seven Treasures for Hair Teapills"*)

hé shǒu wū (何首乌), Radix Polygoni Multiflori	42.1 %	AB
dāng guī (当归), Radix Angelicae Sinensis	10.6	AB
gǒu qǐ zǐ (枸杞子), Fructus Lycii	10.5	AB
huái niú xī (怀牛膝), Radix Achyranthis Bidentatae	10.5	K
fú líng (茯苓), Poria	10.5	FC
tù sī zǐ (菟丝子), Semen Cuscutae	10.5	AC
bǔ gǔ zhī (补骨脂), Fructus Psoraleae	5.3	AC

Ingredients: (from the standardized *"Seven Treasures Formula"*)

hé shǒu wū (何首乌), Radix Polygoni Multiflori	25.0 %	AB
dāng guī (当归), Radix Angelicae Sinensis	12.5	AB
gǒu qǐ zǐ (枸杞子), Fructus Lycii	12.5	AB
huái niú xī (怀牛膝), Radix Achyranthis Bidentatae	12.5	K
fú líng (茯苓), Poria	12.5	FC
tù sī zǐ (菟丝子), Semen Cuscutae	12.5	AC
bǔ gǔ zhī (补骨脂), Fructus Psoraleae	12.5	AC

Nourishes and invigorates blood, tonifies yin, tonifies kidney yang and qi, nourishes the liver. Use for deficiency of blood causing hair thinning, hair loss, patch balding with shiny bald spots, and for loss of other body hair. Other symptoms include dry skin, cracked fingernails, pale sclera and lips. Applicable for loss of hair due to postpartum, hypothyroid or following chemotherapy or radiation. Can also be used for blood deficiency causing dizziness, insomnia, fatigue, soreness in the muscles and limbs, and poor concentration.

Pulse: Normal, or thin or weak
Tongue: Pale

Comments: *Hé shǒu wū* is the principal herb to nourish the hair by enriching blood, supported by *dāng guī* and *gǒu qǐ zǐ*. In the Plum Flower version, *hé shǒu wū* comprises 42% of the formula, while the Taiwan formulas use 25%. Supportive herbs support the underlying kidney *yang* and *qi* deficiency: *tù sī zǐ, bǔ gǔ zhī* and *huái niú xī.*

Qi Bao Mei Ran Dan can be used following chemotherapy to boost liver *yin* and blood, and for hypothyroid due to deficiency of blood with deficiency of kidney *yang*.

Caution: *Huái niú xī* is contraindicated during pregnancy.

Further Reading:

Bensky et al, p. 409
Chen & Chen, p. 690
Ellis, p. 209

Modern Formulas:

BAN TU WAN

Formula: *bān tū wán* (斑秃丸), "Patchy Baldness Pill"
Source: Modern patent medicine

Availability:

Alopecia Areata Pill (PM)
Ban Tu Wan (PM)

Ingredients: (from Guang Dong Yi Kang Pharmaceutical *"Alopecia Areata Pill"*)

hé shǒu wū (何首乌), Radix Polygoni Multiflori	20. %	AB
shú dì huáng (熟地黄), Radix Rehmanniae Praep.	10	AB
shēng dì huáng (生地黄), Radix Rehmanniae	10	DC
dāng guī (当归), Radix Angelicae Sinensis	10	AB
dān shēn (丹参), Radix/Rhiz. Salviae Miltiorrhizae	10	K
bái sháo (白芍), Radix Paeoniae Alba	10	AB
wǔ wèi zǐ (五味子), Fructus Schisandrae	10	L
dǎng shēn (党参), Radix Codonopsis	10	AA
mù guā (木瓜), Fructus Chaenomelis	5	FA
qiāng huó (羌活), Radix Notopterygii	5	BA

Nourishes and moves blood, tonifies spleen qi, nourishes liver yin. Use for deficiency of blood causing hair loss and patch balding. Applicable for postpartum loss of hair and hair loss following chemotherapy or radiation. Can also be used for blood deficiency causing dizziness, insomnia, fatigue, soreness in the muscles and limbs, and poor concentration.

Pulse: Normal, or thin or weak
Tongue: Pale

Comments: This modern formula addresses hair loss by building blood, with 70% of the formula consisting of blood-building or blood moving herbs: *hé shǒu wū, shú dì huáng, dāng guī, bái sháo, shēng dì huáng,* and *dān shēn*. It differs from *Qi Bao Mei Ran Dan*, above, which also boosts kidney *qi*. Supportive herbs in this formula, instead, tonify spleen *qi* (*dǎng shēn*) while moving the formula throughout the scalp and skin (*mù guā* and *qiāng huó*).

OTHER FORMULAS APPLICABLE FOR THIS CATEGORY:

Modern Formulas:

sheng fa jiao nang

Sheng Fa Capsules (PM)
Sheng Fa Wan (PIM)
Yang Xue Sheng Fa Jiao Nang (PM)

Other:

Polygonum 14 (EV)
Shou Wu Pian - Foti Hair (GC)
Shou Wu Wan - Fo Ti Hair Tonic (TL)
Woman's Hair Formula (DR.J)

14. EYE AND VISION DISORDERS

Classical formulas:

Qi Ju Di Huang Wan	*qǐ jú dì huáng wán* (杞菊地黄丸)

Modern formulas:

Ming Mu Di Huang Wan	*míng mù dì huáng wán* (明目地黄丸)
Ming Mu Shang Qing Pian	*míng mù shàng qīng piān* (明目上清片)
Nei Zhang Yan Ming Wan	*nèi zhàng yǎn míng wán* (内障眼明丸)

Eye disorders have been a specialty in Chinese medicine at least as far back as the 13th century ("Secret Treatise on Eye Diseases, Long-Mu's Discussion", *Mì Chuán Yǎn Kē Lóng Mù Lùn*, 秘传眼科龙木论). A modern Chinese medicine clinical text on ophthalmology, in English, lists forty-one different conditions treatable with Chinese herbal medicine. (*Ophthalmology, Volume 17, English-Chinese Encyclopedia Of Practical Traditional Chinese Medicine*, Xu Xiangcai, Editor. Higher Education Press, Beijing, 1994.)

In Chinese medicine, eye disorders are divided between those due to deficiency or those due to excess. Deficiency presentations are rooted in liver and kidney function. Liver blood and *yin* moisten the eye (including the pure *yin* fluids of the center of the eye as well as the ability to produce tears), and kidney *yin* promotes liver *yin*. Absence of *yin* leads to dryness, blurry or poorly focused vision, atrophy, and hardening of the lens. Excess conditions are due to heat from liver or gallbladder fire, which also deplete *yin.* Symptoms include redness and burning, eye stye and hardening of the lens.

The formulas in this chapter tend to nourish liver *yin* or clear liver heat and fire; many treat root and branch simultaneously. The formulas are applicable for blurry vision, weakening of eyesight, dry eyes, photophobia (sensitivity to light), burning and redness, and eye stye. Some of the formulas are helpful for early stage cataracts, glaucoma, optic neuritis or degeneration. In serious or uncommon problems, one should seek out experienced herbal practitioners as well as medical ophthalmologists.

Quick reference of the formulas in this chapter:

Qi Ju Di Huang Wan	Dry eye, poor vision
Ming Mu Di Huang Wan	Glaucoma, dry eye, poor vision
Ming Mu Shang Qing Pian	Acute red eye and infectio
Nei Zhang Yan Ming Wan	Cataracts, chronic red eye

Classical Formulas:

QI JU DI HUANG WAN

Formula: *qǐ jú dì huáng wán* (杞菊地黄丸)
"Lycium, Chrysanthemum, Rehmannia Pill"
Author: Huá Shòu (滑寿)
Source: *Má Zhěn Quán Shū* (麻疹全书), circa 1350
Literal: "Measles Complete Treatise"
also attributed to:
Author: Wēi Yì-Lín (危亦林)
Source: *Shì Yī Dé Xiào Fāng* (世医得效方), 1345
Literal: "Generations (of) Physicians Obtained Effective Formulas"

Availability:

Lycii Chrysanthemum Teapills (PF)
Lycium & Rehmannia (CC)
Lycium Rehmannia Teapills (MS)
Lycium, Chrysanthemum & Rehmannia Formula (EG)
Qi Ju Di Huang Wan (BP, GC, HT, PM, TL, TZ)

Ingredients: (from the standardized *"Lycium, Chrysanthemum & Rehmannia Formula"*)

shú dì huáng (熟地黄), Radix Rehmanniae Praep.	27.7 %	AB
shān zhū yú (山茱萸), Fructus Corni	13.8	L
shān yào (山药), Rhizoma Dioscoreae	13.8	AA
fú líng (茯苓), Poria	10.3	FC
mǔ dān pí (牡丹皮), Cortex Moutan	10.3	DC
zé xiè (泽泻), Rhizoma Alismatis	10.3	FC
gǒu qǐ zǐ (枸杞子), Fructus Lycii	6.9	AB
jú huā (菊花), Flos Chrysanthemi	6.9	BB

Nourishes kidney yin, nourishes liver yin and blood, benefits the eyes. Use for deficiency of *yin* affecting the eyes causing dryness, blurry vision, and poor night vision. It is used for photophobia (sensitivity to light), early cataract, optic neuritis, retinal detachment, retinitis, and herpes simplex retinitis, and dry eyes due to Sjögren's syndrome. Can be used for dizziness, headaches, and hypertension due to deficiency of *yin*.

Pulse: Thin
Tongue: Normal, or dry

Comments: *Qi Ju Di Huang Wan* treats vision problems rooted in deficiency of liver *yin* without obvious signs of excess *yang* or heat. Symptoms include blurring of vision, or gradual weakening of eyesight. It is the formula of choice for dry eyes, especially when the patient relies on "liquid tears" type products.

This formula is a development of *Liu Wei Di Huang Wan* (1119), a foundation formula for treating deficiency of kidney *yin* (see Chapter 17A). Two herbs are added to the foundation prescription: *gǒu qǐ zǐ* moistens liver *yin* and benefits the eyes, while *jú huā* brings the formula upwards to the eyes and clears wind-heat affecting the eyes.

The idea of "brightening the eyes" involves clearing redness and dryness associated with heat. It also refers to enhancing vision, by nourishing *yin* that benefits the aqueous humor of the eye interior, as well as ability to produce tears to moisten the exterior of the eye. The formula may have been developed to address conjunctivitis and red eye associated with infectious measles.

Further Reading:

Bensky et al, p. 368
Chen & Chen, p. 640
Ellis, p. 210

Modern Formulas:

MING MU DI HUANG WAN

Formula: *míng mù dì huáng wán* (明目地黄丸)
"Brighten Eyes Rehmannia Pill"

Source: Modern patent medicine. Cited in:
Zhōng Huā Rén Mín Gòng Hé Guó Yào Diǎn (中华人民共和国药典), 2005
Literal: "People's Republic of China (Herbal) Medicine Compendium"

Availability:

Bright Eye Rehmannia (K)
Ming Mu Di Huang Teapills (PF)
Ming Mu Di Huang Wan (BP, GC, HT, MS, PIM, PM, TL)
Ming Mu Formula (GF)

Ingredients: (from Herbal Times *"Ming Mu Di Huang Wan"*)

shú dì huáng (熟地黄), Radix Rehmanniae Praep.	18.3 %	AB
shān yào (山药), Rhizoma Dioscoreae	9.1	AA
shān zhū yú (山茱萸), Fructus Corni	9.1	L
shí jué míng (石决明), Concha Haliotidis	9.1	O
bái jí lí (白蒺藜), Fructus Tribuli	6.8	O
bái sháo (白芍), Radix Paeoniae Alba	6.8	AB
dāng guī (当归), Radix Angelicae Sinensis	6.8	AB
fú líng (茯苓), Poria	6.8	FC
gǒu qǐ zǐ (枸杞子), Fructus Lycii	6.8	AB
jú huā (菊花), Flos Chrysanthemi	6.8	BB
mǔ dān pí (牡丹皮), Cortex Moutan	6.8	DC
zé xiè (泽泻), Rhizoma Alismatis	6.8	FC

Nourishes liver and kidney yin, nourishes liver blood, subdues yang, benefits the eyes. Use for eye conditions due to *yin* deficiency compounded with ascendant liver *yang* and deficiency of liver blood. Symptoms include glaucoma and early formation of cataracts, and can also be used for poor vision, night blindness, dry eyes, red and itchy eyes, photophobia, excessive tearing, dryness, or internal pressure. Can be used in chronic optic neuritis, retinitis and dry eyes due to Sjögren's syndrome. Also used for liver *yin* deficiency causing dizziness, tinnitus, and chronic night sweating.

Pulse: Thin; may be wiry or rapid
Tongue: Normal, or reddish with a dry coat

Comments: This modern formula is an enhancement of *Qi Ju Di Huang Wan* (above), adding in *dāng guī* and *bái sháo* to nourish liver blood, and *shí jué míng* and *bái jí lí* to settle ascendant liver *yang*. While addressing the same symptoms as *Qi Ju Di Huang Wan,* namely eye dryness and blurry vision, the enhancements also address glaucoma, pressure behind the eyes and early formation of cataracts. It is popular in China for treating early or moderate glaucoma. It cannot reverse cataracts, but may slow down their development.

***Note**:* A classical formula with the name *Ming Mu Di Huang Wan* exists in the literature, but has a very different formula. It is not available as a product. See Sheid, Bensky et al, p. 369-370.

Caution: *Bái jí lí* is contraindicated during pregnancy.

MING MU SHANG QING PIAN

Formula: *míng mù shàng qīng piān* (明目上清片)
"Brighten Eyes Upper Clearing Tablet"
Source: Modern patent medicine

Availability:

Ming Mu Shang Ching Pien (PM)
Ming Mu Shang Qing Pian (PM)

Ingredients: (from Great Wall Brand, Tianjin Drug Manufactory, "*Ming Mu Shang Ching Pien*")

zhī zǐ (栀子), Fructus Gardeniae	30.0 %	DA
dāng guī (当归), Radix Angelicae Sinensis	20.3	AB
huáng lián (黄连), Rhizoma Coptidis	6.4	DB
jú huā (菊花), Flos Chrysanthemi	6.4	BB
dà huáng (大黄), Radix/Rhizoma Rhei	6.4	PA
huáng qín (黄芩), Radix Scutellariae	6.4	DB
lián qiào (连翘), Fructus Forsythiae	4.0	DD
bái jí lí (白蒺藜), Fructus Tribuli	4.0	O
chán tuì (蝉蜕), Periostracum Cicadae	4.0	BB
mài mén dōng (麦门冬), Radix Ophiopogonis	4.0	AD
shí gāo (石膏), Gypsum Fibrosum	4.0	DA
chē qián cǎo (车前草), Herba Plantaginis	4.0	FC

Clears liver heat, resolves heat toxins, dispels wind, nourishes liver blood and yin, benefits eyes, stops pain. Use for acute eye infections marked by redness, burning, tearing, or producing exudate. Applicable for conjunctivitis, eye stye, and to promote healing in the area in or around the eye. Discontinue once infection and heat symptoms have cleared.

Pulse: Normal, or wiry, floating, rapid
Tongue: Normal, or reddish with a yellow coat

Comments: This extraordinary formula is the medicine of choice for red eye, conjunctivitis, and stye. It is applicable for red eye due to endogenous liver heat, as well as topical infection. It can also be used to clear sclera hemorrhage following trauma. Given its composition, it would also be appropriate for any localized infection of the face or head.

Heat-clearing herbs include *zhī zǐ, huáng lián, jú huā, dà huáng, huáng qín, lián qiào, chán tuì,* and *shí gāo*, and make up 68% of the formula. The lead herb, *zhī zǐ*, makes up 30%, and clears liver heat, the underlying source of most redness of the sclera and conjunctiva. Other herbs moisten liver blood and *yin* (*dāng guī, mài mén dōng*), clear wind-heat (*chán tuì*), and settle ascendant *yang* (*bái jí lí*). *Jú huā* takes the formula to the eyes. *Chē qián cǎo* helps lead heat downwards to be excreted in the urine.

Caution 1: Bacterial conjunctivitis is contagious, and sanitary precautions should be taken. Also, this formula is drying, and should not be used for the treatment of cataracts or chronic eye dryness.

Caution 2: *Dà huáng* and *bái jí lí* are contraindicated during pregnancy.

Caution 3: This formula is cold. Use only for duration of event involving heat, inflammation or infection. Discontinue or reduce dosage if epigastric pain or diarrhea occurs.

NEI ZHANG YAN MING WAN

Formula: *nèi zhàng yǎn míng wán* (内障眼明丸)
"Cataract Eye Brighten Pill"
Source: Modern patent medicine

Availability:

Tribulus & Chrysanthemum Combo (PM)
Vision A Formula (PM)

Ingredients: (from KGS *"Vision A Formula"*)

màn jīng zǐ (蔓荆子), Fructus Viticis	21.0 %	FA
bái jí lí (白蒺藜), Fructus Tribul	15.8	O
dāng guī (当归), Radix Angelicae Sinensis	15.8	AB
chuān xiōng (川芎), Rhizoma Ligustici Chuanxiong	15.8	K
jīng jiè (荆芥), Herba Schizonepetae	10.4	BA
jú huā (菊花), Flos Chrysanthemi	5.3	BB
bò hé (薄荷), Herba Menthae	5.3	BB
huáng lián (黄连), Rhizoma Coptidis	5.3	DB
tiān huā fěn (天花粉), Radix Trichosanthis	5.3	CB

Tonifies qi, nourishes blood and yin, clears heat, dispels wind, brightens the eyes. Use for cataract at the early and middle stages, as well as vision symptoms due to aging, including poor or blurred vision, myopia, and eyes strained from reading. Also applicable in eye disorders due to heat, including red eye, stye, or chronic eye inflammation. The formula can be used for retinal disorders including degeneration of the retina and recovery from eye surgery.

Pulse: Normal, or thin, floating
Tongue: Normal, or thin dry coat

Comments: This modern formula is intended to stop or slow further development of cataracts, and therapy should begin as early as possible. Cataracts are due to deficiency of liver *yin* or blood with excessive heat, which dry out the surface of the eye. This formula inhibits cataract development by nourishing *yin* and blood and clearing heat. The formula can also be used for chronic inflammation affecting the eyes, and for eye dryness. *Ming Mu Shang Qing Pian*, above, is preferred for acute inflammation.

Màn jīng zǐ is the lead herb. It dispels wind-heat attacking the liver channel, supported by *jú huā*, *jīng jiè*, and *bò hé*. *Bái jí lí* has a dual function of anchoring ascendant liver *yang*, and "brightening the eyes", that is clearing redness and heat. *Jú huā* leads the formula to the eyes and clears heat.

Caution: *Bái jí lí* and *tiān huā fěn* are contraindicated during pregnancy.

OTHER PRODUCTS APPROPRIATE FOR THIS CATEGORY:

Modern Formulas:

For eye infection:

Huang Lian Shang Qing Pian

See Chapter 3A

Other:

Shi Hu Ye Guang Wan (PM)
Celosia 10 (SF)
Chien-Li Tablets (SF)

15. MISCELLANEOUS DISORDERS

15A. WASTING-THIRST
Diabetes, Metabolic Syndrome

Classical Formulas:

Yu Quan Wan	*yù quán wán* (玉泉丸)

Modern Formulas:

Xiao Ke Wan	*xiāo kě wán* (消渴丸)

Diabetes as a disease entity has been recognized in the literature of Chinese herbal medicine at least by the second century (Zhāng Zhòng-Jǐng, 张仲景, in the *Jīn Guì Yào Lüè*, 金匮要略, 220**).** The disease is known as *xiāo kě* (消渴) "emaciation-thirst disease", indicating two of the primary symptoms. Other symptoms include turbid and frequent urination, dry mouth and hunger. In this regard, Zhang was referring to type 1 diabetes mellitus.

Today, modern medicine divides diabetes mellitus into two types, both of which show elevated blood sugar. Type I, or juvenile-onset diabetes, usually appears before age 20. It is a genetically influenced autoimmune disorder that may be triggered by viral exposure. In this type, blood sugar is elevated because insulin-making beta cells in the pancreas have been irreversibly destroyed; the patient requires insulin by injection for the rest of their life. Although Chinese doctors attempted to address this condition with herbal medicine, it is unlikely that they had a significant effect in preventing an inevitable and rapid death.

Type II, or adult-onset diabetes, usually attacks people in their middle years, and is brought about by over-consumption of sugars and carbohydrates coupled with a sedentary lifestyle. In this type, beta cells produce insulin, but cell walls turn-off insulin receptors so as not to bring too much sugar into the cell, raising the total levels of blood sugar. This is called insulin-resistance. Sugar in the blood forms triglycerides, which is then stored as fat. In the West, type II diabetes is treated with blood sugar-reducing drugs such as metformin.

Type II diabetes, also known as metabolic syndrome, is at epidemic levels in developed countries due to high caloric and high glycemic diets. Control is possible with a low caloric/low carbohydrate diet to control and reduce blood sugar and insulin resistance, and exercise (aerobic and weight-bearing), which utilizes accumulated blood sugar and reduces insulin resistance at the cellular wall level.

In Chinese medicine, both types I and II are seen as a disease of *yin* and *qi* deficiency with excessive heat and dryness, affecting the lung, stomach and kidney. The blood becomes sticky, and advanced cases lead to blood stasis. Both types are aggravated by poor diet or excessive sexual activity.

Although designed for type I diabetes to control symptoms of hunger and thirst, the herbal formulas offered in this chapter can be helpful for patients with type II - metabolic syndrome and insulin resistance. Herbs that nourish *yin* and spleen *qi* can help restore the spleen-pancreas to its normal regulation of insulin and glycogen. By moistening *yin* the herbal combinations are beneficial in clearing sticky sugar accumulating in the blood and causing cellular glycosylation. By dispersing heat, the herbs can reduce the inflammatory effects that elevated insulin has on blood vessel epithelia.

The formulas included here are also helpful for chronic throat dryness, including Sjögren's syndrome.

Classical Formulas:

YU QUAN WAN

Formula: *yù quán wán* (玉泉丸), "Jade Spring Pills"
Author: Yáng Shì-Yíng (杨士瀛) *aka* Yáng Rén-Zhāi (杨仁斋)
Source: *Rén Zhāi Zhí Zhǐ Fāng* (仁斋直指方), 1264
Literal: "Ren-Zhai's Straight Indications Formula Discussion"

also discussed in:

Author: Shěn Jīn-Ào (沈金鳌)
Source: *Shěn Shì Zūn Shēng Shū* (沈氏尊生书), 1773
Literal: "Shen Shi's Venerate Life Books"

Availability:

Jade Fluid Decoction (AL)
Jade Source Combination (KP)
Jade Source Formula (GF)
Jade Spring Nourishing Formula (K)
Jade Spring Teapills (PF)
Trichosanthes And Pueraria Formula (EG)
Yu Quan Wan (PM)

Ingredients: (from Plum Flower's *"Jade Spring Teapills"*)

tiān huā fěn (天花粉), Radix Trichosanthis	13.5 %	CB
gé gēn (葛根), Radix Puerariae Lobatae	13.5	BB
dǎng shēn (党参), Radix Codonopsis	10.0	AA
huáng qí (黄芪), Radix Astragali	9.0	AA
fú líng (茯苓), Poria	9.0	FC
shēng dì huáng (生地黄), Radix Rehmanniae	9.0	AB
mài mén dōng (麦门冬), Radix Ophiopogonis	9.0	AD
wū méi (乌梅), Fructus Mume	9.0	L
wǔ wèi zǐ (五味子), Fructus Schisandrae	9.0	L
gān cǎo (甘草), Radix Glycyrrhizae	9.0	AA

Ingredients: (from KP *"Jade Source Combination"*)

huáng qí (黄芪), Radix Astragali	14.3 %	AA
tài zǐ shēn (太子参), Radix Pseudostellariae	14.3	AA
shú dì huáng (熟地黄), Radix Rehmanniae Praep.	14.3	AB
tiān huā fěn (天花粉), Radix Trichosanthis	11.4	CB

mài mén dōng (麦门冬), Radix Ophiopogonis	11.4	AD
wǔ wèi zǐ (五味子), Fructus Schisandrae	11.4	L
gé gēn (葛根), Radix Puerariae Lobatae	8.6	BB
gēng mǐ (粳米), Semen Oryzae (rice)	8.6	
shān zhū yú (山茱萸), Fructus Corni	5.7	L

Nourishes kidney yin, clears heat, generates fluid to stop thirst, tonifies spleen qi, astringes jing. Use for emaciation-thirst syndrome (diabetes), with symptoms of thirst, frequent urination, excessive hunger, weight loss, fatigue or turbid urine. Also for metabolic syndrome, with lab values of elevated blood sugar, fasting insulin and elevated triglycerides, and symptoms of fatigue, hunger before meals and weight gain. May be helpful in Sjögren's syndrome.

Pulses: Thin, sometimes rapid, or may be soft and weak
Tongue: Normal, or reddish with cracks and a scanty coat

Comments: "Jade Spring" means spring in the water sense, not the season, and refers to the throat's ability to produce saliva and moisture. Jade is considered a preeminent source of *yin*, and a jade spring constantly provides *yin* and fluid, alleviating thirst, one of diabetes characteristic symptoms. The *Yu Quan* formulas tonify *yin*, replenish fluid and build *qi* while astringing *qi* and *yin* into the organs.

Although *Yu Quan Wan* was formulated for symptoms we associate with type I diabetes (weight loss, thirst, frequent urination), it is currently being used in China and elsewhere for treating type II adult-onset diabetes. The combination of the *tiān huā fěn, mài mén dong, gé gēn* and *dì huáng* helps to remove the blood-dryness associated with sticky sugar, and thereby reduce blood sugar.

There are numerous versions of *Yu Quan Wan* that are available. The Plum Flower version follows the original prescription. KP's *Jade Source Combination* keeps 6 of the original 10 herbs, adding in *gēng mǐ* and *shān zhū yú.* It omits *fú líng, wū méi* and *gān cǎo*, and substitutes *tài zǐ shēn* for *dǎng shēn.* Versions from Golden Flower and Kan also modify the original formula.

Caution: *Tiān huā fěn* is contraindicated during pregnancy.

Further Reading:

Bensky et al, p. 375
Chen & Chen, p. 1052
Ellis, p. 393

Modern Formulas:

XIAO KE WAN

Formula: *xiāo kě wán* (消渴丸), "Diabetes Pills"
Source: Modern patent medicine
Classical antecedent: *yù quán wán* (玉泉丸). See above.

Availability:

Xiao Ke Wan (HT)
Xiao Ke Ning Wan (TL)

Ingredients: (from Herbal Times *"Xiao Ke Wan"*)

shēng dì huáng (生地黄), Radix Rehmanniae	7.3 %	DC
gé gēn (葛根), Radix Puerariae Lobatae	7.3	BB
huáng qí (黄芪), Radix Astragali	7.3	AA
shí gāo (石膏), Gypsum Fibrosum	7.3	DA
tiān huā fěn (天花粉), Radix Trichosanthis	7.3	CB
bái mù ěr (白木耳), Tremella	5.5	AD
fú líng (茯苓), Poria	5.5	FC
shān yào (山药), Rhizoma Dioscoreae	5.5	AA
mǔ dān pí (牡丹皮), Cortex Moutan	5.5	DC
shān zhū yú (山茱萸), Fructus Corni	5.5	L
xuán shēn (玄参), Radix Scrophulariae	5.5	DC
zé xiè (泽泻), Rhizoma Alismatis	5.5	FC
cāng zhú (苍术), Rhizoma Atractylodis	3.6	FB
hǎi jīn shā (海金沙), Spora Lygodii	3.6	DD
huái niú xī (怀牛膝), Radix Achyranthis Bidentatae	3.6	K
rén shēn (人参), Radix Ginseng	3.6	AA
wǔ wèi zǐ (五味子), Fructus Schisandrae	3.6	L
zhī mǔ (知母), Rhizoma Anemarrhenae	3.6	DA
gān cǎo (甘草), Radix Glycyrrhizae	3.4	AA

Nourishes yin, clears heat, generates fluid to stop thirst, boosts spleen qi. Use for emaciation-thirst syndrome, with symptoms of thirst, frequent urination, excessive hunger, weight loss, fatigue or turbid urine. Also for metabolic syndrome, with lab values of elevated blood sugar, fasting insulin and elevated triglycerides, and symptoms of fatigue, hunger before meals and weight gain. May be helpful in Sjögren's syndrome.

Pulses: Thin, sometimes rapid, or may be soft and weak.
Tongue: Normal, or reddish with cracks and a scanty coat

Comments: This formula is an elaboration of *Yu Quan Wan* (above) containing five of the original herbs: *gé gēn, tiān huā fěn, huáng qí, rén shēn, fú líng* and *gān cǎo.* This foundation moistens the throat and boosts *qi*. The formula goes on to include 14 other herbs, including the complete prescription of *Liu Wei Di Huang Wan* to enhance nourishing of *yin: shēng dì huáng, fú líng, shān yào, mǔ dān pí, shān zhū yú, zé xiè* (see Chapter 17A). It also contains herbs to clear heat (*shí gāo, xuán shēn, zhī mǔ*), and herbs to moisten lung *yin* (*bái mù ěr*).

This formula is valuable in treating type II diabetes and metabolic syndrome. Herbs that moisten *yin* can reduce blood stickiness due to sugar; heat-dispelling herbs can reduce inflammatory consequences of elevated insulin; and the overall effect may be to normalize insulin sensitivity on the cellular wall.

Caution: *Tiān huā fěn* and *huái niú xī* are prohibited during pregnancy.

OTHER PRODUCTS APPROPRIATE FOR THIS CATEGORY:

Modern Formulas:

Diaquell (BP)
Equilibrium (EV)
Jiang Tang Pian/Wan (GC)
Myrtle Seng (HC)
Sugar Pearls (CP)

15B. INTERNAL BLEEDING

Classical Formulas:

Shi Hui San — *shí huī sǎn* (十灰散)

Modern Formulas:

Yun Nan Bai Yao Jiao Nang — *yún nán bái yào jiāo náng* (云南白药胶囊)

Chinese herbal formulas can be used to control internal bleeding. They are symptomatic in approach, that is, they use herbs whose properties are known to arrest bleeding. In TCM practice, however, underlying causes should also be addressed, and outside of trauma, may include 14 separate TCM differentiations. Bleeding disorders are further differentiated into disease or symptom categories, and include coughing of blood, vomiting blood, bloody stools, urinary bleeding and subcutaneous bleeding. They can also be used for post-surgical internal bleeding.

The formulas discussed here are symptomatic in approach, and have clinical value. They can be combined with other formulas.

For further discussion of underlying patterns of bleeding disorders, see *Practical Therapeutics of Traditional Chinese Medicine,* Wu and Fischer, Paradigm Publications, 1997 or similar volumes.

Classical Formulas:

SHI HUI SAN

Formula: *shí huī sǎn* (十灰散), "Ten (Herbal) Ash Powder"
Author: Gé Kě–Jiǔ (葛可久) *aka* Gé Qián–Sūn (葛乾孙)
Source: *Shí Yào Shén Shū* (十药神书), 1348
Literal: "Ten Medicines Divine Book"

Availability:

Shi Hui San (HT)

Ingredients: (from Herbal Times *"Shi Hui San"*. All herbs prepared as *tàn,* 炭, charred.)

cè bǎi yè (侧柏叶), Cacumen Platycladi/Biotae	10. %	J
mǔ dān pí (牡丹皮), Cortex Moutan	10	DC
dà huáng (大黄), Radix/Rhizoma Rhei	10	PA
zhī zǐ (栀子), Fructus Gardeniae	10	DA
zōng lǚ pí (棕榈皮), Petiolus Trachycarp	10	J
bái máo gēn (白茅根), Rhizoma Imperatae	10	J
qiàn cǎo (茜草), Radix/Rhizoma Rubiae	10	J
hé yè (荷叶), Folium Nelumbinis	10	DF
xiǎo jì (小蓟), Herba Cirsii	10	J
dà jì (大蓟), Herba Cirsii Japonici	10	J

Cools blood, stops bleeding, subdues fire. Use for bleeding disorders due to heat and dryness, with escape of blood from orifices. Use for lung fire causing coughing or spitting up of blood, including tuberculosis and certain presentations of AIDS. Also for fire in the middle *jiao* causing vomiting of blood or nosebleed, including esophageal or stomach hemorrhage with ulceration. Can be used adjunctively for urinary bleeding or to stop uterine hemorrhage. Applicable in hemorrhagic fever due to heat.

Pulse: Rapid; may be surging or thin
Tongue: Red

***Comments*:** This formula is used for acute bleeding disorders due to internal fire from the liver, lung or stomach. It was originally designed for advanced tuberculosis, but has application in a variety of bleeding disorders. It is applied as the first treatment of bleeding due to internal factors, and accompanied or replaced by appropriate formulas to address the root cause. The name refers to the fact that all ingredients in the original formula were charred by dry stir-frying, to enhance astringent and hemostatic effects. For the Herbal Times version, all ingredients were dry-charred (*tàn*, 炭) according to the traditional preparation.

Caution: This is a cooling formula. Do not use in bleeding disorders due to deficiency with cold.

Further Reading:

Bensky et al, p. 598
Chen & Chen, p. 939

Modern Formulas:

YUNNAN BAI YAO CAPSULE

Formula: *yún nán bái yào jiāo náng* (云南白药胶囊)
"Yunnan (Province) White Medicine Capsule"
Source: Modern patent medicine from Yunnan Baiyao Group, China

Availability:

Yunnan Baiyao Capsule (PM)
Yunnan Paiyao Capsules (PM)
Yunnan Paiyao Powder (PM)

Ingredients: (from Yunnan Baiyao Group "*Yunnan Baiyao Capsule*")

tián qī (田七), Radix Notoginseng	40.0 %	J
sǎn yū cǎo (散瘀草), Herba Ajuga Forrestii	17.0	
huái shān yào (淮山药), Rhizoma Dioscoreae	13.3	AA
chuān shān lóng (穿山龙,) Rhizoma Dioscoreae Nip.	11.5	FA
lǎo hè cǎo (老鹤草), Herba Geranii	7.2	FA
kǔ liáng jiāng (苦良姜), Rhizoma Dioscoreae Parviflora	6.0	
bái niú dǎn (白牛胆), Herba Inulae Cappae	5.0	

Stops bleeding, dispels blood stasis, disperses swelling, relieves pain. Use internally for swelling, bruising or bleeding in acute trauma. Also useful in other bleeding disorders including postpartum hemorrhage, nosebleed, blood in urine or stool, bleeding ulcer, menorrhagia, and post-surgery. Can be used internally for infected wounds or for postpartum blood stasis. Use topically to stop bleeding, and as an antiseptic against infection.

Pulse: Normal, or weak and thin or large and rapid
Tongue: Normal, or pale or dark

Comments: *Yunnan Bai Yao* comes as capsule or powder. The powder form is more appropriate for topical application in traumatic bleeding (see Chapter 5B), while the capsules are meant to be taken internally. It is used for bleeding, including vomiting of blood, blood in the urine or stool, or uncontrollable nosebleed. It can also be used internally for traumatic swelling or bruising, and following surgery. The complete formula has only been revealed recently; outside of *tián qī*, the main ingredient, and a strong hemostatic agent, and also *shān yào,* all the other ingredients are little known plants from Yunnan province.

Caution: In general, do no take internally for more than three or four days. *Tián qī* is cautioned internally during pregnancy, and should not be used for a prolonged period.

OTHER FORMULAS APPROPRIATE FOR THIS CATEGORY:

tián qī (田七), Radix/Rhizoma Notoginseng
- Pseudoginseng Capsules, Raw (HT)
- Raw Tienchi Capsules (PF)
- San Qi Tablets (GF)
- Tian Qi Teapills (PF)
- Tien-Chi Ginseng Tablets (PIM)

16. QI AND BLOOD TONICS

16A. QI TONICS

Single herb:

Feng Wang Jiang (Royal Jelly)	*fēng wáng jiāng* (蜂王浆)
Huang Qi (Astragalus)	*huáng qí* (黄芪)
Ren Shen (Ginseng)	*rén shēn* (人参)
Xi Yang Shen (American Ginseng)	*xī yáng shēn* (西洋参)

Two herb combination:

Ren Shen Feng Wang Jiang (Ginseng Royal Jelly)	*rén shēn fēng wáng jiāng* (人参蜂王浆)

Classical Formulas:

Yu Ping Feng San	*yù píng fēng sǎn* (玉屏风散)

Modern Formulas:

Shen Qi Wu Wu Wei Zi Wan	*shēn qí wu wǔ wèi zǐ wán* (参芪五味子丸)

The Chinese word *qì* (气), for TCM, describes a bioenergy that circulates and infiltrates through the body via the acupuncture network. In Chinese medicine, various kinds of *qi* are described, including the *qi* of the acupuncture network and the *qi* of various organs. Most of the formulas in this category nourish spleen and lung *qi*, which are necessary to produce the healthy *qi* of the whole body (*zhèng qì*, 正气). One of the formulas also tonifies heart *qi* - *Shen Qi Wu Wei Zi Wan*.

The spleen and lung work to extract *qi* from the environment – from food and air. The spleen channel has an upward-moving direction, and its function is to extract *qi* and fluid from food in the small intestine and send it to the upper *jiao*. There it combines with *qi* from the air. Kidney *qi* (including constitutional *yuán jīng*, 原精) is also utilized, circulating though the eight extraordinary channel network, and acting as a catalyst to merge the three types of energy into *zōng qì* (宗气).

Zong qi circulates through the blood vessels and the acupuncture network. The heart is responsible for pumping the blood, while the lung pumps and circulates *qi* through the meridian sequence. In the acupuncture channels, the concentric aspect of *zong qi* is called *yíng qì* (营气), which nourishes the internal organs and allows them to function normally. The more active centripetal energy emanating off the concentric *ying qi* is called *wèi qì* (卫气), which infiltrates tissue and interstitial fluids surrounding the acupuncture channels and is responsible for cellular function and immune modulation.

Deficiency of the spleen, lung or kidney can lead to deficiency of *ying qi* and *wei qi*. This interferes with organ function and immune response, and can account for generalized fatigue as well as act as the root cause of many illnesses. Deficiency of *qi* can also lead to deficiency of blood.

The herbs and formulas in this category boost *qi* to treat spleen, lung and heart deficiency. Symptoms of lung weakness include difficulty breathing, weak voice, spontaneous sweating, and susceptibility to allergies. Deficiency of spleen can cause poor digestion, loose stool and weak limbs. Deficiency of heart *qi* leads to fatigue, difficulty breathing, poor concentration and palpitations.

Qi tonics tend to be warming, and are used cautiously in deficiency heat presentations.

Formulas that tonify *qi* for proper digestion can also be found in *Chapter 5A. Spleen Qi Deficiency* and *Chapter 5B. Spleen Yang Deficiency.* Formulas that address stagnation of *qi* can be found in *7A. Liver Stagnation* and *6C. Food Stagnation.* Additional tonic herbs can be found in *Chapter 18B. Single Herb Tonics.*

Single herb:

FENG WANG JIANG
ROYAL JELLY

Herb: *fēng wáng jiāng* (蜂王浆), Lac Regis Apis (Royal Jelly)
Source: Modern use

Availability:

Capsules
Liquid Vials

Combination Products:

Astragalus Royal Jelly (PM)
Birds' Nest Lingzhi Pollen Royal Jelly Oral Liquid (PM)
Cordyceps Royal Jelly (PM)
Ginseng Royal Jelly (PM)
Huahuangbao Chinese Pollen Royal Jelly (PM)
Notoginseng Royal Jelly (PM)
Peking Lingchih Royal Jelly (PM)
Reshi & Royal Jelly Extract (PM)

Tonifies spleen, heart and kidney qi, tonifies ying and wei qi. Use as a general tonic for *ying* and *wei qi*, for preventing illness, recovering from illness, childbirth, or surgery, and enhancing the immune system. Use to improve appetite and to treat senility, poor sleep, dizziness, palpitation and fatigue. Helpful as a general tonic for wasting diseases such as chronic hepatitis, tuberculosis, AIDS, and declining health.

Pulse: Weak, soft
Tongue: Normal, or pale, swollen

Comments: Royal jelly is not listed in the traditional materia medica, but has become popular in China as a longevity tonic. It is a special food made from bee saliva, honey and pollen, and, when given to a common drone bee, allows it to become a queen, able to lay thousands of eggs in a single day. The queen bee, raised exclusively on royal jelly, lives sixteen times longer than the average bee. Royal jelly tonifies spleen, heart and kidney *qi*, and supporting both digestion and sexual function. It is used for infertility, low energy and to promote vitality and longevity. It is very helpful for malnutrition, poor appetite, and weight loss.

Caution: May cause colic in nursing infants.

HUANG QI
ASTRAGALUS

Herb: *huáng qí* (黄芪), Radix Astragali
Properties: Sweet, slightly warm
Channels: Spleen, Lung
Source: *Shén Nóng Běn Cǎo Jīng* (神农本草经), 300 BCE – 200 CE
Literal: "Shen Nong's Materia Medica Classic"
Author: Unknown

Availability:

Liquid vials
Powder capsules

Tonifies qi, raises yang, tonifies wei qi, secures the exterior, discharges pus, benefits the movement of water. Use as a tonic for *ying qi* and *wei qi* and to help build blood. Use to prevent illness, and to help recovery from chronic illness, surgery or childbirth. Applicable in fatigue, poor appetite, spontaneous sweating, slow healing wounds, prolapsed organs, frequent colds and deficiency edema. Useful during allergy season to fortify the *qi.* Useful to heal wounds and discharge accumulated pus.

Pulse: Normal, or weak, soft
Tongue: Normal, or pale, swollen

Comments: Astragalus *huáng qí* enhances the immune system by boosting *wei qi*. The actions of the herb allow *qi* to radiate out from the channels that activates the immune system in the lymphatics, the interstitial fluids and the blood. It can help promote healing in slow-healing wounds, or after surgery, and is helpful during and following chemotherapy and radiation therapy. It is often prescribed to help expel pus in wounds.

Astragalus *huáng qí* can be taken as capsules, but the more common method are glass vials where *huáng qí* is combined with honey and water, to be taken with a small straw. Because of its availability as a liquid, it is particularly useful as an immune tonic for young children recovering from illness, or preventing common cold or allergy. .

Further Reading:

Bensky, Clavey, Ströger, *Materia Medica*, p. 718
Chen & Chen, *Medical Herbology*, p. 847

REN SHEN
CHINESE GINSENG

Herb: *rén shēn* (人参), Radix Ginseng
Properties: Sweet, slightly bitter, slightly warm
Channels: Lung, Spleen
Source: *Shén Nóng Běn Cǎo Jīng* (神农本草经), 300 BCE–200 CE
Literal: "Shen Nong's Materia Medica Classic"
Author: Unknown

Availability:

Capsules
Powder

Tonifies spleen, lung and heart qi, tonifies yuan and ying qi, generates fluid, calms shen. Use as a general tonic for *ying qi*, and to tonify lung, heart, and spleen. Enhances and improves digestive function, including poor appetite and loose stools, and to support deficient heart and lung *qi* causing palpitation, shortness of breath, insomnia, or fatigue with exertion. Other symptoms include spontaneous sweating, poor memory, insomnia, restlessness or anxiety, poor circulation, anemia, or poor sexual function. Use for recovery from illness, prostration, shock, surgery and childbirth and to enhance the immune system.

Pulse: Normal, or weak, soft
Tongue: Normal, or pale, swollen

Comments: Ginseng *rén shēn* is an excellent general *qi* tonic. In China, people over the age of 40 commonly use it to promote digestion or to nourish heart or lung *qi*. It is also used for recovery from surgery or childbirth. *Rén shēn* is not much benefit to kidney *qi*, and its reputation for enhancement of sexual function is not accurate. Red ginseng has been heat-treated to make it more *yang* and warming than white, natural ginseng. As a *yang* and *qi* tonic, it is more indicated for men then women, although women can use it when there is a clear deficiency of *yang* or *qi*. For example, it is given during labor.

There are two kinds of ginseng used in TCM. Besides *rén shēn*, which is a *qi* and *yang* tonic, there is American Ginseng *xī yáng shēn* (西洋参, Radix Panacis Quinquefolii), a *qi* and *yin* tonic, described below. So-called Siberian Ginseng (*cì wŭ jiā,* 刺五加, Radix Acanthopanacis), is not really a ginseng, and is described in *Chapter 18B. Single Herb Tonics*.

Caution: Discontinue during colds and flu, as *rén shēn* tends to pull pathogenic factors into the interior. Do not use *rén shēn* or *rén shēn* formulas in cases of *yin* deficiency with heat, or in real heat such as fever. Ginseng *rén shēn* can raise blood pressure; caution for patients with hypertension. Discontinue if it causes headache, insomnia or palpitation.

Further Reading:

Bensky, Clavey, Ströger, *Materia Medica*, p. 710
Chen & Chen, *Medical Herbology*, p. 835

XI YANG SHEN
AMERICAN GINSENG

Herb: *xī yáng shēn* (西洋参), Radix Panacis Quinquefolii
Properties: Sweet, bitter, cold
Channels: Kidney, Heart, Lung
Source: *Běn Cǎo Cóng Xīn* (本草从新), 1751
Literal: "Materia Medica From (the) New"
Author: Wú Yí-Luò (吴仪洛) *aka* Wú Zūn-Chéng (吴遵程)

Availability:

Capsules
Powder

Tonifies qi, nourishes yīn, clears lung fire, generates fluid, relieves cough. Use for deficiency of *yin* and *qi* causing low voice or loss of voice, fatigue, dry cough, thirst, and irritability. Also used for lung fire with coughing up of blood. Use to replace *qi* and *yin* during acute and chronic fever.

Pulse: Normal, or weak, soft, or thin or rapid
Tongue: Normal, or pale with a dry coat

Comments: American ginseng *xī yáng shēn* is one of the few foreign herbs that have been absorbed into the Chinese materia medica. It provides a *qi* tonic that is cooling, and thereby useful for replenishing *qi* during fevers. The herb was sought after when tuberculosis, a disease that consumes lung *qi* and *yin*, proved to be a great plague during China's nineteenth century. For similar reasons, it is appropriate in fever due to AIDS or other causes of protracted fever with deficiency of *qi*, including following radiation therapy. It can also be used as a general *qi* tonic, or when the warm Chinese ginseng is not tolerated.

Further Reading:

Bensky, Clavey, Ströger, *Materia Medica*, p. 820
Chen & Chen, *Medical Herbology*, p. 841

Two-herb combination:

GINSENG AND ROYAL JELLY

Formula: *rén shēn fēng wáng jiāng* (人参蜂王浆)
Source: Chinese patent medicine

Availability:

Vials
Capsules

Ingredients:

rén shēn (人参), Radix Ginseng	AA
fēng wáng jiāng (蜂王漿), Lac Regis Apis (Royal Jelly)	AA
fēng mì (蜂蜜), Mel (honey)	PB

Tonifies spleen qi, tonifies lung qi, tonifies heart qi, tonifies ying and wei qi. Use as a general tonic for *ying* and *wei qi*, for preventing illness, recovering from illness, surgery and childbirth, and enhancing the immune system. Benefits digestive function and appetite. Use for fatigue, lassitude, low sexual energy, palpitation, and weak heart function. Can fight residual or chronic infection including chronic liver disease; also for anemia, and preventing degenerative effects of aging.

Pulse: Normal, or weak, soft
Tongue: Normal, or pale

Comments: This popular tonic combines Ginseng *rén shēn* with Royal Jelly *fēng wáng jiāng*. It comes is a box of ten vials of liquid, with accompanying straws. Royal jelly is considered an excellent longevity tonic in China, and *rén shēn* is valued as a general tonic for spleen, heart and lung *qi* (see above). It is helpful following chronic illness or surgery where there is reduced vitality or appetite, or when there is low weight gain.

Caution: May cause colic in nursing infants. Discontinue during acute colds and flu, as *rén shēn* tends to pull pathogenic factors into the interior.

Classical Formulas:

YU PING FENG SAN

Formula: *yù píng fēng sǎn* (玉屏风散)
"Jade Screen (against the) Wind Powder"
Author: Zhū Zhèn-Hēng (朱震亨) *aka* Zhū Dān-Xī (朱丹溪)
Source: *Dān Xī Xīn Fǎ* (丹溪心法), 1481
Literal: "Dan-Xi's Heart Method" (eg, "Personal Insights")

Availability:

Astragalus & Siler Formula (EG)
Children's Jade Defense (GF)
Jade Screen (JD, TT)
Jade Screen Formula (CC)
Jade Screen Tablets (SF)
Jade Screen Teapills (PF)
Jade Windscreen Formula (GF, HS)
Yu Ping Feng San (BP, TZ)
Yu Ping Feng Wan (HT, JD, TL)
* Astra C (HC)
* Jade Windscreen (K)

Ingredients: (from the standardized *"Astragalus & Siler Formula"*)

huáng qí (黄芪), Radix Astragali	60. %	AA
bái zhú (白术), Rhizoma Atractylodis Macrocephalae	20	AA
fáng fēng (防风), Radix Saposhnikov./Ledebouriellae	20	BA

Replenishes qi, tonifies wei qi, consolidates the exterior, stops sweating. Use for deficiency of *wei qi* causing spontaneous sweating, catching cold easily, or before or during allergies. Symptoms can include sensitivity to cold and wind, fatigue, pale or puffy complexion, low voice, and poor appetite. Use for pediatric cold, chronic hay fever allergies and chronic nasal discharge of white or clear mucus. Used adjunctively in the treatment of chronic disease, including AIDS, tuberculosis, and weakened liver due to cirrhosis or hepatitis. Taken preventatively for the common cold, to boost immune responsiveness, and to prevent allergy.

Pulse: Normal, or floating and soft
Tongue: Normal, or pale

Comments: This is a valuable formula for building a weakened immune system, especially when the symptoms include perspiring easily or sensitivity to wind or cold. It is valuable in pediatric conditions for chronic runny nose and as a *qi* tonic before and during hay fever allergies. It is also useful for patients following hospitalization, childbirth, or prolonged illness.

A simple formula, it uses *bái zhú* to build and astringe *ying qi, huáng qí* to build *wei qi,* and *fáng fēng* to disperse *wei qi* to the surface. Most manufacturers follow the standardized formula, with 60% belonging to *huáng qí.*

Further Reading:

Bensky et al, p. 326
Chen & Chen, p. 773
Ellis, p. 392

Modern Formulas:

SHEN QI WU WEI ZI WAN

Formula: *shēn qí wu wǔ wèi zǐ wán* (参芪五味子丸)
"Ginseng, Astragalus, Schisandra Pill"
Source: Modern patent medicine

Availability:

Abundant Qi Plus Teapills (PF)
Shen Qi Wu Wei Zi Wan (MS)

Ingredients: (from Minshan *"Shen Qi Wu Wei Zi Wan"*)

wǔ wèi zǐ (五味子), Fructus Schisandrae	46.1 %	L
huáng qí (黄芪), Radix Astragali	30.8	AA
dǎng shēn (党参), Radix Codonopsis	15.4	AA
suān zǎo rén (酸枣仁), Semen Ziziphi Spinosae	7.7	N

Tonifies heart and lung qi, astringes sweating, calms shen. Use for deficiency of heart or lung *qi* causing fatigue, shortness of breath following exertion, spontaneous sweating, palpitation, insomnia, low voice volume, lack of vitality. Also for anxiety and restlessness due to *qi* deficiency. Useful as a heart *qi* tonic and preventative in aging patients. Can also be used as a lung *qi* tonic in chronic asthma and chronic cough.

Pulse: Normal, or thin, weak, soft
Tongue: Normal, or pale or swollen

Comments: This formula addresses heart and *shen* problems due to deficiency of heart *qi*. Due to the inclusion of *suān zǎo rén*, the formula targets the heart. Otherwise, the three lead herbs could also benefit the spleen, lung, liver or kidney. *Wǔ wèi zǐ*, the main herb, has astringing properties that bring the formula into the interior. This herb astringes spontaneous sweating, especially when enhanced by combining with the *qi* tonics *huáng qí* and *dǎng shēn*. The formula is valuable for strengthening heart *qi* in the aging population.

OTHER PRODUCTS APPLICABLE TO THIS CATEGORY:

Classical Formulas:

Bu Fei Tang

See Chapter 3F

Huang Qi Gui Zhi Wu Wu Tang

See Chapter 4C

Si Jun Zi Wan

See Chapter 6A

Modern Formulas:

Shen Qi Da Bu Wan

Abundant Qi Teapills (PF)
Shen Qi Da Bu Wan (MS, TL)

Other:

Abundant Qi Teapills (PF)
Cordyceps 3 (EV)
Five Mushroom Formula (GF)
Full Force with Astragalus (HC)
Ginseng and Royal Jelly (PF, PM)
Ginseng Endurance Formula (GF)
Ginseng Tonic Capsules (PM)
Immune Plus (DRJ)
Licorice 25 (HC)
Power Mushrooms (HC)
Reshi & Royal Jelly Extract (PF)
Tonify Qi (CMS)
Vibrant (EV)

16. QI AND BLOOD TONICS

16B. BLOOD TONICS

Single herb:

Dang Gui (Angelica)	*dāng guī* (当归)
He Shou Wu (Polygonum)	*hé shǒu wū* (何首乌) i

Classical Formulas:

Si Wu Tang	*sì wù tāng* (四物汤)

Modern Formulas:

Dang Gui Jing (Tang Kwe Gin)	*dāng guī jīng* (当归精)
Fu Fang Dang Gui Wan	*fù fāng dāng guī wán* (复方当归丸)
Shou Wu Zhi	*shǒu wū zhī* (首乌汁)

Products in this category nourish the blood. Because blood nourishes every cell in the body, blood deficiency particularly affects the function of the brain, heart, liver, uterus and skin. In TCM, the heart dominates the blood vessels, the liver stores the blood, and the spleen controls the blood. Deficiency can affect all three *zang-fu* organs.

Blood deficiency includes that which can be measured by laboratory analysis, including low counts of red blood cells, white blood cells, platelets or hematocrit. Blood deficiency can exist even when lab tests appear normal, indicating weak blood vitality. Devitalized red blood cells have the tendency to clump together, because they cannot repel each other electromagnetically. This also affects its ability to bind with oxygen and carbon dioxide.

Signs and symptoms of blood deficiency are a more important indicator than blood counts. They include thin or weak pulse, pale tongue and lips, pale conjunctiva in the eyes, dry or itchy skin, pale complexion, dry hair or hair that falls out easily, fatigue, poor concentration, amenorrhea or irregular menses, floaters in the eyes, dry brittle finger nails and low body temperature. Blood deficiency in the liver can also lead to dry, brittle tendons, and is found in stiffness and inflexibility associated with aging. Deficiency of heart blood can cause insomnia, palpitation, dizziness and irregular heart beat, as well as poor memory and concentration. Blood tonics are also used to nourish and moisten the intestines in the treatment of constipation. For these reasons, blood tonics are often employed to treat or prevent problems of aging.

In China, blood-tonifying formulas are popular with women to compensate for blood lost during menses, and to prevent dryness of the skin and hair loss. Chinese women often take a blood tonic for the two weeks following every period. Blood deficiency is also evident following childbirth, major surgery, hemorrhagic loss of blood due to trauma, and excessive uterine bleeding. They are also necessary to compensate for blood damage due to radiation therapy. Problems of infertility often involve a blood deficiency, in addition to deficiency of kidney or stagnation of liver.

Causes of nontraumatic blood deficiency are often due to an underlying deficiency of *qi*, which in turn may be due to dysfunction of the spleen (digestive ability), lung (including air pollution or smoking) or kidney. People on kidney dialysis, for example, show all the signs of blood deficiency. Hemophilia, a constitutional kidney deficiency in Chinese medicine, is also seen as a problem of blood deficiency, as are other platelet disorders. Underlying conditions need to be addressed, and successful nourishment of the blood usually requires concurrent tonification of *qi*, *yin* and *jing*.

The products offered in this chapter may be used alone, or to reinforce other prescriptions. Alone, they may be cloying and stagnating in nature and affect digestion. Caution is advised in terms of nausea, indigestion or loose stools. Caution is also advised during menses so as not to cause excessive bleeding. Also, formulas for blood tonification are often discontinued during early stages of exogenous wind invasions (colds and flu), as they tend to drive pathogenic wind deeper into the body.

Blood tonics can also be found in section *Chapter 16C. Qi and Blood Tonics*. Blood tonics specific to gynecological disorders can be found in chapter *8A. Gynecological Tonics.*

Tonification of blood may require combining with formulas to tonify *qi* (Chapters *6A. Spleen Qi Tonics* or *Chapter 16A. Qi Tonics*) or formulas that tonify kidney *jing* (*Chapter 17B. Kidney Yang and Jing Tonics*).

Single Herb:

DANG GUI
ANGELICA DANG GUI, TANG KWEI

Herb:	*dāng guī* (当归), Radix Angelicae Sinensis
Properties:	Sweet, acrid, warm
Channels:	Heart, Liver, Spleen
Source:	*Shén Nóng Běn Cǎo Jīng* (神农本草经), 300 BCE–200 CE Literal: "Shen Nong's Materia Medica Classic"
Author:	Unknown

Availability:

Angelica Dang Gui Capsules (PF)
Dang Gui Extract Wan (HT)
Dang Gui Su (PM)
Dang Gui Wan (PM, TL)

Nourishes and warms blood, invigorates blood, nourishes liver, moistens intestines, regulates menses. Use for deficiency of blood, affecting vitality, menstruation and vision. Useful for poor memory, palpitations, dizziness, headache, tremor, dry hair, alopecia (hair falling out), dry skin, and cracked nails. Nourishes the liver and kidney to regulate menses, including irregular menses, amenorrhea, and scanty periods. Useful following postpartum bleeding. Also adjunctively to moisten dry intestines to treat constipation.

Pulse: Normal, or thready or wiry
Tongue: Normal, or pale

Comments: *Dāng guī* is valued by the Chinese for nourishing, moving and warming blood. It is used alone or in combination for various gynecological complaints, including regulation of female hormones, irregular menses, amenorrhea or spotting periods, infertility, and as a postpartum tonic. It is commonly taken after the period to enhance blood production and vitality. It is also used to repair damaged liver cells.

Dāng guī is often combined with *huáng qí* (黄芪, Radix Astragali) to boost *qi* and blood. This becomes the formula *Dang Gui Bu Xue Tang* (Chapter 16C), which can be used to raise red and white blood cells during or following chemotherapy and radiation.

Note: Correct pronunciation is "dahng gway". It is often spelled as "tang-kwei" and mispronounced as "taang-kwee" or "taang-kwhy".

Caution: In general, discontinue or reduce dosage during menses, which can lead to a heavier flow. *Dāng guī* may lower prothrombin times when combined with blood thinners such as Coumadin.

Further Reading:

Bensky, Clavey, Ströger, *Materia Medica*, p. 748
Chen & Chen, *Medical Herbology,* p. 918

HE SHOU WU
POLYGONUM HE SHOU WU

Herb: *hé shǒu wū* (何首乌), Radix Polygoni Multiflori
Properties: Sweet, bitter, astringent, slightly warm
Channels: Kidney, Liver
Source: *Rì Huá Zǐ Běn Cǎo* (日华子本草), 713
Literal: "Ri Hua-Zi's Materia Medica"
Author: Rì Huá-Zǐ (日华子)

Availability:

Dr. Shen's Shou Wu Pill (DS)
He Shou Wu Capsules (PF)
He Shou Wu Tablets (GF)
Nourish Hair (JD)
Shou Wu Chih (PM)
Shou Wu Essence (PM)
Shou Wu Formula (CC)
Shou Wu Pian (PF)
Shou Wu Wan (HT)

Nourishes blood, consolidates and strengthens jing, benefits kidney, strengthens tendon and bone, boosts marrow, moistens the intestines. Use for chronic deficiencies of liver blood and *yin* affecting vitality, fertility, menstruation, skin and hair, memory and vision. Counters liver fire due to deficiency, with accompanying symptoms of headache, eye pain, dizziness, and tinnitus. Benefits lower back and painful joints, stops spermatorrhea and vaginal discharge, treats constipation.

Useful for dry hair, alopecia (hair falling out), dry skin, and cracked nails. Also used for blurred vision, numbness or tingling of the limbs, poor concentration and poor memory, restless sleep, fatigue or anxiety due to deficiency of blood and *jing*. Also for le*aka*ge of sperm (spermatorrhea) and depletion from excessive sexual activity in males. Can be beneficial following radiation therapy.

Pulse: Normal, or thready or wiry
Tongue: Normal, or pale

Comments: *Hé shǒu wū*, also called *Fo-Ti,* is valued by the Chinese for graying hair, dry skin and male sexual depletion. Similar in function to *shú dì huáng* (熟地黄, Radix Rehmanniae Praep.), it is less cloying and easier on the digestion, and can be used on a daily basis. *Hé shǒu wū* helps boost marrow, aiding in blood production. In this regard, it also helps memory, concentration and brain fog, where the brain is also considered in TCM to be marrow. Clinical research indicates its ability to reduce blood lipids and cholesterol and regulate blood glucose levels.

Further Reading:

Bensky, Clavey, Ströger, *Materia Medica*, p. 747
Chen & Chen, *Medical Herbology*, p. 927

Classical Formulas:

SI WU TANG

Formula: *sì wù tāng* (四物汤), "Four Substance Decoction"
Author: Imperial Medical Bureau (*tài yī jú*, 太医局);
revised by Chén Shī-Wén (陈师文)
Source: *Tài Píng Huì Mín Hé Jì Jú Fāng* (太平惠民和剂局方), 1078
Literal: "(Era of) Great Peace, Benefit People Harmonious Medicines, Office (of) Formulas"

also attributed to:
Author: Lìn Dào Rén (Lin the Daoist) (蔺道人)
Source: *Xiān Shòu Lǐ Shāng Xù Duàn Mì Fāng* (仙授理伤续断秘方), 846
Literal: "Immortal Instructs Management (of) Injuries (and) Repair (of) Fractures, Secret Formulas"

Availability:

Four Substances (K)
Four Substances For Women Teapills (PF)
Four-Substance Formula (HS)
Si Wu Tang (TZ)
Si Wu Tang Pian/Wan (GC)
Si Wu Wan (HT, PM, TL)
Tangkuei Four Combination (EG)

Ingredients: (from the standardized formula *"Tangkuei Four Combination"*)

shú dì huáng (熟地黄), Radix Rehmanniae Praep.	25. %	AB
dāng guī (当归), Radix Angelicae Sinensis	25	AB
bái sháo (白芍), Radix Paeoniae Alba	25	AB
chuān xiōng (川芎), Rhizoma Ligustici Chuanxiong	25	K

Ingredients: (from Herbal Times *"Si Wu Wan"*)

shú dì huáng (熟地黄), Radix Rehmanniae Praep.	31.2 %	AB
dāng guī (当归), Radix Angelicae Sinensis	25.0	AB
bái sháo (白芍), Radix Paeoniae Alba	25.0	AB
chuān xiōng (川芎), Rhizoma Ligustici Chuanxiong	18.8	K

Nourishes and regulates blood, invigorates blood, regulates menses. Use for deficiency of blood affecting vitality, menstruation, and vision. Useful for poor memory, palpitations, dizziness, headache, tremor, dry hair, alopecia (hair falling out), anemia, dry or pale skin, and cracked nails. Regulates liver and kidney to regulate menses, treating irregular menses, amenorrhea, and scanty periods. Use for postpartum fatigue, restless fetus syndrome and depression. Also adjunctively to moisten dry intestines to treat constipation.

Pulse: Normal, or thready or wiry
Tongue: Normal, or pale

Comments: This is an important foundation formula for blood deficiency, combining four herbs acting synergistically. *Dāng guī* and *bái sháo* work together to build and circulate liver blood; *chuān xiōng* moves blood; and *shú dì huáng* builds blood while strengthening kidney *jing*. The formula can be used alone or to reinforce other products. If there is underlying *qi* deficiency, it is important to combine with a *qi* tonic. When combined with *Si Jun Zi Tang* (Chapter 6A), it becomes *Ba Zhen Tang* (Chapter 16C), a tonic formula for deficiency of *qi* and blood. *Si Wu Tang* is a popular postmenstrual and postpartum tonic for women.

Further Reading:

Bensky et al, p. 333
Chen & Chen, p. 562
Ellis, p. 297

Modern Formulas:

DANG GUI JING
TANG KWEI GIN

Formula: *dāng guī jīng* (当归精), "Angelica *Dang Gui* Essence"
Source: Modern patent medicine

Availability:

Dang Gui Jing (PM)
Tang Kwei Gin (PF, PM)
Tankwe Gin (PM)

Ingredients: (from Chung Lien Drug Works; Wuhan *"TanKwe Gin"*)

dāng guī (当归), Radix Angelicae Sinensis	69.0 %	AB
fú líng (茯苓), Poria	4.5	FC
ē jiāo (阿胶), Colla Corii Asini	4.5	AB
bái sháo (白芍), Radix Paeoniae Alba	4.5	AB
dǎng shēn (党参), Radix Codonopsis	4.5	AA
huáng qí (黄芪), Radix Astragali	4.5	AA
shú dì huáng (熟地黄), Radix Rehmanniae Praep.	4.5	AB
chuān xiōng (川芎), Rhizoma Ligustici Chuanxiong	2.0	K
gān cǎo (甘草), Radix Glycyrrhizae	2.0	AA
Alcohol, Sugar		

Packing and Dosage:

Bottles of 200 cc (7 fl. oz.). Take 1-2 teaspoons (5 cc), 1-3 x day.

Nourishes blood, tonifies qi, regulates liver and kidney. Use for deficiency of blood presenting with pale complexion, fatigue, cracked, brittle nails, dry skin and hair, blurring of vision and visual disturbances. Also for numbness or tingling of the limbs, lightheadedness, dizziness, palpitations, poor memory and concentration, bruising easily. Use for gynecological disorders including scanty, irregular menses or amenorrhea, post-menstrual fatigue, and infertility. Also for chronic non-healing ulcers and sores.

Pulse: Normal, or thready or wiry
Tongue: Normal, or pale

Comments: *Dang Gui Jing* is a popular liquid tonic for nourishing blood and regulating female hormones. It is mostly used as a gynecological tonic, particularly post-menses and post-partum. It can also be used for low blood lab values, and is beneficial following chemotherapy or radiation. It can be used for long periods of time.

This formula reinforces *dāng guī* (69% of the formula) with the other blood tonics of *Si Wu Tang* (*bái sháo, shú dì huáng* and *chuān xiōng*) as well as *ē jiāo* so that the blood tonics contribute 83% of the formula. Another 11% of the formula tonifies *qi* (*dǎng shēn, huáng qí* and *gān cǎo*), which is necessary to adequately build blood.

The Plum Flower version is similar to the original Chung Lian formula, omitting *ē jiāo*.

Caution: Discontinue or reduce dosage during menses to avoid excessive bleeding. Also, discontinue during colds and flu, as tonics tend to drive pathogenic factors into the interior.

FU FANG DANG GUI WAN

Formula: *fù fāng dāng guī wán* (复方当归丸)
"Compound Angelica *Dang Gui* Pill"
Source: Modern patent medicine

Availability:

Angelica Compound Wan (HT)
Angelica Dang Gui Pills (MS)
Dong Quai Tablet (PM)

Ingredients: (from Herbal Times *"Angelica Compound Wan"*)

dāng guī (当归), Radix Angelicae Sinensis	70. %	AB
chuān xiōng (川芎), Rhizoma Ligustici Chuanxiong	10	K
bái zhú (白术), Rhizoma Atractylodis Macrocephalae	10	AA
dà zǎo (大枣), Fructus Jujubae	10	AA

Nourishes blood, tonifies qi, nourishes the liver, regulates menses, moistens intestines. Use for deficiency of blood, affecting vitality, menstruation, and vision. Useful for poor memory, palpitations, dizziness, headache, tremor, dry hair, alopecia, dry skin and cracked nails. Nourishes the liver and kidney to regulate menses, treating irregular menses, amenorrhea, and scanty periods. Use for postpartum fatigue, restless fetus syndrome (threatened miscarriage) and depression due to deficiency. Also used adjunctively to moisten intestines to treat constipation, especially in the elderly.

Pulse: Normal, or thready or wiry
Tongue: Normal, or pale

Comments: This formula consists of 70% *dāng guī* with 10% *chuān xiōng* to move blood and 20% to tonify *qi* (*bái zhú* and *dà zăo*). It is a good tonic for building blood as well as helpful in regulating female hormones. It is a popular post-menstrual and postpartum tonic for women, and can be used following chemotherapy or radiation.

SHOU WU ZHI

Formula: *shǒu wū zhī* (首乌汁), "Polygonum *He Shou Wu* Juice"
Source: Modern patent medicine

Availability:

Shou Wu Chih (PM)
Shou Wu Essence (PF)

Ingredients: (from United Pharmaceutical Manufactory; Guangzhou *"Shou Wu Chih"*)

hé shǒu wū (何首乌), Radix Polygoni Multiflori	25.0 %	AB
dāng guī (当归), Radix Angelicae Sinensis	25.0	AB
huáng jīng (黄精), Rhizoma Polygonati	20.0	AA
shēng dì huáng (生地黄), Radix Rehmanniae	10.0	DC
chuān xiōng (川芎), Rhizoma Ligustici Chuanxiong	10.0	K
bái zhǐ (白芷), Radix Angelicae Dahuricae	6.7	BA
gān cǎo (甘草), Radix Glycyrrhizae	1.6	AA
dīng xiāng (丁香), Flos Caryophylli	.8	E
jú hé (橘核), Semen Citri Reticulatae	.8	G
Sugar and distilled water		

Ingredients: (from Plum Flower *"Shou Wu Essence"*. Ingredient percentages not given.)

jīn yīng zǐ (金樱子), Fructus Rosae Laevigatae	L
hé shǒu wū (何首乌), Radix Polygoni Multiflori	AB
huáng jīng (黄精), Rhizoma Polygonati	AA
tù sī zǐ (菟丝子), Semen Cuscutae	AC
bǔ gǔ zhī (补骨脂), Fructus Psoraleae	AC
dāng guī (当归), Radix Angelicae Sinensis	AB
chén pí (陈皮), Pericarpium Citri Reticulatae	G
Sugar, Distilled water	

Packing and Dosage:

Bottles of 200 cc (7 fl. oz.) (Plum Flower); or 500 cc (16 fl. oz) (United Pharmaceutical). Take 1-3 teaspoons (5 cc), 1-3 x day.

Tonifies blood, invigorates blood, moves qi, nourishes liver and benefits kidney, nourishes jing and yang. Use for chronic deficiencies of blood and *jing*, including those due to heavy menses, childbirth, or aging. Symptoms may include infertility, poor male sexual function, amenorrhea or irregular menses, dry hair and skin, thinning hair, cracked fingernails, poor memory and fatigue. Useful in alopecia (hair falling out), male sexual depletion, and stiff tendons. Also as a post-menstrual tonic, and to increase female fertility, and as a general geriatric tonic. Useful following radiation therapy.

Pulse: Normal, or thready or wiry-thin
Tongue: Normal, or pale

Comments: This is an excellent tonic for blood and *jing*, available in liquid form. Both versions listed here contain *hé shǒu wū, dāng guī* and *huáng jīng*. The product from United Pharmaceutical devotes 70% of the formula to these 3 herbs. *Hé shǒu wū* tonifies kidney and liver, and promotes both liver blood and kidney *jing*. *Dāng guī* supports liver blood, and *huáng jīng* supports kidney *jing*.

The formula can be used as a general blood tonic, and is particularly good for enhancing male sexual function and female fertility. It is also used a variety of gynecological conditions due to blood deficiency; for men, it can be used for fatigue and depletion following sexual activity.

Plum Flower does not list the ingredient percentages. Its lead herb is *jīn yīng zǐ,* an astringent used to arrest spermatorrhea in men, and for deficiency leukorrhea in women. It also contains *tù sī zǐ* and *bǔ gǔ zhī*, herbs that further enhance tonification of kidney *yang* and *jing*.

OTHER FORMULAS APPROPRIATE FOR THIS CATEGORY:

Classical Formulas:

Ba Zhen Tang
See Chapter 16C

Bu Xue Tiao Jing Tang
See Chapter 6A

Dang Gui Bu Xue Tang
See Chapter 16C

Jiao Ai Tang
See Chapter 6A

Qi Bao Mei Ran Dan
See Chapter 13B

Tao Hong Si Wu Tang
See Chapter 6C

Wen Jing Tang
See Chapter 6A

Wu Ji Bai Feng Wan
See Chapter 6A

Zhong Zi Wan
See Chapter 6A

tián qī (田七), Radix/Rhizoma Notoginseng
Pseudoginseng Capsules, Cooked (HT)
Steamed Tienchi Capsules (PF)
Tien-Chi Ginseng Tablets (PM)

Modern Formulas:

Ban Tu Wan

See Chapter 13B

Others:

Angelica Restorative Formula (K)
Dang Gui Pian/Wan – Hemovigor (GC)
Marrow Plus (HC)
Millettia 9 (SF)
Shou Wu Tablets (SF)
Tang Kuei and Salvia Formula (GF)
Tang-Kuei 18 (SF)
Tonify Blood (CMS)
Woman's Hair Formula (DRJ)

16C. COMBINED QI AND BLOOD TONICS

Classical Formulas:

Ba Zhen Tang	*bā zhēn tāng* (八珍汤)
Dang Gui Bu Xue Tang	*dāng guī bǔ xuè tāng* (当归补血汤)
Ren Shen Yang Rong Tang	*rén shēn yǎng róng tāng* (人参养荣汤)
/ Yang Ying Tang	*yǎng yíng wán* (养营丸)

Modern Formulas:

Ren Shen Shou Wu Wan (Ginseng and Polygonum)
rén shēn shǒu wū wán (人参首乌丸)

Formulas that tonify both *qi* and blood are used in China following surgery, radiation chemotherapy, childbirth, or an extended illness. A number of TCM diseases or *zang-fu* syndromes include *qi* and blood deficiency as one of their differentiations; in these cases formulas from this chapter can be combined with other formulas. These include gynecological diseases (dysmenorrhea, amenorrhea, heavy menstrual periods, menstrual spotting, difficult labor or pregnancy, vaginal itching), heart and *shen* patterns (depression, insomnia, anxiety), liver patterns (dizziness, tremors), blood disorders (subcutaneous bleeding, nosebleed), skin disorders (wind rash, alopecia, slow healing wounds), eye disorders (optic atrophy, diminished vision), *wei* syndrome (tremors, post-stroke), and *bi* syndrome (deficiency joint and muscle pain).

The formulas in this chapter typically combine herbs that tonify *qi* with herbs that nourish blood, adding in other herbs to move *qi* or blood so as to prevent cloying. Nourishing blood usually is more successful when *qi* is tonified at the same time.

A more detailed description of *qi* tonics can be found in the introductions to chapters *6A. Spleen Qi Deficiency* and *16A. Qi Tonics*. A description of blood tonics can be found in the introduction to *16B. Blood Tonics*.

Formulas that tonify *qi* and blood use warming herbs. Caution is advised in heat conditions and deficiency of *yin*. Also, it is recommended that tonics not be used during early stages of colds and flu, as they tend to drive pathogenic factors deeper into the body.

Classical Formulas:

BA ZHEN TANG

Formula: *bā zhēn tāng* (八珍汤), "Eight Treasures Decoction"
Author: Xuē Jǐ (薛己) *aka* Xuē Xīn-Fǔ (薛新甫) *aka* Xuē Li-Zhāi (薛立斋)
Source: *Zhèng Tǐ Lèi Yào* (正体类要), 1529
Literal: "Standardized Category Essentials"

Origin:
Formula: *shí quán dà bǔ tang* (十全大补汤) (see Chapter 18A)
Author: Wú Yàn-Kuí (吴彦夔)
Source: *Chuán Xìn Shì Yòng Fāng* (传信适用方), 1180
Literal: "Transmitted Suitable (and) Useable Formulas"

Availability:

Ba Zhen Tang (BP, TZ)
Ba Zhen Wan (GC, HT, JD, PIM, TL)
Dr. Shen's Women's Precious Pill (DS)
Eight-Treasures (HC)
Nu Ke Ba Zhen Wan (MS)
Tangkuei & Ginseng Eight Combination (EG)
Women's Precious Formula (CC)
Women's Precious Teapills (PF)
Women's Treasure (JD)
* Ba Zhen Yi Mu Wan (TL)
* Tang-Kuei Tablets (SF)
* Women's Precious (K)
* Women's Precious Formula (GF)

Ingredients: (from the standardized *"Tangkuei & Ginseng Eight Combination"*)

dāng guī (当归), Radix Angelicae Sinensis	10.9 %	AB
chuān xiōng (川芎), Rhizoma Ligustici Chuanxiong	10.9	K
bái sháo (白芍), Radix Paeoniae Alba	10.9	AB
shú dì huáng (熟地黄), Radix Rehmanniae Praep.	10.9	AB
rén shēn (人参), Radix Ginseng	10.9	AA
fú líng (茯苓), Poria	10.9	FC
bái zhú (白术), Rhizoma Atractylodis Macrocephalae	10.9	AA
shēng jiāng (生姜), Rhizoma Zingiberis Recens	10.9	E
dà zǎo (大枣), Fructus Jujubae	7.3	AA
gān cǎo (甘草), Radix Glycyrrhizae	5.5	AA

Ingredients: (from Herbal Times *"Ba Zhen Wan"*)

shú dì huáng (熟地黄), Radix Rehmanniae Praep.	18.2 %	AB
dāng guī (当归), Radix Angelicae Sinensis	18.2	AB
bái sháo (白芍), Radix Paeoniae Alba	12.1	AB
bái zhú (白术), Rhizoma Atractylodis Macrocephalae	12.1	AA
dǎng shēn (党参), Radix Codonopsis	12.1	AA
fú líng (茯苓), Poria	12.1	FC
chuān xiōng (川芎), Rhizoma Ligustici Chuanxiong	9.1	K
gān cǎo (甘草), Radix Glycyrrhizae	6.1	AA

Nourishes blood, tonifies qi. Use for deficiency of *qi* and blood causing fatigue, dry hair and skin, pale complexion, cracked nails, dizziness, poor memory or concentration. Use for the menstrual disorders of amenorrhea, scanty or irregular periods or following heavy periods, and to promote fertility. Also, anemia, dizziness, heart palpitations, optic atrophy and slow healing of wounds when due to deficiency of *qi* and blood. Use following childbirth, surgery, radiation and prolonged illness.

Pulse: Thready and weak
Tongue: Pale with thin white coat

Comments: *Ba Zhen Wan* is a popular in China to tonify blood following menses, surgery or radiation, or as a general tonic. The prescription combines two foundation formulas, each with four herbs. The first is *Si Jun Zi Tang* (Chapter 6A), which tonifies *qi* using *rén shēn* (or *dǎng shēn*), *fú líng*, *bái zhú* and *gān cǎo*. The second is *Si Wu Tang* (Chapter 16B) to nourish blood, using *dāng guī*, *bái sháo*, *shú dì huáng* and *chuān xiōng*. The herbs *gān jiāng* and *dà zǎo* are often added to the formula to boost *qi* and warm the stomach.

The author, Xue Ji, may have been inspired by the formula *Shi Quan Da Bu Wan*, created in 1180 (see *Chapter 18A*).

Caution: Discontinue during colds and flu, as tonics tend to drive pathogenic factors into the interior.

Further Reading:

Bensky et al, p. 346
Chen & Chen, p. 604
Ellis, p. 9

DANG GUI BU XUE TANG

Formula: *dāng guī bǔ xuè tāng* (当归补血汤)
"Angelica *Dang Gui* Tonify Blood Decoction"
Author: Lǐ Gǎo (李杲) *aka* Lǐ Dōng-Yuán (李东垣)
Source: *Nèi Wài Shāng Biàn Huò Lùn* (内外伤辨惑论), 1247
Literal: "Internal External Injury, Clarify False-Notions Discussion"

Availability:

Dang Gui Bu Xue Tang (EG, TZ)
Dang Gui Bu Xue Wan (PM)
Tangkuei & Astragalus Combination (EG)

Ingredients: (from the standardized *"Tangkuei & Astragalus Combination"*)

huáng qí (黄芪), Radix Astragali	83.3 %	AA
dāng guī (当归), Radix Angelicae Sinensis	16.7	AB

Ingredients: (from Lanzhou Traditional Herbs/KGS "Dang Gui Bu Xue Wan")

huáng qí (黄芪), Radix Astragali	71.1 %	AA
dāng guī (当归), Radix Angelicae Sinensis	28.8	AB

Tonifies qi, nourishes blood, consolidates the exterior, harmonizes yin and yang. Use to replenish *qi* and blood following fever or during deficiency fever, excessive blood flow during menses, or blood loss due to surgery, trauma or postpartum. Also to heal sores and wounds, deficiency *bì* patterns causing weakness and flaccidity, scanty menses or amenorrhea, irregular periods, and to build *wèi qi* to protect against cold and allergy.

Pulse: Weak or soft or thin
Tongue: Pale or swollen or moist

Comments: This two-herb formula understands that the key to building blood is to build *qi*, according to the TCM axiom "visible blood originates from invisible *qi*". Here, the *qi* tonic *huáng qí* comprises the lion's share of the formula, with a smaller amount of the blood tonic *dāng guī*. It was originally created to treat low-grade fever due to exhaustion with an underlying etiology of blood deficiency, and in this regard it is useful for low-grade postpartum fever. In modern times, it is also used to replenish blood following trauma, surgery, childbirth, heavy menses, and radiation/chemotherapy.

The combination of *huáng qí* and *dāng guī* promotes the healing of wounds and sores. *Huáng qí* brings *wèi qi* to the surface to promote healing, while *dāng guī* helps to regenerate flesh and tissue.

Further Reading:

Bensky et al, p. 338
Chen & Chen, p. 580
Ellis, p. 67

REN SHEN YANG RONG TANG / YANG YING WAN

Formula: *rén shēn yǎng róng tāng* (人参养荣汤)
"Ginseng Nourish Luxuriant-Growth Decoction"
aka: *yǎng yíng wán* (养营丸), "Nourish *Ying-Qi* Pills"
Author: Imperial Medical Bureau (*tài yī jú,* 太医局);
revised by Chén Shī-Wén (陈师文)
Source: *Tài Píng Huì Mín Hé Jì Jú Fāng* (太平惠民和剂局方), 1078
Literal: "(Era of) Great Peace, Benefit People Harmonious Medicines, Office (of) Formulas"

Availability:

Using the *Ren Shen Yang Rong Wan* formula:

Ginseng & Rehmannia Combination (EG)
Ginseng Nourishing Formula (GF)
Ren Shen Yang Rong Tang (BP, TZ)

Using the *Yang Ying Wan* Formula:

Fu Ke Yang Rong Wan (PM)
Renshen Yang Ying Wan (PM)
Yang Ying Teapills (PF)
Yang Ying Wan (MS, PM)

The *Ren Shen Yang Rong Wan* formula:

Ingredients: (from Blue Poppy *"Ren Shen Yang Rong Tang"*)

bái sháo (白芍), Radix Paeoniae Alba	23.7 %	AB
dāng guī (当归), Radix Angelicae Sinensis	7.8	AB
chén pí (陈皮), Pericarpium Citri Reticulatae	7.8	G
huáng qí (黄芪), Radix Astragali	7.8	AA
ròu guì (肉桂), Cortex Cinnamomi	7.8	E
rén shēn (人参), Radix Ginseng)	7.8	AA
bái zhú (白术), Rhizoma Atractylodis Macrocephalae	7.8	AA
zhì gān cǎo (炙甘草), Radix Glycyrrhizae Praep.	7.8	AA
shú dì huáng (熟地黄), Radix Rehmanniae Praep.	5.9	AB
wǔ wèi zǐ (五味子), Fructus Schisandrae	5.9	L
fú líng (茯苓), Poria	5.9	FC
yuǎn zhì (远志), Radix Arillus Longanlae	4.0	N

Ingredients: (from the standardized *"Ginseng & Rehmannia Combination"*)

bái sháo (白芍), Radix Paeoniae Alba	12.0 %	AB
shēng jiāng (生姜), Rhizoma Zingiberis Recens	9.0	BA
bái zhú (白术), Rhizoma Atractylodis Macrocephalae	7.6	AA
huáng qí (黄芪), Radix Astragali	7.6	AA
zhì gān cǎo (炙甘草), Radix Glycyrrhizae Praep.	7.6	AA
chén pí (陈皮), Pericarpium Citri Reticulatae	7.6	G
guì zhī (桂枝), Ramulus Cinnamomi	7.6	E
dāng guī (当归), Radix Angelicae Sinensis	7.6	AB
rén shēn (人参), Radix Ginseng	7.6	AA
wǔ wèi zǐ (五味子), Fructus Schisandrae	6.1	L
fú líng (茯苓), Poria	6.1	FC
shú dì huáng (熟地黄), Radix Rehmanniae Praep.	6.1	AB
yuǎn zhì (远志), Radix Polygalae	4.5	N
dà zǎo (大枣), Fructus Jujubae	3.0	AA

The *Yang Ying Wan* formula:

Ingredients: (From Minshan "Yang Ying Wan" and Plum Flower "Yang Ying Teapills")

dǎng shēn (党参), Radix Codonopsis	15.1 %	AA
bái zhú (白术), Rhizoma Atractylodis Macrocephalae	7.6	AA
huáng qí (黄芪), Radix Astragali	7.6	AA
gān cǎo (甘草), Radix Glycyrrhizae	7.5	AA
ròu guì (肉桂), Cortex Cinnamomi	7.5	E
chén pí (陈皮), Pericarpium Citri Reticulatae	7.5	G
dāng guī (当归), Radix Angelicae Sinensis	7.5	AB
dà zǎo (大枣), Fructus Jujubae	7.5	AA
bái sháo (白芍), Radix Paeoniae Alba	7.5	AB
shú dì huáng (熟地黄), Radix Rehmanniae Praep.	5.7	AB
wǔ wèi zǐ (五味子), Fructus Schisandrae	5.7	L
fú líng (茯苓), Poria	5.7	FC
yuǎn zhì (远志), Radix Polygalae	3.8	N
shēng jiāng (生姜), Rhizoma Zingiberis Recens	3.8	BA

continued

Tonifies qi, nourishes blood, invigorates blood, nourishes yin and assists yang, benefits spleen, heart and lung, calms shen. Use for systemic deficiencies of *qi*, blood, *yin* and *yang* with root deficiency in the spleen, heart or kidney. Symptoms include fatigue, poor concentration or memory, insomnia, palpitations, restlessness, cold or heavy limbs and spontaneous sweating. Can be used as a post-menstrual and post-partum tonic. Valuable as a general tonic for the aged, recovery from surgery or prolonged illness, and for treating chronic non-healing sores.

Pulse: Thin, weak, deep
Tongue: Normal, or pale or wet, swollen

Comments: This formula was developed for patients recovering from tuberculosis and other serious illness. It is now popular in China as a general tonic for aging patients, as well as post-partum or following a prolonged illness. Using herbs to tonify *qi* and blood, it also benefits the heart using directional herbs such as *yuǎn zhì* and *wǔ wèi zǐ*. In this regard, it is good for diminished memory and concentration, anxiety, and palpitations.

There are several variations of the formula, based on differing ingredient percentages. The original formula, which has been reproduced by Blue Poppy, contains 24% *bái sháo*, a cooling blood tonic. This signifies the intention of boosting while cooling heart blood in order to calm the mind. The Taiwan (EG) manufacturers use 12% *bái sháo*.

Another group of products follow Minshan's modern version, called *Yang Ying Wan*. This formulation prioritizes spleen and heart *qi* rather than cooling heart blood and calming *shen*. It also adds *shēng jiāng* to the original formula.

Ren Shen Yang Rong Wan and *Yang Ying Wan* are similar to *Shi Quan Da Bu Wan* (Chapter 18A), but that formula is better for boosting kidney *yang* and spleen *qi*, while these formulas are better for tonifying spleen and heart in order to calm *shen*.

Note: The name *Ren Shen Yang Rong Wan* is often confused with *Yang Rong Wan*, a modern formula used for gynecological complaints related to blood deficiency (see Chapter 8A).

Further Reading:

Bensky et al, p. 350
Chen & Chen, p. 615
Ellis, p. 242

Modern Formulas:

REN SHEN SHOU WU WAN
GINSENG AND POLYGONUM

Formula: *rén shēn shǒu wū wán* (人参首乌丸), "Ginseng Polygonum Pills"
Source: Modern patent medicine

Availability:

Ginseng & Fo Ti Extract (PM)
Ginseng With Polygonum Mulliflorium (PM)
Ren Shen Shou Wu Jing (PM)

Ingredients: (from Kwangchow Pharmaceutical Industry *"Ginseng with Polygonum Mulliflorum"*)

hé shǒu wū (何首乌), Radix Polygoni Multiflori	60. %	AB
rén shēn (人参), Radix Ginseng	40	AA

Nourishes blood, tonifies qi, benefits jing, strengthens tendon and bone. Use for chronic deficiencies of *qi* and blood affecting vitality, menstruation and mental clarity. Benefits lower back, painful joints, blurred vision, poor memory and concentration. Also for dry hair, dry skin and cracked nails. A general tonic for *qi* and blood, it can be used following radiation, postpartum and surgery and for sexual depletion, and as a geriatric tonic.

Comments: *Ren Shen Shou Wu Wan* combines Polygonum *hé shǒu wū* with Ginseng *rén shēn. Hé shǒu wū* (also known in the West, erroneously, as *Fo-Ti*) is used as a blood tonic following male sexual depletion, by women to support hair growth, and to moisten and increase tendon elasticity. *Rén shēn* is a tonic for spleen and heart *qi* (see description in Chapter 16A). The combination is a very good general tonic for *qi* and blood, strengthening the heart and mind, and keeping tendons and ligaments moist and supple. It is used to slow the effects of aging, and is valued as a longevity tonic.

Caution: Discontinue during colds and flu, as tonics tend to drive pathogenic factors into the interior. Also, this is a warming formula. Caution if heat or dry symptoms occur.

OTHER FORMULAS APPROPRIATE FOR THIS CATEGORY:

Classical Formulas:

Gui Pi Tang

See Chapter 9

Shi Quan Da Bu Wan

See Chapter 18A

Modern Formulas:

Thyro-Forte (EV)

17. KIDNEY TONICS

17A. KIDNEY YIN TONICS

Classical Formulas:

Liu Wei Di Huang Wan	*liù wèi dì huáng wán* (六味地黄丸)
Zuo Gui Wan	*zuǒ guī wán* (左归丸)

Kidney *yin* resides in the TCM energetic kidney. It is a purified moistening mist that is derived from fluid as it passes through the kidney. *Yin* is a cool liquid in distinction to blood, which is a warm liquid. Kidney *yin* is used to moisten and cool other *zang-fu* organs, particularly the liver, heart and lung. It moistens all of the mucosal membranes of the respiratory and digestive tract from the nose and throat to the anus, as well as eye and vagina. It also provides the liquid used inside the eye, in synovial joints, and in cerebral spinal fluid.

Yin can be deficient constitutionally, or diminish with age. It can also be consumed by exposure to heat, with prolonged stress or over-study, chronic disease, and overconsumption of spicy food. An overactive sex life, or giving birth many times, can exhaust kidney *yin*. There are modern contributors also: use of pharmaceutical drugs can deplete *yin*, as evidenced by common reported side effects of dry mouth, dizziness, or palpitation. Electric magnetic fields, such as clock radios, photocopiers, fluorescent lights, and hybrid cars can also deplete *yin*. In fact, Chinese medicine historically focused of deficiencies of kidney *yang*, due to pervasive cold and damp or physically hard work. Ironically, modern Western societies are more afflicted by *yin* deficiencies, due to drugs and electromagnetic fields.

Chronic deficiencies of *yin* of the liver, heart, stomach or lung are rooted in a deficiency of kidney *yin*. Sometimes, tonification of kidney *yin* is sufficient to correct a disorder. Other times, concurrent tonification of kidney *yin* as well as liver, heart or lung *yin* are required.

Deficiency of *yin* is responsible for abnormal dryness, manifesting as dry eyes, nose, throat, mouth or vagina. (Dry skin and hair on the other hand is due to blood deficiency.) It can also exhibit as deficiency heat, showing as deficiency fever, menopausal hot flashing or night sweats. Other signs may include dizziness, ear ringing, weak lumbar area, weak knees, impotence or reduced sexual drive, spermatorrhea, poor eyesight, anxiety, palpitations and insomnia.

Diseases and symptoms due to kidney *yin* deficiency include diabetes, chronic kidney disease, menstrual disorders, hyperthyroidism, chronic hepatitis and some cases of hypertension. It is not uncommon to have concurrent deficiencies of *yin* and blood, or even both *yin* and *yang.*

Kidney *yin* tonics may be helpful in treating modern stress disorders with symptoms of restlessness and anxiety. They help reduce elevated cortisol levels found in adrenal stress presentations.

This chapter includes formulas for treating kidney *yin* deficiency at its root. Other products that address *yin* deficiency can be found in the following chapters:

3E. Lung *Yin* Deficiency
8E. Menopausal Disorder and Deficiency Fire
9. Disturbed *Shen*
14. Eye and Vision Disorders

Classical Formulas:

LIU WEI DI HUANG WAN

Formula: *liù wèi dì huáng wán* (六味地黄丸), "Six Flavor Rehmannia Pill"
Author: Qián Yǐ (钱乙)
Source: *Qián Shì Xiǎo Ér Yào Zhèng Zhí Jué* (钱氏小儿药证直), 1119
Literal: "Qian's Key (to) Children's Medicines (and) Patterns, Straight Secrets"

Origin:
Formula: *jīn guì shèn qì wán* (金匮肾气丸), "Golden Cabinet Kidney Qi Pill"
Author: Zhāng Zhòng-Jǐng (张仲景)
Source: *Jīn Guì Yào Lüè* (金匮要略), 220
Literal: "Golden Cabinet Essential Summary"

Availability:

Liu Wei Di Huang Wan (BP, HT, JD, MS, PIM, PM, TL)
Rehmannia 6 Formula (CC)
Rehmannia Six Formula (EG, GF)
Six Flavor Rehmannia (PM)
Six Flavor Tea (JD)
Six Flavor Teapills (MS, PF)
* Jade Moon Phase 2 (JW)
* Nine Flavor Tea (HC)
* Quiet Contemplative (K)

Ingredients: (from the standardized *"Rehmannia Six Formula"*)

shú dì huáng (熟地黄), Radix Rehmanniae Praep.	32. %	AB
shān zhū yú (山茱萸), Fructus Corni	16	L
shān yào (山药), Rhizoma Dioscoreae	16	AA
mǔ dān pí (牡丹皮), Cortex Moutan	12	DC
fú líng (茯苓), Poria	12	FC
zé xiè (泽泻), Rhizoma Alismatis	12	FC

Benefits the kidney, nourishes kidney and liver yin, cools deficiency heat, consolidates jing. Use for deficiency of *yin* affecting kidney or liver, with symptoms of dryness in the eyes, mouth, nose, throat or vagina; also weak lumbar area and knees, deficiency headache, dizziness, tinnitus, hypertension, insomnia, anxiety and fatigue. It is used in diabetes, chronic nephritis, infantile underdevelopment, hyperthyroidism, menopausal disorder, and some cases of hypertension. The formula can be taken for long periods of time.

Pulse: Normal, or thin
Tongue: Normal, or reddish and dry

Comments: The original application of *Liu Wei Di Huang Wan* in 1119 CE was as a pediatric formula, to treat the five "delays" of standing, walking, hair growth or fontanel closure, teeth development, and speech. Since the Ming dynasty (1368–1644), it has been used as a formula for *yin* deficiency affecting the kidney, liver, lung, stomach or heart. Modern applications include kidney *yin* deficiency leading to infertility, chronic nephritis, chronic hepatitis and diabetes, as well as addressing dryness in the mucus membranes (eye, throat, vagina). *Yin* tonics are useful for normalizing elevated cortisol produced by stress, alleviating anxiety, tension and poor sleep.

Shú dì huáng is the lead herb (32%), moistening and benefiting *yin* and blood. *Shān zhū yú* astringes the formula into the kidney, moistens kidney and liver *yin,* boosts *jing*, and clears deficiency heat. *Shān yào* replenishes spleen *yin*, and also benefits the kidney. As a relative of the Mexican yam, it has beneficial affects on the adrenal gland function. *Mǔ dān pí* clears deficiency heat in the kidney and real heat in the liver. *Fú líng* and *zé xiè* free dampness, which is astringed into the kidney to increase kidney *yin*, and helps to mitigate the greasiness of *shú dì huáng*.

Qian Yi's formula, created in 1119, is based on *Jin Gui Shen Qi Wan* (see Chapter 17B), a *Shang Han Lun* formula (220 CE). It takes the original formula and removes the two *yang*-boosting herbs, *ròu guì* (肉桂, Cortex Cinnamomi) and *fù zǐ* (炙附子, Radix Aconiti Lateralis).

continued

Liu Wei Di Huang Wan has served as the foundation formula for important classical prescriptions, each of which adds 2 herbs to the original formula to either help guide to a specific location or to enhance a new function:

1350	*Qi Ju Di Huang Wan* (Chapter 14. Eye and Vision Disorders)
1584	*Zhi Bai Di Huang Wan* (Chapter 8E. Menopausal Disorder and Deficiency Fire)
1615	*Ba Xian Chang Shou Wan* (Chapter 3E. Lung *Yin* Deficiency)
1774	*Er Long Zuo Ci Wan* (Chapter 7B. Liver *Yang* and Internal Wind)

The following modern formulas also use *Liu Wei Di Huang Wan* as their foundation:

Ming Mu Di Huang Wan (Chapter 14. Eye and Vision Disorders)
Xiao Ke Wan (Chapter 15A. Wasting-Thirst)

Further Reading:

Bensky et al, p. 365
Chen & Chen, p. 627
Ellis, p. 188

ZUO GUI WAN

Formula: *zuǒ guī wán* (左归丸), "Left Restore Pill"
Author: Zhāng Jiè-Bīn (张介宾) *aka* Zhāng Jǐng-Yuè (张景岳)
Source: *Jǐng Yuè Quán Shū* (景岳全书), 1624
Literal: "Jing-Yue's Complete Writings"

Availability:

Cyathula & Rehmannia Formula (EG)
Left-Side Replenishing Teapills (PF)
Replenish The Left (K)
Zho Kwei Pills (PM)
Zuo Gui Wan (BP, HT, PM, TL)
Zuo Gui Yin (BP, TZ)
* True Yin Formula (GF)

Ingredients: (from Herbal Times *"Zuo Gui Wan"*)

shú dì huáng (熟地黄), Radix Rehmanniae Praep.	26. %	AB
shān yào (山药), Rhizoma Dioscoreae	11	AA
gǒu qǐ zǐ (枸杞子), Fructus Lycii	11	AB
shān zhū yú (山茱萸), Fructus Corni	11	L
tù sī zǐ (菟丝子), Semen Cuscutae	11	AC
lù jiǎo jiāo (鹿角胶), Colla Cornus Cervi	11	AC
guī bǎn jiāo (龟板胶), Plastrum Testudinis/Chinemys	11	AD
chuān niú xī (川牛膝), Radix Cyathulae	8	K

Ingredients: (from Kwangchow Pharmaceceutical *"Zho Kwei Pills"*)

shú dì huáng (熟地黄), Radix Rehmanniae Praep.	20. %	AB
fú líng (茯苓), Poria	16	FC
shān zhū yú (山茱萸), Fructus Corni	15	L
gǒu qǐ zǐ (枸杞子), Fructus Lycii	15	AB
shān yào (山药), Rhizoma Dioscoreae	15	AA
tù sī zǐ (菟丝子), Semen Cuscutae	10	AC
huái niú xī (怀牛膝), Radix Achyranthis Bidentatae	8	K

Nourishes kidney qi and yin, consolidates and increases jing, strengthens tendon and bone. Use for kidney deficiency causing weak lumbar area, lower legs or knees, dizziness, insomnia, anxiety and fatigue. Can be used for menopausal disorder, hypertension, and fatigue. Also, deficiency headache, dizziness, tinnitus, hypertension, insomnia, anxiety and fatigue. It is used in chronic nephritis, hyperthyroidism, menopausal disorder, and some cases of hypertension. The formula can be taken for long periods of time.

Pulse: Normal, or thin
Tongue: Normal, or reddish and dry

Comments: *Zuo Gui Wan* is a Ming dynasty formula (1368–1644) for nourishing kidney *yin*. "Returning the left" refers to the left kidney, which the author, Zhang Jie-Bin, believes belongs to the *yin*. (It is complemented by Zhang's *You Gui Wan*, Chapter 17B.) In clinical practice, *Zuo Gui Wan* is preferred for general kidney weakness or deficiency, while *Liu Wei Di Huang Wan* (above) is preferred for dryness patterns.

The chief herb is *shú dì huáng*, which is used to moisten *yin* and promote blood. The original *Zuo Gui Wan* employs animal parts, including turtle bone (*guī bǎn*) to enhance *yin* and *jing* available from bone marrow, combined with the *yang* tonifying aspects of deer antler (*lù jiǎo jiāo*). Compared with *Liu Wei*, it also adds *gǒu qǐ zǐ* to benefit *yin* and *jing*, and *tù sī zǐ*, to boost kidney *yang* and *jing*. *Niú xī* strengthens the tendons, and benefits the knees. In general, the formula strengthens kidney *qi*, leaning slightly to the *yin* aspect.

The original formula calls for the animal parts *lù jiāo* and *guī bǎn*. Herbal Times and the standardized Taiwan prescription (EG), for example, follow the original formula. Some manufacturers choose to omit *lù jiāo* and *guī bǎn*, including Plum Flower and Kwangchow Pharmaceutical.

The formula has no herbs to mitigate the cloying and dampening effects of some of the ingredients, and is recommended for a limited duration. *Liu Wei Di Huang Wan*, above, is preferred for longer-term use.

Caution: Both *guī bǎn* and *chuān niú xī* are contraindicated during pregnancy. Also, *shú dì huáng* can cause bloating, nausea, or loose stools. Reduce dosage if necessary.

Further reading:

Bensky et al, p. 372
Chen & Chen, p. 647
Ellis, p. 426

OTHER FORMULAS APPROPRIATE FOR THIS CATEGORY:

Yin deficiency with heat, see Chapter 8E

Da Bu Yin Wan
Qing Gu San
Zhi Bai Di Huang Wan
Geng Nian An Wan

Liver *yin* deficiency, See Chapter 7A

Yi Guan Jian

Lung *yin* deficiency, See Chapter 3E

Ba Xian Chang Shou Wan / Mai Wei Di Huang Wan
Bai He Gu Jin Tang
Sha Shen Mai Men Dong Tang
Sheng Mai San
Gu Ben Wan

Heart *yin* deficiency, See Chapter 9

Bai Zi Yang Xin Tang
Gan Mai Da Zao Tang
Tian Wang Bu Xin Dan
Gan Mai Da Zao Tang
Suan Zao Ren Tang

Modern Formulas:

Anemarrhena Tablets (SF)
Nourish Essence Formula (GF)
Rehmannia 16 (SF)
Rehmannia Cool Blood Formula (GF)
Restorative Tablets (SF)
Supplement Yin (BP)
Tonify Moisture (CMS)
Tortoise Shell Tablets (SF)

17. KIDNEY TONICS

17B. KIDNEY YANG AND JING TONICS

Classical Formulas:

Jin Gui Shen Qi Wan	*jīn guì shèn qì wán* (金匮肾气丸)
/ Ba Wei Di Huang Wan	*bā wèi dì huáng wán* (八味地黄丸)
Wu Zi Yang Zong Wan	*wǔ zǐ yǎn zōng wán* (五子衍宗丸)
You Gui Wan	*yòu guī wán* (右归丸)

Modern Formulas:

Cong Rong Bu Shen Wan	*cōng róng bǔ shèn wán* (苁蓉补肾丸)
Ge Jie Bu Shen Wan	*gé jiè bǔ shèn wán* (蛤蚧补肾丸)
/ Ge Jie Da Bu Wan	*gé jiè dà bǔ wán* (蛤蚧大补丸)
Gui Ling Ji (Kwei Ling Chi)	*guī líng jí* (龟龄集)

Kidney *yang,* if we include *mingmen* fire, is the energy and heat source for the whole body. *Jing* is the essence of *yang*; it is stored in kidney, the extraordinary channels, and in bone marrow, which In TCM includes the brain. In modern physiology, kidney *yang* and *jing* empower the adrenal glands, testes and ovaries, as well as influence the entire endocrine system.

Kidney *yang* extends to all organs. First, it pumps *qi* and *yang* to the upper burner, affecting heart and lung. Kidney *yang* keeps the heart beating and keeps the blood warm. If kidney *yang* is weak, the heart gets cold, leading to congestive heart failure. Kidney *yang* also roots the lungs, allowing the diaphragm to descend on inhalation. Weakness can precipitate asthma. When the *yang* of the upper *jiao* is affected, fatigue and low vitality follow, as well as poor concentration or forgetfulness.

Second, kidney *yang* provides the energy for digestive peristalsis, helping food move through the digestive tract. It also warms and nurtures stomach fire and spleen *yang*, directly boosting hydrochloric acid, and thereby aiding digestive strength. Deficiency can contribute to sluggish metabolism, constipation, and poor absorption of nutrients. In extreme cases of *yang* deficiency, the intestines lose their contractile strength, causing diarrhea or cramping upon waking ("daybreak diarrhea").

Third, kidney *yang* and *jing* affect urogenital function. It governs the ability to constrict the urethra, and deficiency can lead to urinary dribbling or frequency. *Yang* deficiency often contributes to swollen prostate and lower leg edema. It also controls erection and ejaculation, and deficiency leads to impotence or poor sexual function for men. In extreme cases, spontaneous le*aka*ge of semen without erection or ejaculation can occur, called spermatorrhea. For these reasons, *yang* and *jing* tonics are used to enhance male sexual performance. Also, because kidney *yang* warms the uterus, it can underlie cases of female infertility, amenorrhea and other menstrual issues. These formulas can also be useful for postpartum fatigue.

Fourth, weakness of kidney *yang* is often the cause of weak lumbar area, chronic back problems, degeneration of spinal discs, and knee pain or degeneration. As kidney nourishes and controls the bone, osteoporosis is usually due to kidney deficiency (*yang, yin* and *jing*.)

Fifth, kidney *yang*, along with kidney *yin,* helps to regenerate marrow and create blood, and some cases of blood deficiency are due to kidney deficiency. Radiation depletes kidney *yang*, and tonification of *yang, yin* and blood is often required following radiation. *Yang, yin* and *jing* deficiencies can lead to dementia and other brain degenerative illnesses.

Kidney *yang* and *mingmen* strength is initially determined by one's constitution. As we age, we use up our supply of *yang* and *jing,* leading to diminished organ function and becoming cold from poor circulation. Lowered warmth and fire can lead to blood stagnation, and many diseases of the aged are due to blood stagnation rooted in deficiency of *yang* and *mingmen* fire. It is quite common for Chinese, especially men, to take kidney *yang* tonics as they age. The *yang* can also be depleted by prolonged illness, surgery, etc.

It is recommended that tonics, including formulas that tonify *yang*, not be used during the early stages of pathogenic wind (common cold), as they tend to drive pathogenic wind deeper into the body. Because of the warming and drying nature of these formulas, they should not be used in cases of deficiency fire or deficiency of *yin*.

Classical Formulas:

JIN GUI SHEN QI WAN

Formula: *jīn guì shèn qì wán* (金匮肾气丸), "Golden Cabinet Kidney *Qi* Pill"
aka: *shèn qì wán* (肾气丸), "Kidney *Qi* Pill"
aka: *bā wèi dì huáng wán* (八味地黄丸), "Eight Flavor Rehmannia Pill"
Author: Zhāng Zhòng-Jǐng (张仲景)
Source: *Jīn Guì Yào Lüè* (金匮要略), 220
Literal: "Golden Cabinet Essential Summary"

Availability:

Dynamic Warrior (K)
Golden Book Herbal (PM)
Golden Book Teapills (MS, PF)
Golden Cabinet Kidney Formula (JD)
Jin Gui Shen Qi Wan (BP, HT, PIM, PM, TL, TZ)
Kidney Qi Formula From The Golden Cabinet (HS)
Rehmannia 8 (HC)
Rehmannia Eight Formula (EG, HS)
* Essential Yang Formula (GF)

Ingredients: (from the standardized *"Rehmannia Eight Formula"*)

shú dì huáng (熟地黄), Radix Rehmanniae Praep.	29.7 %	AB
shān yào (山药), Rhizoma Dioscoreae	14.8	AA
shān zhū yú (山茱萸), Fructus Corni	14.8	L
fú líng (茯苓), Poria	11.1	FC
mŭ dān pí (牡丹皮), Cortex Moutan	11.1	DC
zé xiè (泽泻), Rhizoma Alismatis	11.1	FC
ròu guì (肉桂), Cortex Cinnamomi	3.7	E
zhì fù zǐ (炙附子), Radix Aconiti Lateralis Praeparata	3.7	E

Tonifies kidney yang, warms mingmen fire, benefits kidney qi. Use for chronic deficiency of kidney *qi* and *yang* causing lower back pain or weakness, weak knees, coldness in the abdomen, lumbar region or legs, and urinary dysfunction. Also for *yang* deficiency causing male impotence, female infertility, cold limbs, or edema. Used in polyuria due to diabetes, toxemia during pregnancy, hypothyroid, bladder prolapse, chronic nephritis and chronic prostatitis.

Pulse: Normal, or deep, thready
Tongue: Normal, or pale or swollen

Comments: This classical formula from Zhang Zhong-Jing, dating to the early 3rd century, is considered one of the basic prescriptions for tonifying kidney *qi* and *yang*. The foundation of the formula supports kidney *yin*, and later became isolated as *Liu Wei Di Huang Wan* to support kidney *yin* (see *Chapter 17A*). In *Jin Gui Shen Qi Wan*, two warming herbs are used, *zhì fù zǐ* and *ròu guì,* to enhance the tonification of kidney *yang,* dispel cold and remove dampness. Small doses are used so as not to consume *yin* or scatter the *yang*.

Zhang's original formula used *shēng dì huáng* (生地黄, Radix Rehmanniae), which cools and moistens the kidney, but later clinicians and most manufacturers substitute the more warming *shú dì huáng*. Likewise, the original formula used cinnamon twig *guì zhī* (桂枝, Ramulus Cinnamomi), when later formulators substituted cinnamon bark *ròu guì*. The combination of *ròu guì* and *zé xiè* helps to circulate and regulate water metabolism, addressing edema and water retention due to deficiency of *mingmen* fire.

Compared with *You Gui Wan* (below), *Shen Qi Wan* is gentler and can be used for longer periods.

Caution: *Zhì fù zǐ* is contraindicated during pregnancy.

Further Reading:

Bensky et al, p. 395 (as *Shen Qi Wan*)
Chen & Chen, p. 668 (as *Jin Gui Shen Qi Wan*)
Ellis, p. 7 (as *Bai Wei Di Huang Wan*)

WU ZI YAN ZONG WAN

Formula: *wǔ zǐ yǎn zōng wán* (五子衍宗丸)
"Five Seed Develop Family Pill"
Author: Lǐ Chān (李梴) *aka* Lǐ Tǐng (李挺) *aka* Lǐ Jiàn-Zhāi (李健齋)
Source: *Yī Xué Rù Mén* (医学入门), 1575
Literal: "Medical Studies Introduction"

Availability:

Five Ancestors Teapills (PF)
Wu Zi Yan Zong Wan (GC, HT, PM)
* Jiu Zi Hui Chun Wan - Nine Seeds Return To Spring (TL)

Ingredients: (from Herbal Times *"Wu Zi Yan Zong Wan"*)

gǒu qǐ zǐ (枸杞子), Fructus Lycii	34.8 %	AB
tù sī zǐ (菟丝子), Semen Cuscutae	34.8	AC
fù pén zǐ (覆盆子), Fructus Rubi	17.4	L
chē qián zǐ (车前子), Semen Plantaginis	8.7	FC
wǔ wèi zǐ (五味子), Fructus Schisandrae	4.3	L

Ingredients: (from Plum Flower *"Five Ancestors Teapills"*)

gǒu qǐ zǐ (枸杞子), Fructus Lycii	34.7 %	AB
tù sī zǐ (菟丝子), Semen Cuscutae	34.7	AC
fù pén zǐ (覆盆子), Fructus Rubi	17.6	L
chē qián zǐ (车前子), Semen Plantaginis	8.8	FC
wǔ wèi zǐ (五味子), Fructus Schisandrae	4.2	L

Tonifies kidney yang, tonifies blood and yin, benefits and consolidates jing. Use for deficiency of kidney *qi*, *yang* and *jing* causing general weakness, sexual dysfunction, impotence, premature ejaculation, male infertility, low sperm count, urinary dribbling, and lumbar weakness. Useful as a general tonic for aging men, for chronic prostatitis, and chronic kidney disease. Also used for female infertility due to *yang* and *jing* deficiency.

Pulse: Normal, or deep, weak
Tongue: Normal, or pale or swollen

Comments: This formula is used to enhance male fertility, and to counter spermatorrhea or premature ejaculation. It is effective at raising sperm count and increasing sperm motility, and can also be used in female infertility. In the original formula, five herbal seeds were used to astringe and consolidate *jing*. Research has confirmed positive effects for male infertility and uterine hypoplasia. It has also been found to be hepato-protective.

70% of the formula consist of two herbs: *gǒu qǐ zǐ* and *tù sī zǐ*. Together, these two herbs boost kidney *yang*, support kidney *yin* and *jing*. For this reason, the formula can support lumbar weakness, as well as treat infertility and poor male sexual function.

Both Herbal Times and Plum Flower follow the same percentage ingredientss. Tanglong has a version, *Jiu Zi Hui Chun Wan* which expands the original to a 14-ingredient formula, adding herbs to support *yang*, consolidate *jing* and clear heat.

YOU GUI WAN

Formula: *yòu guī wán,* (右归丸), "Right Restoring Pills"
Author: Zhāng Jiè-Bīn (张介宾) *aka* Zhāng Jǐng-Yuè (张景岳)
Source: *Jǐng Yuè Quán Shū* (景岳全书), 1624
Literal: "Jing-Yue's Complete Writings"

Availability:

Eucommia & Rehmannia Formula (EG)
Replenish The Right (K)
Yanourish Remedy (PM)
Yao Kwei Pills (PM)
You Gui Teapills (PF)
You Gui Wan (BP, GC, HT)
You Gui Yin (TZ)
* Jade Moon Phase 4 (JW)
* Strengthen The Root (TT)

Ingredients: (from Herbal Times *"You Gui Wan"*)

shú dì huáng (熟地黄), Radix Rehmanniae Praep.	18. %	AB
shān yào (山药), Rhizoma Dioscoreae	13	AA
lù jiǎo jiāo (鹿角胶), Colla Cornus Cervi	13	AC
dāng guī (当归), Radix Angelicae Sinensis	9	AB
dù zhòng (杜仲), Cortex Eucommiae	9	AC
gǒu qǐ zǐ (枸杞子), Fructus Lycii	9	AB
shān zhū yú (山茱萸), Fructus Corni	9	L
chǎo tù sī zǐ (炒菟丝子), Semen Cuscutae, charred	9	AC
zhì fù zǐ (炙附子), Radix Aconiti Lateralis Praeparata	5	E
ròu guì (肉桂), Cortex Cinnamomi	5	E

Tonifies kidney yang, warms mingmen fire, nourishes kidney yin, nourishes blood, benefits and consolidates jing, strengthens tendon and bone. Use for chronic deficiency of kidney *qi* and *yang* causing fatigue, lower back pain or weakness, weak knees, and urinary dysfunction. Also useful for *yang* deficiency causing male impotence, spermatorrhea, female infertility, cold limbs, edema, poor digestion, abdominal bloating, and loose stools. Applied in osteoporosis, chronic nephritis, chronic prostatitis and Addison's disease. This is a good kidney *qi* tonic for aging patients and following illness, and can be taken for long periods of time.

Pulse: Deep, weak, thready
Tongue: Normal, or pale with white coat

Comments: This classical formula dates back to the late Ming dynasty (1368–1644), and is considered one of the more important prescriptions for tonifying kidney *yang*. "Returning the right" refers to the right, or *yang*, kidney. It actually supports kidney *yang*, *yin* and *jing,* in effect strengthening kidney *qi.* Based on *Jin Gui Shen Qi Wan* (above), it is considered a stronger formula. It has additional herbs to support kidney *yang* (*tù sī zǐ* and *dù zhòng*), which help to support a weak lumbar area, while *dāng guī* and *gǒu qǐ zǐ* support blood and *yin,* which help nourish the tendons. In this regard, *You Gui Wan* is better for lumbar or waist weakness, while *Jin Gui Shen Wi Wan* is preferred for cold patterns with urinary disturbance.

Lù jiāo jiāo, a boiled-down gelatin made from deer antler (*lù róng,* 鹿茸*,* Cornu Cervi Pantotrichum), is an important ingredient used in the original formula for nourishing *yang* and *jing*, and helps male sexual dysfunction. Versions from Herbal Times, Kan, and Blue Poppy contain significant amounts of *lù jiāo jiāo*. Other versions contain small or none. The standardized Taiwan formula contains only 1%, while versions from Kwangchow Pharmaceutical (*Yao Kwei Wan*) and Plum Flower do not contain any. However, these products are still effectivel for supporting kidney *yang* and *jing.*

You Gui Wan is complemented by *Zuo Gui Wan*, also authored by Zhang Jing-Yue (see *Chapter 17A. Kidney Yin Deficiency*).

Caution: *You Gui Wan* can be cloying in patients with weak digestion.

Further Reading:

Bensky et al, p. 401
Chen & Chen, p. 678
Ellis, p. 388

Modern Formulas:

CONG RONG BU SHEN WAN

Formula: *cōng róng bǔ shèn wán* (苁蓉补肾丸), "Cistanche Tonify Kidney Pill"
Source: Modern patent medicine

Availability:

Cong Rong Bu Shen Wan (GC, MS, PM)

Ingredients: (from Minshan *"Cong Rong Bu Shen Wan"*)

ròu cōng róng (肉苁蓉), Herba Cistanches	33.1 %	AC
shú dì huáng (熟地黄), Radix Rehmanniae Praep.	33.1	AB
tù sī zǐ (菟丝子), Semen Cuscutae	33.1	AC
wǔ wèi zǐ (五味子), Fructus Schisandrae	.6	L

Tonifies kidney yang, nourishes kidney yin, consolidates the kidneys, unblocks the bowels. Use as a general kidney tonic for problems including weakness and soreness of the lumber region, poor male sexual function, infertility, and fatigue. Also for cold extremities due to *yang* deficiency, frequent urination or dribbling. Can be used in constipation due to *yang* deficiency, with poor peristalsis.

Pulse: Deep, weak
Tongue: Normal, or pale, swollen or wet

Comments: Basically a three-herb formula, *Cong Rong Bu Shen Wan* is a simple yet effective prescription for kidney deficiency. While supporting kidney *yang* with *ròu cōng róng* and *tù sī zǐ*, it also nourishes kidney *yin* with *shú dì huáng*. The tiny amount of *wǔ wèi zǐ* helps to astringe the formula into the kidney.

The formula is helpful for weakened lumbar area, urinary difficulties, and male sexual dysfunction. In female infertility, *Cong Rong Wan* can be combined with blood tonics to address underlying kidney *yang* deficiency.

GE JIE BU SHEN WAN
GE JIE DA BU WAN

Formula: *gé jiè bǔ shèn wán* (蛤蚧补肾丸), "Gecko Tonify Kidney Pill"
Source: Modern patent medicine

Availability:

Gejie Bu Shing Wan (PM)
Gejie Nourishing Kidney Pill (PM)

Formula: *gé jiè dà bǔ wán* (蛤蚧大补丸); "Gecko Large Tonifying Pill"
Source: Modern patent medicine

Availability:

Gejie Da Bu Wan (PM)
Gekko Tonic Teapills (PF)
* Gecko-A (SF)

Ingredients: (from Yulin Pharmaceutical Factory *"Ge Jie Bu Shen Wan"*)

gé jiè (蛤蚧), Gecko	27.7 %	AC
yín yáng huò (淫羊藿), Herba Epimedii	16.6	AC
ròu cōng róng (肉苁蓉), Herba Cistanches	14.4	AC
bái zhú (白术), Rhizoma Atractylodis Macrocephalae	11.1	AA
huáng qí (黄芪), Radix Astragali	11.1	AA
fú líng (茯苓), Poria	7.8	FC
rén shēn (人参), Radix Ginseng	5.6	AA
dōng chóng xià cǎo (冬虫夏草), Cordyceps	5.6	AC

Ingredients: (from Yulin Pharmaceutical Factory *"Ge Jie Da Bu Wan"*)

gé jiè (蛤蚧), Gecko	21.5 %	AC
shú dì huáng (熟地黄), Radix Rehmanniae Praep.	6.8	AB
huáng jīng (黄精), Rhizoma Polygonati	5.7	AA
shān yào (山药), Rhizoma Dioscoreae	5.3	AA
nǚ zhēn zǐ (女贞子), Fructus Ligustri Lucidi	5.2	AD
bā jǐ tiān (巴戟天), Radix Morindae Officinalis	4.3	AC
bái zhú (白术), Rhizoma Atractylodis Macrocephalae	4.3	AA
dǎng shēn (党参), Radix Codonopsis	4.3	AA
dù zhòng (杜仲), Cortex Eucommiae	4.3	AC
huáng qí (黄芪), Radix Astragali	4.3	AA
fú líng (茯苓), Poria	5.0	FC
xù duàn (续断), Radix Dipsaci	4.8	AC
gǒu jǐ (狗脊), Rhizoma Cibotii	4.8	AC
mù guā (木瓜), Fructus Chaenomelis	4.7	FA
gǒu qǐ zǐ (枸杞子), Fructus Lycii	4.1	AB
gǔ suì bǔ (骨碎补), Rhizoma Drynariae	4.0	AC
dāng guī (当归), Radix Angelicae Sinensis	3.8	AB
gān cǎo (甘草), Radix Glycyrrhizae	2.8	AA

Ingredients: (from Plum Flower *"Gecko Tonic Pills"*)

shú dì huáng (熟地黄), Radix Rehmanniae Praep.	8.3 %	AB
dù zhòng (杜仲), Cortex Eucommiae	7.1	AC
xù duàn (续断), Radix Dipsaci	7.1	AC
gǔ suì bǔ (骨碎补), Rhizoma Drynariae	7.1	AC
nǚ zhēn zǐ (女贞子), Fructus Ligustri Lucidi	7.1	AD
huáng jīng (黄精), Rhizoma Polygonati	7.1	AA
dǎng shēn (党参), Radix Codonopsis	6.2	AA
gé jiè (蛤蚧), Gecko	5.9	AC
dāng guī (当归), Radix Angelicae Sinensis	5.9	AB
gǒu qǐ zǐ (枸杞子), Fructus Lycii	5.9	AB
huáng qí (黄芪), Radix Astragali	5.9	AA
fú líng (茯苓), Poria	5.9	FC
shān yào (山药), Rhizoma Dioscoreae	5.9	AA
bā jǐ tiān (巴戟天), Radix Morindae Officinalis	4.4	AC
mù guā (木瓜), Fructus Chaenomelis	4.4	FA
gān cǎo (甘草), Radix Glycyrrhizae	2.9	AA
bái zhú (白术), Rhizoma Atractylodis Macrocephalae	2.9	AA

Tonifies yang, tonifies qi, nourishes blood. Use for systemic deficiencies of kidney *qi, yang* and *jing* causing fatigue, cold limbs, weak lower back, poor circulation, shortness of breath and lowered sex drive. Helps to strengthen kidney, lung, spleen and heart, and can be used for frequent urination, insomnia, ear ringing, and palpitation. Excellent in chronic deficiency asthma. Useful following debilitating illness, surgery, or childbirth.

Pulse: Deep, weak, slow
Tongue: Normal, or pale, swollen or wet

Comments: Yulin Pharmaceutical makes two products employing the gecko lizard *gé jiè*. Like most house lizards, the gecko is fast and agile, and is considered very *yang* in nature. The first formula, *Gejie Bu Shen Wan*, contains 28% *gé jiè*, reinforced with another 36% herbs to boost kidney *yang* (*yín yáng huò, ròu cōng róng* and *dōng chóng xià cǎo*). The rest of the formula, another 36.6%, tonifies *qi* (*bái zhú, huáng qí, fú líng* and *rén shēn*). Unlike *Ge Jie Da Bu Wa*n, it does not contain herbs to boost blood.

Ge Jie Da Bu Wan, the larger formula, acts in a similar manner, although it only contains one herb of the first formula, namely *gé jiè* (21%). Having 18 herbs versus 8 herbs, we find that 44% of the formula tonifies *yang*, while another 32% tonifies *qi* and 15% boosts blood. Plum Flower's *Gekko Tonic Teapills* contains the same ingredients as Yulin's *Ge Jie Da Bu Wan*, omitting *gǒu jǐ* (狗脊, Rhizoma Cibotii), and reducing *gé jiè* to 6% of the formula.

All three versions are used for treating deficiency asthma and labored breathing aggravated by exertion. They are also used for lowered sex drive, impotence, as a *qi* and *yang* tonic for the aging, and to boost cortisol levels in weak adrenals.

The gecko formulas are helpful for chronic asthma patients with a history of prednisone use, and can help asthma patients slowly wean off prednisone. They are also a good kidney tonic for male or female infertility due to *yang* and blood deficiency.

Caution 1: Discontinue during colds and flu, as tonics tend to drive pathogenic factors into the interior.

Caution 2: Caution in hypertension.

GUI LING JI

Formula: *guī líng jí* (龟龄集), "Tortoise Age Collection"
Source: Modern patent medicine.
Originally created for Emperor Jiā Jìng (嘉靖), (1521–1567), Ming dynasty. Prescription recorded in 1541.

Availability:

Gui Ling Zhi (PM)
Kwei Ling Chi (PM)

Ingredients: (from Shanxi Traditional Chinese Medicine Works *"Kwei Ling Chi"*)

lù róng (鹿茸), Cornu Cervi Pantotrichum	25. %	AC
rén shēn (人参), Radix Ginseng	20	AA
hǎi mǎ (海马), Hippocampus	8	AC
shú dì huáng (熟地黄), Radix Rehmanniae Praep.	6	AB
ròu cōng róng (肉苁蓉), Herba Cistanches	6	AC
gǒu qǐ zǐ (枸杞子), Fructus Lycii	3	AB
huái niú xī (怀牛膝), Radix Achyranthis Bidentatae	3	K
shā rén (砂仁), Fructus Amomi	3	FB
qiāo nǎo (雀脑), Passeris	2	AC
suǒ yáng (锁阳), Herba Cynomorii	2	AC
dīng xiāng (丁香), Flos Caryophylli	2	E
dù zhòng (杜仲), Cortex Eucommiae	2	AC
dà qīng yán (大青盐), Halitum	2	R
chuān shān jiǎ (穿山甲), Squama Manitis	2	K
tù sī zǐ (菟丝子), Semen Cuscutae	2	AC
bǔ gǔ zhī (补骨脂), Fructus Psoraleae	2	AC
yín yáng huò (淫羊藿), Herba Epimedii	2	AC
gān cǎo (甘草), Radix Glycyrrhizae	2	AA
tiān mén dōng (天门冬), Radix Asparagi	1	AD
shí yān (石燕), Fossilla Spiraferae	1	

Ingredients: (from Herba Enterprise *"Kwei Ling Chi"*. Ingredient dosages not given.)

rén shēn (人参), Radix Ginseng	AA
gǒu qǐ zǐ (枸杞子), Fructus Lycii	AB
huái niú xī (怀牛膝), Radix Achyranthis Bidentatae	K
suǒ yáng (锁阳), Herba Cynomorii	AC
shā rén (砂仁), Fructus Amomi	FB
dà qīng yán (大青盐), Halitum	R
tù sī zǐ (菟丝子), Semen Cuscutae	AC
yín yáng huò (淫羊藿), Herba Epimedii	AC
tiān mén dōng (天门冬), Radix Asparagi	AD
hǎi mǎ (海马), Hippocampus	AC
shú dì huáng (熟地黄), Radix Rehmanniae Praep.	AB
dīng xiāng (丁香), Flos Caryophylli	E
dù zhòng (杜仲), Cortex Eucommiae	AC
ròu cōng róng (肉苁蓉), Herba Cistanches	AC
bǔ gǔ zhī (补骨脂), Fructus Psoraleae	AC
gān cǎo (甘草), Radix Glycyrrhizae	AA
shí yān (石燕), Fossilla Spiraferae	

Tonifies kidney yang, tonifies spleen qi, benefits jing, nourishes the brain. Use for deficiency of *yang, jing*, and *mingmen* fire causing mental or physical fatigue, general weakness, frequent urination, weak lungs, lumbar pain or weakness, cold extremities, poor memory or concentration, poor digestion and poor circulation. Indicated for impotence and male sexual dysfunction including premature ejaculation, and fatigue and poor memory following ejaculation or with aging. Also useful in women where deficiency of kidney *yang* and *jing* is contributing to infertility, amenorrhea, cold uterus, cold damp vaginal discharges, postpartum fatigue, and certain cases of menopausal disorder. Can be used for "daybreak diarrhea" due to kidney *yang* deficiency.

Pulse: Normal, or deep, weak, thin
Tongue: Normal, or pale or swollen

continued

Comments: This formula was developed for the Ming dynasty Emperor Jia Jing (*Jiā Jìng*, 嘉靖) in 1541 as a health, fertility and longevity tonic. Although not recorded in any of the medical classics, the formula was discovered in the second half of the 20th century by medical researchers looking at the herbal prescriptions of the various rulers in Beijing's Forbidden Palace. It has been made available as a popular patent medicine. Its name, "Tortoise Age Collection", refers to the mythical longevity of great land tortoises. *Gui Ling Ji* was declared a "National Protected Prescription" in 2004.

In the main, the formula boosts kidney *yang*, mingmen fire, and *jing*. In the Shanxi version, 45% of the formula consists of ginseng *rén shēn* and deer horn *lù róng*, with an additional 8% of seahorse *hǎi mǎ*. Another 35% uses herbs that nourish blood, *yin* and *yang*. It seems to be the only prescription using sparrow brain (*qiāo nǎo*) as an ingredient; the sparrow is considered to be very *yang*, not needing to migrate from Beijing during the winter. A newer version from Herba Enterprise contains neither *lù róng* nor *qiāo nǎo*.

Caution: Discontinue during colds and flu, as tonics tend to drive pathogenic factors into the interior. Caution during pregnancy and in hypertension.

OTHER FORMULAS APPROPRIATE FOR THIS CATEGORY:

YANG TONICS

Yao Tong Pian

See Chapter 4F

Zhuang Yao Jian Shen Pian

See Chapter 4F

Other:

Adrenoplex (EV)
Adrenosen (HC)
Cord Tablets (SF)
Epimedium 8 (SF)
Eucommia 18 (SF)
Forever Yang Formula (PH)
Huan Shao Zhuang Yang (GC)
Purge Cold (CMS)
Strengthen Water (CMS)
Vitality Pearls (CP)

YANG AND JING TONICS

Classical Formulas:

Huan Shao Dan
See Chapter 18A

Shi Quan Da Bu Tang
See Chapter 18A

Modern Formulas:

Shou Wu Chih (PM)
See Chapter 16B

Shou Wu Essence (Pf)
See Chapter 16B

Ren Shen Bu Wan (Ginseng Tonic Pills)
See Chapter 18A

Ren Shen Lu Rong Wan (Ginseng Antler Pilll)
See Chapter 18A

Other:

Boost Essence Formula (PH)
Deer Tail Extract (PM)
Huan Shao Zhuang Yang (GC)
Jade Treasure Clear (K)
Jade Treasure Cool (K)
Jade Treasure Support (K)
Kang Wei Ling (PM)
Love Pearls (CP)
Man's Treasure (SF)
Nan Bao Capsules (PM)
Nourish Essence Formula (GF)
Pantocrin (PM)
Replenish Essence (CMS)
Tzepao Sanpien Extract (PM)
Virility Tabs (HC)
Vital Treasure Formula (GF)
Vitality for Men (EV)
Zhuang Yang Wan (GC, PM)

18. COMBINATION AND SINGLE HERB TONICS

18A. COMBINATION TONICS

Classical Formulas:

Huan Shao Dan	*huán shào dān* (还少丹)
Shi Quan Da Bu Tang	*shí quán dà bŭ tāng* (十全大补汤)
Zhi Gan Cao Tang	*zhì gān căo tāng* (炙甘草汤)

Modern Formulas:

Ren Shen Bu Wan (Ginseng Tonic Pills)
rén shēn bŭ wán (人参补丸)

Ren Shen Lu Rong Wan (Ginseng Antler Pills)
rén shēn lù róng wán (人参鹿茸丸)

Formulas that combine various tonic herbs to treat major systems of the body - *qi*, blood, *yin and yang* - are commonly self-prescribed in China, especially as people pass the age of 50. The formulas address the effects of aging, including fatigue, slowing down of metabolism, aching of joints or muscles, poor tendon flexibility, poor concentration or memory, and loss of hair or skin tone. Some formulas may also address specific *zang-f*u organs, such as heart or lung. In addition to applications for aging, one also uses up reserves of *qi,* blood*, yin* and *yang* following childbirth, surgery, chemotherapy, radiation or prolonged illness.

The formulas in this chapter address these combination deficiencies. They are also used to enhance both male and female fertility, and to regulate the menses. The formulas take individual tonic herbs (*qi,* blood*, yin* and *yang*) and combine them, or combine small formulas.

In general, one can take systemic formulas on a regular basis to enhance vitality and longevity, or for a shorter course following illness or surgery. If formulas lead to restlessness, insomnia, overheating or abdominal bloating, reduce dosage or discontinue. Also, it is best to discontinue tonics during pathogenic wind events such as a common cold, as tonic herbs and formulas tend to pull pathogenic energy deeper into the body.

Inexperienced practitioners in North America like to use tonic formulas with any complaint of fatigue. This is a mistake. Tonic formulas are basically intended for people as they age past 50 years, or following a serious and prolonged illness, following major surgery, or following childbirth. In other cases of fatigue, there is often accompanying stagnation – either of *qi* or blood, or both. In those cases, priority should be given to clearing excess stagnation first. Go to the appropriate chapters: *Chapter 4B. Blood Stagnation Bi Syndrome; Chapter 6C. Food Stagnation; Chapter 7A. Liver Stagnation; Chapter 8C. Uterine Blood Stasis;* and *Chapter 10. Heart Blood Stasis.*

Other tonification formulas can be found in the following chapters:

Chapter 6A.	Spleen *Qi* Deficiency
Chapter 6B.	Spleen *Yang* Deficiency
Chapter 16A.	*Qi* Tonics
Chapter 16B.	Blood Tonics
Chapter 16C.	*Qi* and Blood Tonics
Chapter 17A.	Kidney *Yin* Tonics
Chapter 17B.	Kidney *Yang* and *Jing* Tonics
Chapter 18B.	Single Herb Tonics

A Comparison:

Huan Shao Dan	*Qi*, blood, *yang* and *jing*
Shi Quan Da Bu Tang	*Qi*, blood and *yang*
Zhi Gan Cao Tang	Heart weakness or irregularity
Du Zhong Bu Tian Wan	*Qi*, blood and *yang*
Ren Shen Bu Wan (Ginseng Tonic Pills)	Spleen and kidney *qi*
Ren Shen Lu Rong Wan (Ginseng Antler Pills)	*Qi*, blood, *yin, yang*

Classical Formulas:

HUAN SHAO DAN

Formula: *huán shào dān* (还少丹), "Restore Youth Elixir"
Author: Hóng Zūn (洪遵) *aka* Hóng Jǐng-Píng (洪景平)
Source: *Hóng Shì Jí Yàn Fang* (洪氏集验方), 1170
Literal: "Hong's Collection (of) Examined Formulas"

Availability:

Huan Shao Wan (HT, TL)
Lycium Formula (EG)
Return To Spring Teapills (PF)
Youth Again (PM)

Ingredients: (from KPC *"Lycium Formula"*)

shān yào (山药), Rhizoma Dioscoreae	10.8 %	AA
chuān niú xī (川牛膝), Radix Cyathulae	10.8	K
shān zhū yú (山茱萸), Fructus Corni	7.1	L
fú ling (茯苓), Poria	7.1	FC
dù zhòng (杜仲), Cortex Eucommiae	7.1	AC
yuǎn zhì (远志), Radix Polygalae	7.1	N
wǔ wèi zǐ (五味子), Fructus Schisandrae	7.1	L
chǔ shí zǐ (楮实子), Fructus Broussonetiae	7.1	AD
xiǎo huí xiāng (小茴香), Fructus Foeniculi	7.1	E
bā jǐ tiān (巴戟天), Radix Morindae Officinalis	7.1	AC
ròu cōng róng (肉苁蓉), Herba Cistanches	7.1	AC
shú dì huáng (熟地黄), Radix Rehmanniae Praep.	3.7	AB
gǒu qǐ zǐ (枸杞子), Fructus Lycii	3.6	AB
shí chāng pú (石菖蒲), Rhizoma Acori Tatarinowii	3.6	M
dà zǎo (大枣), Fructus Jujubae	3.6	AA

Ingredients: (from Herbal Times *"Huan Shao Wan"*)

dà zǎo (大枣), Fructus Jujubae	9.1 %	AA
shú dì huáng (熟地黄), Radix Rehmanniae Praep.	9.1	AB
fú ling (茯苓), Poria	9.1	FC
shān yào (山药), Rhizoma Dioscoreae	9.1	AA
bā jǐ tiān (巴戟天), Radix Morindae Officinalis	6.1	AC
dù zhòng (杜仲), Cortex Eucommiae	6.1	AC
gǒu qǐ zǐ (枸杞子), Fructus Lycii	6.1	AB
huái niú xī (怀牛膝), Radix Achyranthis Bidentatae	6.1	K
huáng jīng (黄精), Rhizoma Polygonati	6.1	AA
shān zhū yú (山茱萸), Fructus Corni	6.1	L
wǔ wèi zǐ (五味子), Fructus Schisandrae	6.1	L
xiǎo huí xiāng (小茴香), Fructus Foeniculi	6.1	E
zhǐ shí (枳实), Fructus Aurantii Immaturus	6.1	G
yuǎn zhì (远志), Radix Polygalae	6.1	N
shí chāng pú (石菖蒲), Rhizoma Acori Tatarinowii	3.0	M

Ingredients: (from Plum Flower *"Return To Spring Teapills"*)

dà zǎo (大枣), Fructus Jujubae	22.3 %	AA
shú dì huáng (熟地黄), Radix Rehmanniae Praep.	6.5	AB
gǒu qǐ zǐ (枸杞子), Fructus Lycii	6.5	AB
bì xiè (萆薢), Rhizoma Dioscoreae Hypoglaucae	6.5	FC
fú ling (茯苓), Poria	6.5	FC
ròu cōng róng (肉苁蓉), Herba Cistanches	6.5	AC
xiǎo huí xiāng (小茴香), Fructus Foeniculi	6.5	E
bā jǐ tiān (巴戟天), Radix Morindae Officinalis	6.5	AC
dù zhòng (杜仲), Cortex Eucommiae	6.5	AC
huái niú xī (怀牛膝), Radix Achyranthis Bidentatae	6.5	K
wǔ wèi zǐ (五味子), Fructus Schisandrae	6.4	L
shān zhū yú (山茱萸), Fructus Corni	6.4	L
chǔ shí zǐ (楮实子), Fructus Broussonetiae	6.4	AD

Tonifies spleen, kidney and heart, nourishes yin, blood and jing, strengthens yang, strengthens tendons and ligaments. Use as a systemic tonic with symptoms of fatigue, poor concentration, stiff tendons and joints, and weakness and soreness of the lumber region and knees. Also for poor male sexual function, weakness or dizziness following ejaculation, and male infertility. Also for female infertility, postpartum fatigue, and clear vaginal discharge due to yang deficiency. Helpful in general deficiencies in aging, with symptoms of fatigue, memory loss, poor vision, short breath, palpitation or insomnia.

Pulse: Normal, or deep, weak
Tongue: Normal, or pale or swollen

Comments: *Huan Shao Dan* is a complex tonic that nourishes kidney, spleen and heart. It is particularly useful for kidney *yang* deficiency causing weaken back, knees and legs. By tonifying blood and *yin* as well as *yang*, the tendons and ligaments are nourished and strengthened. Because it also tonifies spleen *qi* and heart blood, the formula is useful for the elderly when *yang, qi* and blood have become depleted.

Three variations of *Huan Shao Dan* are offered here. The version from KPC most approximates the original formula, with *shān yào* and *niú xī* being the lead herbs. This is most appropriate for weakened back and knees. In the Herbal Times version, *shān yào, dà zǎo, shú dì huáng* and *fú ling* are the lead herbs, benefiting kidney, spleen and heart *qi* as well as kidney *yang*. In the Plum Flower version, *dà zǎo* occupies 22% of the formula, lending strong support to spleen *qi* while the other herbs support the kidney. The Plum Flower version does not include Dioscorea *shān yào*, instead using *bì xiè* (萆薢, Rhizoma Dioscoreae Hypoglaucae).

Caution: *Niú xī* is contraindicated during pregnancy.

Further Reading:

Bensky et al, p. 404
Chen & Chen, p. 681
Ellis, p. 140

SHI QUAN DA BU TANG

Formula: *shí quán dà bǔ tāng* (十全大补汤)
"Ten Ingredients Great Tonifying Decoction"
Author: Wú Yàn-Kuí (吴彦夔)
Source: *Chuán Xìn Shì Yòng Fāng* (传信适用方), 1180
Literal: "Transmitted Suitable (and) Useable Formulas"
also attributed to:
Author: Imperial Medical Bureau (*tài yī jú*, 太医局);
revised by Chén Shī-Wén (陈师文)
Source: *Tài Píng Huì Mín Hé Jì Jú Fāng* (太平惠民和剂局方), 1078
Literal: "(Era of) Great Peace, Benefit People Harmonious Medicines, Office (of) Formulas"
Origin:
Formula: *nèi bǔ huáng qí tāng* (内补黄芪汤)
"Internal Tonification (with) Astragalus Decoction"
Author: Liú Juān-Zǐ (刘涓子); Revised by Gōng Qìng-Xuān (龚庆宣)
Source: *Liú Juān Zǐ Guǐ Yí Fāng* (刘涓子鬼遗方), 499
Literal: "Li Juan-Zi's Ghost-Bequeathed Formulas"

Availability:

All-Inclusive Great Tonifying Formula (HS)
General Tonic Formula (GF)
Ginseng & Tangkuei Ten Combination (EG)
Shi Quan Da Bu Tang/Wan (BP, TZ/HT, MS, PM, TL)
Ten Flavor Tea Extract (PM)
Ten Flavor Teapills (PF)
Ten Treasures (K)

Ingredients: (from Herbal Times *"Shi Quan Da Bu Wan"*)

dāng guī (当归), Radix Angelicae Sinensis	16.2 %	AB
shú dì huáng (熟地黄), Radix Rehmanniae Praep.	16.2	AB
bái sháo (白芍), Radix Paeoniae Alba	10.8	AB
bái zhú (白术), Rhizoma Atractylodis Macrocephalae	10.8	AA
dǎng shēn (党参), Radix Codonopsis	10.8	AA
fú líng (茯苓), Poria	10.8	FC
huáng qí (黄芪), Radix Astragali	10.8	AA
chuān xiōng (川芎), Rhizoma Ligustici Chuanxiong	5.8	K
zhì gān cǎo (炙甘草), Radix Glycyrrhizae Praep.	5.4	AA
ròu guì (肉桂), Cortex Cinnamomi	2.8	E

Nourishes blood, warms and tonifies qi, assists yang. Use for deficiency of *qi* and blood causing fatigue, dry hair and skin, cracked nails, poor concentration or memory, dizziness, palpitation, spontaneous perspiration, or weak limbs. Use as a general tonic following childbirth, surgery, prolonged illness, or in the elderly. Can also be useful in non-healing sores. Use for gynecological disorders of amenorrhea, scanty periods, or profuse menses.

Pulse: Normal, or deep, weak, thin
Tongue: Normal, or pale or swollen

Comments: *Shi Quan Da Bu Wan* boosts *qi* and blood, and warms *yang*. It is used by the aged as a general tonic, and for patients following surgery, chemotherapy, radiation or chronic illness. It is often used by women following menses as a general tonic and to warm the uterus. In the modern clinic, it has been found effective for promoting microcirculation, adrenal function, immunological function, and repair of gastric ulcer.

Shi Quan Da Bu Wan contains the two formulas *Si Jun Zi Tang* (Chapter 6A), which tonifies *qi*, and *Si Wu Tang* (Chapter 16B), which nourishes blood, plus two warming herbs, *huáng qí* and *ròu guì*. *Huáng qí* reinforces the building of *qi* and blood, while cinnamon bark *ròu guì* boosts kidney *yang*.

The formula is similar to *Ren Shen Yang Rong Wa*n (Chapter 16C). That prescription is better for boosting spleen and heart in order to calm *shen*, while this formula is better for boosting kidney *yang* and spleen *qi.*

Caution 1: Discontinue during colds and flu, as tonics tend to drive pathogenic factors into the interior.

Caution 2: *Ròu guì* is contraindicated during pregnancy.

Further Reading:

Bensky et al, p. 348
Chen & Chen, p. 609
Ellis, p. 281

ZHI GAN CAO TANG

Formula: *zhì gān cǎo tāng* (炙甘草汤), "Prepared Glycyrrhiza Decoction"
Author: Zhāng Zhòng-Jǐng (张仲景)
Source: *Shāng Hán Lùn* (伤寒论), 220
Literal: "Injury (by) Cold, Discussion"

Availability:

Licorice Combination (EG)
Zhi Gan Cao Tang (BP, TZ)
Zhi Gan Cao Teapills (PF)
Zhi Gan Cao Wan (HT)

Ingredients: (from the standardized *"Licorice Combination"*)

shú dì huáng (熟地黄), Radix Rehmanniae Praep.	38.2 %	AB
huǒ má rén (火麻仁), Fructus Cannabis	9.5	PB
zhì gān cǎo (炙甘草), Radix Glycyrrhizae Praep.	9.5	AA
dà zǎo (大枣), Fructus Jujubae	9.5	AA
guì zhī (桂枝), Ramulus Cinnamomi	7.9	BA
mài mén dōng (麦门冬), Radix Ophiopogonis	7.9	AD
shēng jiāng (生姜), Rhizoma Zingiberis Recens	7.9	BA
rén shēn (人参), Radix Ginseng	4.8	AA
ē jiāo (阿胶), Colla Corii Asini	4.8	AB

Tonifies and warms qi, nourishes blood, nourishes yin, warms the heart. Use for deficiency of *qi,* blood, and *yin* affecting the heart, with symptoms of heart palpitation, irregular heartbeat, fatigue, shortness of breath, anxiety, and insomnia. Also used for intermittent fevers associated with deficiency disorders, or as a general tonic for recovery from chronic illness, childbirth or surgery, including tuberculosis and hepatitis, viral myocarditis and rheumatic heart disease.

Pulse: Thin, weak, may be irregular or knotted
Tongue: Normal, or pale, swollen, dry or wet

Comments: This is an important formula for treating irregular pulse, heart palpitation or arrhythmia due to deficiency of *qi,* blood and *yin.* It is also commonly given as a tonic to strengthen and regulate the heart in older patients, and is also used for recovery after a prolonged illness.

Zhì gān cǎo boosts *qi* of the heart, and is supported by *rén shēn* and *dà zǎo. Shú dì huáng*, the primary herb, nourishes and warms the blood and boosts heart *yin*, and is supported by *mài mén dōng, huǒ má rén* and *ē jiāo*. *Guì zhī* and *shēng jiāng* warms the heart and allows the heart *yin* and *yang* to circulate; it also mitigates the cloying effects of the tonic herbs.

Caution: Reduce dosage if diarrhea develops.

Further Reading:

Bensky et al, p. 356
Chen & Chen, p. 589
Ellis, p. 408

Modern Formulas:

REN SHEN BU WAN
GINSENG TONIC CAPSULES

Formula: *rén shēn bŭ wán* (人参补丸), "Ginseng Tonic Pill"
Source: Modern patent medicine

Availability:

Ginseng Tonic Capsules (PM)

Ingredients: (from Central Medical Manufactory; Tianjin *"Ginseng Tonic Pills"*)

rén shēn (人参), Radix Ginseng	69.2 %	AA
ròu cōng róng (肉苁蓉), Herba Cistanches	9.2	AC
nán shā shēn (南沙参), Radix Adenophorae	6.9	AD
shān zhū yú (山茱萸), Fructus Corni	6.9	L
huái niú xī (怀牛膝), Radix Achyranthis Bidentatae	4.6	K
fú líng (茯苓), Poria	2.7	FC
hăi mă (海马), Hippocampus	.5	AC

Tonifies spleen and heart qi, warms kidney yang, strengthens tendon and bone. Use for deficiency of kidney *yin* and *yang* coupled with deficiency of spleen *qi* causing weak digestion, weakened vitality, poor memory or concentration, and weak lower back or knees. Use as tonic for people as they age, or following childbirth, surgery, or prolonged illness.

Pulse: Normal, or deep, weak, thin
Tongue: Normal, or pale or swollen

Comments: 69% of this popular patent medicine consists of *rén shēn*, an herbal tonic for heart and spleen *qi*. It is reinforced with medicinals to support both kidney *yang* (*ròu cōng róng, hăi mă*) and kidney *yin* (*nán shā shēn, huái niú xī*), which together boost kidney *qi*. *Shān zhū yú* astringes the formula into the kidney. The formula is a good tonic for aging patients, as well as those with diminished kidney fire affecting digestion and vitality.

Caution 1: Discontinue during colds and flu, as tonics tend to drive pathogenic factors into the interior.

Caution 2: *Niú xī* is contraindicated during pregnancy.

REN SHEN LU RONG WAN
JEN SHEN LU JUNG WAN

Formula: *rén shēn lù róng wán* (人参鹿茸丸), "Ginseng, Deer Antler Pills"
Source: Modern patent medicine

Availability:

Jen Shen Lu Yung Wan (PM)
Ren Shen Lu Rong Wan (PM)

Ingredients: (from Tianjin Lerentang Pharmaceutical, Great Wall Brand *"Jen Shen Lu Yung Wan"*)

rén shēn (人参), Radix Ginseng	15. %	AA
lù róng (鹿茸), Cornu Cervi Pantotrichum	15	AC
huáng qí (黄芪), Radix Astragali	15	AA
gǒu qǐ zǐ (枸杞子), Fructus Lycii	15	AB
chén xiāng (沉香), Lignum Aquilariae Resinatum	10	G
dōng chóng xià cǎo (冬虫夏草), Cordyceps	10	AA
hǎi mǎ (海马), Hippocampus	10	AC
shēng dì huáng (生地黄), Radix Rehmanniae	5	AD
huái niú xī (怀牛膝), Radix Achyranthis Bidentatae	5	K

Tonifies spleen and heart qi, warms kidney, benefits kidney yang, yin, qi and jing, tonifies blood, strengthens tendons. Use for systemic deficiencies of *qi*, *yang* and blood causing fatigue, weak lower back or knees, shortness of breath, poor digestion, weakened vitality, poor hearing, and poor memory or concentration. Also helpful for mental restlessness, insomnia, heart palpitations, poor memory, and male sexual depletion. Useful in amenorrhea and female infertility.

Pulse: Normal, or deep, weak, thin
Tongue: Normal, or pale or swollen

Comments: This combined tonic for *qi,* blood, *yin, yang* and *jing* is useful to compensate for the effects of aging, and for people who are recovering from illness or childbirth. It is also a useful fertility tonic for both men and women. The formula contains 30% *rén shēn* and *huáng qí* to tonify *qi*. Deer Antler *lù róng* (15%) nourishes blood and kidney *yang*. An additional 20% from *dōng chóng xià căo* and *hăi mă* support the *yang,* and *gŏu qǐ zǐ* and *shēng dì huáng* (20%) tonify blood and *yin*.

Caution 1: Discontinue during colds and flu, as tonics tend to drive pathogenic factors into the interior.

Caution 2: *Niú xī* is contraindicated during pregnancy.

OTHER FORMULAS APPROPRIATE FOR THIS CATEGORY:

Classical Formulas:

Ba Zhen Tang

See Chapter 16C

Dang Gui Bu Xue Tang

See Chapter 16C

Gui Pi Tang

See Chapter 9.

Jin Gui Shen Qi Wan / Ba Wei Di Huang Wan

See Chapter 17B

Ren Shen Yang Rong Tang / Yang Ying Wan

See Chapter 16C

Modern Formulas:

Fu Fang Shou Wu Wan

See Chapter 4C

Gui Ling Ji - Kwei Ling Chi

See Chapter 17B

Other:

Alrodeer Pills (PM)
Antler 8 (SF)
Astra Essence (HC)
Astragalus & Ganoderma (CC)
Astragalus 10+ (SF)
Astragalus And Ligustrum Formula (GF)
Astragalus-Shitake-Reishi Formula (PH)
Compound-Gl (SF)
Cordyceps Tablets (PIM)
Cordyseng (HC)
Du Zhong Bu Tian Wan (HT)
Eleuthero 10+ (SF)
Five Ginsengs Formula (PH)
Five Mushroom Formula (PH)
Ganoderma 18 (SF)
Ginseng 6 (SF)
Ginseng Endurance Formula (GF)
Immune Plus (DRJ)
Imperial Tonic (EV)
Jing Qi Formula (GF)
Longevitabs (HC)
Nourish Jade Yang (K)
Restorative Formula (GF)
Sea of Qi Formula (GF)

18B. SINGLE HERB TONICS

Ci Wu Jia (Eleutherococcus) *cì wŭ jiā* (刺五加)
Dong Chong Xia Cao (Cordyceps) *dōng chóng xià căo* (冬虫夏草)
Ling Zhi (Ganoderma) *líng zhī* (灵芝)

Other Single Herb Tonics:

See *Chapter 16A. Qi Tonics:*

fēng wáng jiāng (蜂王浆) (Royal Jelly)
huáng qí (黄芪) (Astragalus)
rén shēn (人参) (Ginseng)
xī yáng shēn (西洋参) (American Ginseng)

See *Chapter 16B. Blood Tonics:*

dāng guī (当归) (Angelica Dang Gui, Tang Kwei)
hé shŏu wū (何首乌) (Polygonum)

During the long history of China, many exceptional tonic herbs have been discovered and applied. In the folk medicine tradition, a certain region in China would find a single herb or substance that was observed to contribute powerful effects on one's health and longevity. These include Ginseng *rén shēn*, Ganoderma *líng zhī,* Polygonum *hé shŏu wū*, Astragalus *huáng qí* and Notoginseng *tián qī* (田七). Over the course of time, several individual medicinal substances were also considered to tonify the body systemically, including Cordyceps *dōng chóng xià căo*, human placenta *zĭ hé chē* (紫河车) and Acanthopanax *cì wŭ jiā*.

These single herbs were often combined with other herbs, or added into existing prescriptions to strengthen the effects. Practitioners may do likewise, although patients often enjoy taking isolated herbal tonics such as Cordyceps or Acanthopanax.

Single Herbs:

CI WU JIA / WU JIA SHEN
ACANTHOPANAX, ELEUTHERO, SIBERIAN GINSENG

Herb: *cì wŭ jiā* (刺五加), Radix Acanthopanacis Senticosi
aka: *wŭ jiā shēn* (五加参)
Properties: Spicy, slightly bitter, warm
Channels: Spleen, Kidney, Heart
Source: Modern. The bark is described in:
Shén Nóng Bĕn Căo Jīng (神农本草经), 300 BCE – 200 CE
Literal: "Shen Nong's Materia Medica Classic"

Availability:

Acanthopanax Capsule (PM)
Eleuthero Ginseng (PF)
Eleuthero Ginseng Extract (PM)
Wuchaseng Tablets (PM)

Also as:

Liquid Vials
Liquid Tincture
Capsules

Tonifies spleen and kidney qi, boosts kidney yang and jing, calms shen. Use for deficiency of spleen and kidney *qi* causing fatigue, poor appetite, weak lower back, insomnia, poor memory, or palpitation. Also for depletion of kidney *jing* causing impotence, poor sexual vitality, spermatorrhea or dizziness. Can be used for stagnation of *qi* and blood causing oppression of the chest, chest pain, sore limbs or painful joints. Often taken as a tonic during recovery or rehabilitation; it is used as a *qi* tonic following radiation, chemotherapy and surgery.

Pulse: Weak, sunken
Tongue: Normal, or swollen and pale

Comments: *Cì wǔ jiā* is also known as eleuthero-ginseng or Siberian ginseng, although it is not really a part of the ginseng species. Traditionally, the Chinese have used the bark (*wǔ jiā pí,* 五加皮, Cortex Acanthopanacis) rather than the root, for treating rheumatism and arthritis in wind-damp *bi* conditions. In the 1950s and 60s, Soviet Russians used the root to enhance athletic performance, catching the attention of the Chinese.

Clinically, it is used to enhance vitality, treat leukopenia following chemotherapy or radiation, and to regulate adrenal imbalance, regulating cortisol levels produced during stress. It is recognized as a tonic for kidney *qi* (both *yin* and *yang*) and is recommended following childbirth or surgery and in the aged. It has been shown to enhance the effects of antibiotics, probably by boosting the body's innate immune system. It is commonly given to athletes to improve endurance.

Caution: *Cì wǔ jiā* may potentiate anti-hypertensive pharmaceuticals, promoting too far a drop in blood pressure.

Further Reading:

Bensky, Clavey, Ströger, *Materia Medica,* p. 735
Chen & Chen, *Medical Herbology,* p. 864

DONG CHONG XIA CAO
CORDYCEPS

Herb:	*dōng chóng xià cǎo* (冬虫夏草), Cordyceps
Source:	*Běn Cǎo Cóng Xīn* (本草从新), 1751
	Literal: "Materia Medica From (the) New"
Author:	Wú Yí-Luò (吴仪洛)
Properties:	Sweet, warm
Channels:	Lung, Kidney

Availability:

Capsules
Liquid vials

Tonifies kidney qi and yang, benefits jing, tonifies heart, nourishes lung, dissolves phlegm. Use as a general tonic for *qi*, *yang* and *jing* following childbirth, prolonged illness, surgery, radiation and chemotherapy. Used to relieve cough and phlegm in chronic bronchitis, asthma or emphysema; to treat weakened kidney function causing chronic nephritis, sexual exhaustion, weak lower back and lumbar region, and insomnia; and in chronic hepatitis and cirrhosis. Also for heart deficiency characterized by arrhythmia, palpitation, and shortness of breath. Useful for symptoms of fatigue, general weakness or feebleness, lowered sex drive or performance, female infertility and male impotence.

Pulse: Deep, weak
Tongue: Normal, or swollen, pale

Comments: *Dōng chóng xià cǎo* is a medicinal substance made from the dried carcass of dead caterpillar larva (Hepialus varians) with the fungus that grows on it. It was recorded in Tibetan medical texts in the 15th century, and entered the Chinese *materia medica* in 1751. Cordyceps is considered a tonic for the lung, liver, heart and kidney, and is used to treat asthma, arrhythmia, and shortness of breath. In the last century it was sought after in the treatment of tuberculosis. It has also been prescribed for infertility and impotence. Chinese athletes use it for sports enhancement before and during competitive events.

Cordyceps *dōng chóng xià cǎo* is currently being used to offset the side effects of radiation and chemotherapy, benefiting bone marrow, rebuilding white blood cells and plasma proteins, and repairing liver cells. It is also being investigated for anti-cancer properties. The herbal substance has also been shown to lower cholesterol and blood pressure.

Dōng chóng xià cǎo can be taken alone, or with other herbs. Traditionally, the whole substance is mixed and cooked with dishes made with chicken, duck or lean meat.

Caution: If stomach upset occurs, take with meals. Some patients may respond with heat signs; in such cases, reduce the dosage or discontinue.

Further Reading:

Bensky, Clavey, Ströger, *Materia Medica,* p. 770
Chen & Chen, *Medical Herbology,* p. 883

LING ZHI
GANODERMA, REISHI

Herb: *líng zhī* (灵芝), Ganoderma; "Spirit Mushroom"
Source: *Shén Nóng Běn Cǎo Jīng* (神农本草经), 300 BCE – 200 CE
Literal: "Shen Nong's Materia Medica Classic"
Author: Unknown
Properties: Sweet, bitter, neutral
Channels: Heart, Liver, Lung, Kidney, Spleen

Availability:

Reishi (PF, PM)

also as:

Capsules
Liquid Vials
Pills

Tonifies qi, tonifies blood, nourishes heart, calms shen, nourishes yin and blood, nourishes lung qi, stops cough, stops wheezing. Use to tonify heart, lung and spleen for symptoms of insomnia, poor concentration, fatigue, chronic cough, wheezing. Use as a general tonic following childbirth, surgery, or prolonged illness, or during and following chemotherapy or radiation. Can reduce cholesterol, raise white blood cells, and repair damaged liver cells.

Pulse: Deep, weak
Tongue: Normal, or swollen, pale

Comments: *Líng zhī*, known as Ganoderma or reishi, is a large wood-decaying mushroom; it is wildcrafted as well as cultivated. *Líng zhī* has been valued as a longevity tonic in folk medicine for 2000 years. It is found in ancient Chinese paintings in the hands of famous Daoists, and is known as the "mushroom of immortality".

Modern research confirms its ability to enhance immune function and raise white blood cells, repair damaged liver cells, and reduce cholesterol. It is also being applied in autoimmune diseases such as lupus, scleroderma and alopecia, and is being investigated for inhibiting cancer metastasis. It has been shown to have antiviral and antibacterial properties.

Further Reading:

Bensky, Clavey, Ströger, *Materia Medica,* p. 993
Chen & Chen, *Medical Herbology,* p. 770

EXPLANATION OF TCM TERMS

The following words appear in *italics* throughout the text, and indicate TCM concepts that are best left in their original language. Simple definitions are provided.

***bi* syndrome** (*bì zhèng*, 痹证). *Bi* means obstruction or blockage. A *bi* syndrome involves obstruction of *qi*, blood and dampness in the channels, and includes various patterns of rheumatism, arthritis and trauma.

jiao (*jiāo*, 焦). Indicates one of three areas of the torso, namely the upper (lungs and heart), middle (liver, spleen, pancreas and stomach) and the lower (intestines, kidney, bladder, uterus, and genitals). *Jiao* is often translated as "burner", indicating different metabolic and energetic functions per area.

jing (*jīng*, 精) and ***jing q*i** (*jīng qì*, 精气). The primordial essence responsible for sexual reproduction, growth and development; it also helps strengthen *zheng qi*. It is stored in the kidney, testicles and ovaries.

mingmen (*mìng mén*, 命门) or ***mingmen* fire** (*mìng mén zhī huǒ*, 命门之火). Literally "vitality gate" or "life gate", *mingmen* is the source of primordial fire energy and is responsible for kidney and heart *yang*. It resides in the area between the kidneys and the lumbar spine. *Mingmen* fire warms the body and the blood, and provides energy for the heart and the digestive tract.

qi (*qì*, 气). The life-force energy of the physical universe. In the body, it is known as "vital energy"; it circulates through the acupuncture channels, and nourishes and invigorates the *zang-fu* organs. *Qi* is obtained from food and air and is combined with constitutional reserves. It is also obtained through the interaction of *yang* and *yin* energies in the acupuncture channels, and torso energy centers.

shen (*shén*, 神). The spirit and vitality that resides in the heart center. It is responsible for mental functioning; disturbances can affect sleep, mood and mental focus.

***wei* syndrome** (*wěi zhèng*, 痿证). *Wei* means flaccid, and *wei* syndromes are patterns that include muscle weakness, atrophy or flaccid paralysis.

wei qi (*wèi qì*, 卫气). Literally, "protective energy". The *wei qi* radiates out from the *ying qi* in the channels, energizing the tissue and fluid as it moves from the channel out to the surface. It is responsible for empowering immune function within the blood and fluid.

continued

wen bing (*wēn bìng*, 温病). Literally, "warm diseases", this was a movement in Chinese medicine that developed during the late 18th century, and addressing contagious diseases such as influenza, smallpox, and tuberculosis. Wú Jū-Tōng (吴鞠通) was a principal formulator.

yang (*yáng*, 阳). *Yang* energy is warming, drying and invigorating. Its source in the natural world comes from the sun, and it transverses from the sky to the earth through the *yang* acupuncture channels. In the body, *yang* is generated from *mingmen* fire, which warms and invigorates the kidneys, heart, blood and digestive tract.

yin (*yīn*, 阴). *Yin* energy is cooling and moistening. Its source in the natural world comes from the earth, and it moves from the earth to the sky through the *yin* acupuncture channels. In the body, *yin* is rooted in kidney *yin,* from which it moistens the liver, heart and lungs. *Yin* also provides moistening fluids for the body.

ying qi (*yíng qì*, 营气). Commonly translated as "nutritive energy" or "nourishing energy". This is the centripetal denser aspect of the *zong qi* that goes through the acupuncture channels to nourish the various *zang-fu* organs.

zang-fu (*zàng fǔ*, 脏腑). These are the internal organs, encompassing both the physiological organ as well as the energetic attributes of TCM. The *zang* are the dense or solid organs, and include the heart, spleen-pancreas, lung, kidney and liver. The *fu* are the hollow organs, and include the small intestine, stomach, large intestine, urinary bladder and the gallbladder.

zheng qi (*zhèng qì*, 正气). The "true" or "righteous" energy of the body. Abundant *zheng qi* indicates health and vitality, while weakened *zheng qi* leads to difficulty fighting disease factors.

zong qi (*zōng qì*, 宗气). The source of *ying qi* and *wei qi*, it is the totality of energy that flows through the acupuncture network. It is dependent on *qi* from air, food, and constitutional reserves, and is formed in the upper *jiao*. The name is often translated as "ancestral energy".

THE SIX STAGES AND SIX DIVISIONS

The Six Stages refer to the stages and locations of disease progression. As the ***Six Divisions,*** they refer to classical hand-foot pairings of the acupuncture channels.

Taiyang (*tài yáng*, 太阳). The *taiyang* stage is the first stage of an exogenous pathogenic event, with symptoms in the surface or the respiratory tract. The *Hand Taiyang* is the Small Intestine channel; the *Foot Taiyang* is the Urinary Bladder channel. These channels are the first to be affected by exogenous cold.

shaoyang (*shào yáng*, 少阳). The *shaoyang* stage is when the pathogen is moved towards the interior, and is considered "half-out and half-in". This includes a pathogen lodging in the lymphatics or muscles, and is marked by alternating fever with chills. The *Hand Shaoyang* refers to the Triple Burner channel; the *Foot Shaoyang* is the Gallbladder channel.

yangming (*yáng míng,* 阳明). The *yangming* stage is where the pathogen has proceeded into the channel network. Because the *yang* and *wei qi* energy is strong, this stage exhibits high fever, or heat in the stomach and large intestine. The *Hand Yangming* refers to the Large Intestine channel; the *Foot Yangming* is the Stomach channel.

taiyin (*tài yīn*, 太阴). The *taiyin* stage indicates that exogenous cold has penetrated a weakened spleen or stomach. The *Hand Taiyin* refers to the Lung channel; the *Foot Taiyin* is the Spleen channel.

shaoyin (*shào yīn*, 少阴). The *shaoyin* stage indicates exogenous cold has penetrated a weakened heart or kidney, or that fever has exhausted the heart or kidney. The *Hand Shaoyin* refers to the Heart channel; the *Foot Shaoyin* is the Kidney channel.

jueyin (*jué yīn*, 厥阴). The *jueyin* stage indicates that the pathogen has lodged in the Pericardium or Liver. At this stage, the body is exhausted. The *Hand Jueyin* refers to the Pericardium channel; the *Foot Jueyin* is the Liver channel.

CLASSICAL TEXT REFERENCES
Alphabetically by Text with Date

Detailed information follows on page 606; search by date.

Běn Cǎo Cóng Xīn (本草从新), 1751
Běn Cǎo Gāng Mù (本草纲目), 1578 or 1590
Běn Cǎo Yǎn Yì (本草衍义), 1116

Chéng Fāng Biàn Dú (成方便读), 1904
Chuán Xìn Shì Yòng Fāng (传信适用方)*, 1180*

Dān Xī Xīn Fǎ (丹溪心法), 1481
Dōng Héng Shì Xiào Fāng (东恒试效方), 1266
Dōng Yuán Shì Xiào Fāng (东垣试效方), 1266

Fāng Shì Mài Zhèng Zhèng Zōng (方氏脉症正宗), 1749
Fù Rén Liáng Fāng (妇人良方), 1237
Fù Shì Yǎn Kē Shěn Shì Yáo Hán (傅氏眼科审视瑶函), 1644

Guǎng Wēn Yì Lùn (广瘟疫论), 1774

Hóng Shì Jí Yàn Fang (洪氏集验方), 1170
Huáng Dì Sù Wèn Xuán Míng Lùn Fāng (黄帝素问宣明论方), 1172

Jì Shēng Fāng (济生方), 1253
Jì Yīn Gāng Mù (济阴纲目), 1620
Jiǎn Yaò Jǐ Zhòng Fāng (简要济众方), 1051
Jiào Zhù Fù Rén Liáng Fāng (校注妇人良方), mid-16th c.
Jīn Guì Yào Lüè (金匮要略), 220
Jǐng Yuè Quán Shū (景岳全书), 1624

Lán Shì Mì Cáng (兰室秘藏), date unknown, published 1276
Liáng Fāng Jí Yè (良方集腋), 1842
Liú Juān Zǐ Guǐ Yí Fāng (刘涓子鬼遗方), 499

Má Zhěn Quán Shū (麻疹全书), circa 1350
Mì Chuán Yǎn Kē Lóng Mù Lùn (秘传眼科龙木论), 13th century
Míng Yī Fāng Lùn (名医方论), 1675

Nèi Kē Zhāi Yào (内科摘要), circa 1530
Nèi Wài Shāng Biàn Huò Lùn (内外伤辨惑论), 1247

Pí Wèi Lùn (脾胃论), 1249

Qiān Jīn Yào Fāng (千金要方), 652
Qián Shì Xiǎo Ér Yào Zhèng Zhí Jué (钱氏小儿药证直), 1119
Quán Guó Zhōng Yào Chéng Yào Chù Fāng Jí (全国中药成药处方集), 1962

Rén Zhāi Zhí Zhǐ Fāng (仁斋直指方), 1264
Rì Huá Zǐ Běn Cǎo (日华子本草), 713
Rú Mén Shì Qīn (儒门事亲), 1228

Sān Yīn Jí Yī Bìng Zhèng Fāng Lùn (三因极一病证方论), 1174
Shāng Hán Liù Shū (伤寒六书), 1445
Shāng Hán Lùn (伤寒论), 220
Shāng Hán Quán Shēng Jí (伤寒全生集), 1445
Shè Shēng Zhòng Miào Fāng (摄生众妙方), 1550
Shén Nóng Běn Cǎo Jīng (神农本草经), 300 BCE – 200 CE
Shěn Shì Yáo Hán (审视瑶函), 1642
Shèn Zhāi Yí Shū (慎斋遗书), 1573
Shí Fāng Gē Kuò (时方歌括), 1801
Shí Yào Shén Shū (十药神书), 1348
Shì Yī Dé Xiào Fāng (世医得效方), 1345
Shòu Shì Bǎo Yuán (寿世保元), 1615

Tài Píng Huì Mín Hé Jì Jú Fāng (太平惠民和剂局方), 1078
Tǐ Rén Huì Biān (体仁汇编), 1549
Tóng Shòu Lù (同寿录), 1762

Wài Kē Zhèng Zōng (外科正宗), 1617
Wài Tái Mì Yào (外台秘要), 752
Wàn Bìng Huí Chūn (万病回春), 1587
Wèi Shēng Bǎo Jiàn (卫生宝鉴), 1281
Wēn Bìng Tiáo Biàn (温病条辨), 1798

Xiān Shòu Lǐ Shāng Xù Duàn Mì Fāng (仙授理伤续断秘方), 846
Xiān Xǐng Zhāi Yī Xué Guǎng Bǐ Jì (先醒斋医学广笔记), 1613
Xù Míng Yī Lèi Àn (续名医类案), 1770

Yáng Shì Jiā Cáng Fāng (杨氏家藏方), 1178
Yáng Yī Dà Quán (疡医大全), 1760
Yī Fāng Jí Jiě (医方集解), 1682
Yī Fāng Kǎo (医方考), 1584
Yī Lêi Yuán Róng (医垒元戎), 1291
Yī Lín Gǎi Cuò (医林改错), 1830
Yī Mén Fǎ Lǜ (医门法律), 1658
Yī Xué Qǐ Yuán (医学启源), 1186
Yī Xué Rù Mén (医学入门), 1575
Yī Xué Xīn Wù (医学心悟), 1732
Yī Xué Zhèng Chuán (医学正传), 1515
Yī Xué Zhōng Zhōng Cān Xī Lù (医学衷中参西录), 1918-1934
Yī Zōng Jīn Jiàn (医宗金鉴), 1742
Yông Lèi Qián Fāng (永类钤方), 1331

Zá Bìng Zhèng Zhì Xīn Yì (杂病证治新义), 1958
Zhèng Hé Shèng Jì Zông Lù (政和圣济总录), 1117
Zhèng Tǐ Lèi Yào (正体类要), 1529
Zhèng Zhì Zhǔn Shéng (证治准绳), 1602
Zhōng Guó Guó Yào Gù Yǒu Chéng Fāng Xuǎn Jí (中国国药故有成方选集), 1967
Zhōng Huā Rén Mín Gòng Hé Guó Yào Diǎn (中华人民共和国药典), 2005
Zhōng Yī Fāng Jì Lín Chuáng Shǒu Cè (中医方剂临床手册), 1950s
Zhōng Zàng Jīng (中藏经), 2nd c.

CLASSICAL TEXT REFERENCES
Alphabetically by Author with Date

Detailed information follows on page 606; search by date.

Chén Niàn-Zǔ *aka* Chén Xiū-Yuán (陈念祖 / 陈修园), 1801
Chén Shí-Gōng (陈实功), 1617
Chén Shī-Wén (陈师文), 1078
Chén Yán (陈言) *aka* Chén Wú-Zé (陈无择), 1174
Chén Zì-Míng (陈自明), 1237
Chéng Guó-Péng (程国彭), 1732

Dài Tiān-Zhāng (戴天章), 1774

Fāng Zhào-Quán (方肇权), 1749
Fù Rén-Yǔ (傅仁宇), 1644

Gé Kě–Jiǔ (葛可久) *aka* Gé Qián–Sūn (葛乾孙), 1348
Gōng Qìng-Xuān (龚庆宣), 499
Gōng Tíng-Xián (龚廷贤), 1587, 1615
Gù Shì-Chéng (顾世澄), 1760

Hóng Jī (洪基) *aka* Hóng Jiǔ-Yǒu (洪九有), 1638
Hóng Zūn (洪遵) *aka* Hóng Jǐng-Píng (洪景平), 1170
Hú Guāng-Cí (胡光慈), 1958
Huá Shòu (滑寿), 1350
Huà Tuó (华佗), 2nd c.

Imperial Medical Bureau (*tài yī jú*, 太医局); 1078
Kòu Zōng-Shì (寇宗奭), 1116

Li Chān (李梴) *aka* Lǐ Tǐng (李挺) *aka* Lǐ Jiàn-Zhāi (李健齋), 1575
Lǐ Gǎo (李杲) *aka* Lǐ Dōng-Yuán (李东垣), 1247, 1249, 1276
Lǐ Gǎo (李杲) *aka* Lǐ Dōng-Yuán (李东垣), edited by Luō Tān-Yì (罗天益), 1266
Lǐ Shí-Zhēn (李时珍) *aka* Lǐ Dōng-Bì (李东壁), 1578 or 1590
Lǐ Zhòng-Nán (李仲南), 1331
Lìn Dào Rén (Lin the Daoist) (蔺道人), 846
Liú Juān-Zǐ (刘涓子), 499
Liú Wán-Sù (刘完素), 1172
Luō Měi (罗美), 1675
Luó Tiā-Yì (羅天益), 1281
Miào Xī-Yōng (缪希雍), 1613

CLASSICAL TEXTS REFERENCE

with Formulas and Alternative Translations

Text in the book uses literal character-to-word translations for source texts. Alternative published translations are indicated by the following code letters:

C&C: *Chinese Herbal Formulas and Applications*, John K. Chen and Tina T. Chen, Art of Medicine Press, City of Industry, CA, 2009

F&S: *Formulas and Strategies* (Chinese Herbal Medicine Formulas & Strategies, 2nd Edition, Volker Scheid, Dan Bensky, Andrew Ellis and Randall Barolet, Eastland Press, Seattle, WA, 2009

PMPH: People's Medical Publishing House standardized translations

WESTERN HAN DYNASTY

xī hàn (西汉), 206 BCE – 23 CE
1 book, 4 herbs

Author: Unknown
Source: *Shén Nóng Běn Cǎo Jīng* (神农本草经), 300 BCE – 200 CE
Literal: "Shen Nong's Materia Medica Classic"
C&C, F&S: "Divine Husbandman's Classic of the Materia Medica"
PMPH: "Shen Nong's Classic of the Materia Medica"
Herbs:

huáng qí (黄芪), Radix Astragali (Chapter 16A)
rén shēn (人参), Radix Ginseng (Chapter 16A)
dāng guī (当归), Radix Angelicae Sinensis (Chapter 16B)
líng zhī (灵芝), Ganoderma (Chapter 18B)

EASTERN HAN DYNASTY

dōng hàn (东汉), 25–220 CE
3 books, 27 formulas

Author: Huà Tuó (华佗)
Source: *Zhōng Zàng Jīng* (中藏经), 2nd c.
Literal: "Central Depository Classic"
C&C, F&S: "Treasury Classic"
PMPH: "Central Treasury Classic"
Formula: *wǔ pí yǐn* (五皮饮) (Chapter 12)

Author: Zhāng Zhòng-Jǐng (张仲景)
Source: *Shāng Hán Lùn* (伤寒论), 220
Literal: "Injury (by) Cold, Discussion"
PMPH: "Treatise on Cold Damage"
F&S: "Discussion of Cold Damage"
C&C: "Discussion of Cold-Induced Disorders"
Formulas:
gé gēn tāng (葛根汤) (Chapter 1A)
guì zhī tāng (桂枝汤) (Chapter 1A)
bái hǔ tāng (白虎汤) (Chapter 2B)
dāng guī sì nì tāng (当归四逆汤) (Chapter 4D)
sháo yào gān cǎo tāng (芍药甘草汤) (Chapter 5C)
xiǎo jiàn zhōng tāng (小建中汤) (Chapter 6B)
wū méi wán (乌梅丸) (Chapter 6D)
dà chéng qì tāng (大承气汤) (Chapter 6E)
má zǐ rén wán (麻子仁丸) (Chapter 6E)
xiǎo chái hú tāng (小承气汤) (Chapter 7A)
chái hú jiā lóng gǔ mǔ lì tāng (柴胡加龙骨牡蛎汤) (Chapter 7B)
dà chái hú tāng (大柴胡汤) (Chapter 7C)
wǔ líng sǎn (五苓散) (Chapter 12)
zhēn wǔ tāng (真武汤) (Chapter 12)
zhì gān cǎo tāng (炙甘草汤) (Chapter 18A)

Author: Zhāng Zhòng-Jǐng (张仲景)
Source: *Jīn Guì Yào Lüè* (金匮要略), 220
Literal: "Golden Cabinet Essential Summary"
C&C, F&S, PMPH: "Essentials from the Golden Cabinet"
Formulas:
dà huáng mŭ dān pí tāng (大黄牡丹皮汤) (Chapter 2A)
bàn xià hòu pò tāng (半夏厚朴汤) (Chapter 3C)
huáng qí guì zhī wŭ wù tāng (黄芪桂枝五物汤) (Chapter 4C)
jiāo ài tāng (胶艾汤) (Chapter 8A)
wēn jīng tāng (温经汤) (Chapter 8A)
dāng guī sháo yào săn (当归芍药散) (Chapter 8C)
guì zhī fú líng wán (桂枝茯苓丸) (Chapter 8C)
gān mài dà zăo tāng (甘麦大枣汤) (Chapter 9)
suān zăo rén tāng (酸枣仁汤) (Chapter 9)
fáng jĭ huáng qí tāng (防己黄芪汤) (Chapter 12)
jīn guì shèn qì wán (金匮肾气丸) (Chapter 17B)

SOUTHERN & NORTHERN DYNASTIES

nán běi cháo (南北朝) 386 – 589 CE
1 book, 1 formula

Author: Liú Juān-Zĭ (刘涓子)***;*** Revised by Gōng Qìng-Xuān (龚庆宣)
Source: *Liú Juān Zĭ Guĭ Yí Fāng* (刘涓子鬼遗方), 499
Literal: "Li Juan-Zi's Ghost-Bequeathed Formulas"
F&S: "Formulas Bequeathed by the Unorthodox Genius Liu Juan-Zi"
PMPH: "Liu Juan-Zi's Ghost-Bequeathed Formulas"
Formula: *nèi bŭ huáng qí tāng* (内补黄芪汤) (Chapter 18A)

TANG DYNASTY

táng (唐), 618–907 CE

4 books, 4 formulas, 1 herb

Author: Sūn Sī-Miǎo (孙思邈)
Source: *Qiān Jīn Yào Fāng* (千金要方), 652
Literal: "Thousand Gold (Pieces) Important Formulas"
C&C: "Thousand Ducat Prescriptions"
F&S, PMPH: "Important Formulas Worth a Thousand Gold Pieces"
aka:
Bèi Jí Qiān Jīn Yào Fāng (备急千金要方), 652
Literal: "Prepare (for) Emergency Thousand Gold (Pieces) Important Formulas"
C&C: "Thousands of Golden Prescriptions for Emergencies"
PMPH: "Important Formulas Worth a Thousand Gold Pieces for Emergency"
Formulas:
sū zǐ jiàng qì tāng (苏子降气汤) (Chapter 3C)
dú huó jì shēng tāng (独活寄生汤) (Chapter 4F)

Author: Rì Huá-Zǐ (日华子)
Source: *Rì Huá Zǐ Běn Cǎo* (日华子本草), 713
Literal: "Ri Hua-Zi's Materia Medica"
C&C, F&S: "Materia Medica of Ri Hua-Zi"
PMPH: "Ri Hua-zi's Materia Medica"
Herb: *hé shǒu wū* (何首乌), Radix Polygoni Multiflori (Chapter 16B)

Author: Wáng Tāo (王焘)
Source: *Wài Tái Mì Yào* (外台秘要), 752
Literal: "Outer Platform (Imperial Library) Secret Essentials"
C&C, F&S, PMPH: "Arcane Essentials from the Imperial Library"
Formula: *huáng lián jiě dú tāng* (黄连解毒汤) (Chapter 2A)

Author: Lìn Dào Rén (Lin the Daoist) (蔺道人)
Source: *Xiān Shòu Lǐ Shāng Xù Duàn Mì Fāng* (仙授理伤续断秘方), 846
Literal: "Immortal Instructs Management (of) Injuries (and) Repair (of) Fractures, Secret Formulas"
C&C: "Secret Recipes of Treating Wounds and Bone-Setting Taught by Celestials"
F&S: "Secret Formulas to Manage Trauma and Reconnect Fractures Received from an Immortal"
Formula: *sì wù tāng* (四物汤) (Chapter 16B)

NORTHERN SONG DYNASTY

běi sòng (北宋), 960–1127 CE
2 books, 17 formulas

Author: Zhōu Yìng (周应)
Source: *jiǎn yaò jǐ zhòng fāng* (简要济众方), 1051
Literal: "Simple Important Aid Multitude Formulas"
F&S: "Concise Formulas to Aid the Multitudes"
Formula:
píng wèi sǎn (平胃散) (Chapter 6A)

Author: Imperial Medical Bureau (*tài yī jú,* 太医局*);*
revised by Chén Shī-Wén (陈师文)
Source: *Tài Píng Huì Mín Hé Jì Jú Fāng* (太平惠民和剂局方), 1078
Literal: "(Era of) Great Peace, Benefit People Harmonious Medicines, Office (of) Formulas"
C&C: "Imperial Grace Formulary of the Tai Ping Era"
F&S: "Formulary of the Pharmacy Service for Benefitting the People in the Taiping Era"
PMPH: "Beneficial Formulas from the Taiping Imperial Pharmacy"
Formulas:
chuān xiōng chá tiáo sǎn (川芎茶调散) (Chapter 1A)
liáng gé sǎn (凉膈散) (Chapter 2B)
èr chén tāng (二陈汤) (Chapter 3C)
sū zǐ jiàng qì tāng (苏子降气汤), (Chapter 3C)
xiǎo huó luò dān (小活络丹) (Chapter 4D)
sì jūn zǐ tāng (四君子汤) (Chapter 6A)

píng wèi săn (平胃散) (Chapter 6A)
shēn líng bái zhú săn (参苓白术散) (Chapter 6A)
fù zĭ lĭ zhōng wán (附子理中丸) (Chapter 6B)
huò xiāng zhèng qì săn (藿香正气散) (Chapter 6D)
huái jiăo wán (槐角丸) (Chapter 6F)
xiāo yáo săn (逍遥散) (Chapter 7A)
bā zhèng săn (八正散) (Chapter 11B)
rén shēn yăng róng tāng (人参养荣汤) (Chapter 15C)
sì wù tāng (四物汤) (Chapter 16B)
shí quán dà bŭ tāng (十全大补汤) (Chapter 18A)

SOUTHERN SONG DYNASTY

nán sòng (南宋), 1127–1279 CE
3 books, 3 formulas

Author: Liú Wán-Sù (刘完素)
Source: *Huáng Dì Sù Wèn Xuán Míng Lùn Fāng* (黄帝素问宣明论方), 1172
Literal: "Yellow Emperor's Plain Questions Proclaimed Clear Discussion of Formulas"
C&C, F&S, PMPH: "Formulas from the Discussion Illuminating the Yellow Emperor's Basic Questions"
Formula: *fáng fēng tōng shèng săn* (防风通圣散) (Chapter 2B)

Author: Wú Yàn-Kuí (吴彦夔)
Source: *Chuán Xìn Shì Yòng Fāng* (传信适用方), 1180
Literal: "Transmitted Suitable (and) Useable Formulas"
F&S: "Transmitted Trustworthy and Suitable Formulas"
Formula: *shí quán dà bŭ tang* (十全大补汤) (Chapter 18A)

Author: Zhāng Cóng-Zhèng (张从正) *aka* Zhāng Zĭ-Hé (张子和)
Source: *Rú Mén Shì Qīn* (儒门事亲), 1228
Literal: "Confucians' Duties (to their) Parents"
C&C, F&S, PMPH: "Confucians' Duties to Their Parents"
Formula: *mù xiāng bīng láng wán* (木香槟榔丸) (Chapter 6E)

WESTERN XIA

(*xī xià*, 西夏) 1038–1227 CE

JIN DYNASTY

jīn (金), 1115–1234 CE

13 books, 22 formulas

Author: Kòu Zōng-Shì (寇宗奭)
Source: *Běn Cǎo Yǎn Yì* (本草衍义), 1116
Literal: "Materia Medica Extended Meanings"
C&C, F&S, PMPH: "Extension of the Materia Medica"
Formula:
sāng piāo xiāo sǎn (桑螵蛸散) (Chapter 11C)

Author: Anonymous, Song Imperial Court
Source: *Zhèng Hé Shèng Jì Zǒng Lù* (政和圣济总录), 1117
Literal: "(Era of) Political Harmony, Sagely Assistance, Comprehensive Recording"
C&C: "Comprehensive Recording of Sage-Like Benefit from the Zheng He Era"
F&S: "Comprehensive Recording of Sagely Beneficence from the Zhenghe Era"
PMPH: "Comprehensive Recording of Divine Assistance from the Zhenghe Era"
Formula:
tiān tái wū yào sǎn (天台乌药散) (Chapter 7A)

Author: Qián Yǐ (钱乙)
Source: *Qián Shì Xiǎo Ér Yào Zhèng Zhí Jué* (钱氏小儿药证直), 1119
Literal: "Qian's Children's Medical Patterns, Straight Secrets"
PMPH: "Qian's Key to Diagnosis and Treatment of Children's Diseases"
as:
Xiǎo Ér Yào Zhèng Zhí Jué (小儿药证直), 1119
Literal: "Children's Medical Patterns, Straight Secrets"
C&C: "Craft of Medicinal Treatment for Childhood Disease Patterns"
F&S: "Craft of Medicines and Patterns for Children"
PMPH: "Key to Diagnosis and Treatment of Children's Diseases"

Formulas:

rén shēn bài dú săn (人参败毒散) (Chapter 1A)
dăo chì săn (导赤散) (Chapter 2B)
liù wèi dì huáng wán (六味地黄丸) (Chapter 16A)

Author: Hóng Zūn (洪遵) *aka* Hóng Jǐng-Píng (洪景平)
Source: *Hóng Shì Jí Yàn Fang* (洪氏集验方), 1170
Literal: "Hong's Collection (of) Examined Formulas"
C&C: "Time-Tested Formulas of Hong Family"
F&S: "Hong's Collection of Experiential Formulas"
Formula: *huán shào dān* (还少丹) (Chapter 18A)

Author: Chén Yán (陈言) *aka* Chén Wú-Zé (陈无择)
Source: *Sān Yīn Jí Yī Bìng Zhèng Fāng Lùn* (三因极一病证方论), 1174
Literal: "Three Etiologies Unification (of) Illness, Patterns (and) Formulas Discussion"
C&C, F&S: "Discussion of Illnesses, Patterns, and Formulas Related to the Unification of the Three Etiologies"
PMPH: "Treatise on Diseases, Patterns, and Formulas Related to the Unification of the Three Etiologies"
Formula: *wēn dăn tāng* (温胆汤) (Chapter 7C)

Author: Yáng Tán (杨倓)
Source: *Yáng Shì Jiā Cáng Fāng* (杨氏家藏方), 1178
Literal: "Yang Family Depository (of) Formulas"
C&C: "Collected Formulas of the Yang Family"
F&S: "Yang Family Formulas"
PMPH: "Secret Formulas of the Yang Family"
Formula: *juān bì tāng* (蠲痹汤) – 1 (Chapter 4A)

Author: Zhāng Yuán-Sù (张元素) *aka* Zhāng Jié-Gŭ (张洁古)
Source: *Yī Xué Qĭ Yuán* (医学启源), 1186
Literal: "Medical Studies Informed Origins"
PMPH: "Origins of Medicine"
F&S: "Expounding on the Origins of Medicine"
Formula: *dāng guī niān tòng tāng* (当归拈痛汤) (Chapter 4E)

Author: Chén Zì-Míng (陈自明)
Source: *Fù Rén Liáng Fāng* (妇人良方), 1237
Literal: "Women's Fine Formulas"
C&C, F&S, PMPH: "Fine Formulas for Women"
Formulas:
sān bì tāng (三痹汤) (Chapter 4C)
liù jūn zǐ tāng (六君子汤) (Chapter 6A)
tiān wáng bǔ xīn dān (天王补心丹) (Chapter 9)

Author: Lǐ Gǎo (李杲) *aka* Lǐ Dōng-Yuán (李东垣)
Source: *Nèi Wài Shāng Biàn Huò Lùn* (内外伤辨惑论), 1247
Literal: "Internal External Injury, Clarify False-Notions Discussion"
C&C: "Clarifying Doubts about Injury from Internal and External Causes"
F&S, PMPH: "Clarifying Doubts about Damage from Internal and External Causes"
Formulas:
shēng mài sǎn (生脉散) (Chapter 3E)
liù jūn zǐ tāng (六君子汤) (Chapter 6A)
dāng guī bǔ xuè tāng (当归补血汤) (Chapter 15C)

Author: Lǐ Gǎo (李杲) *aka* Lǐ Dōng-Yuán (李东垣)
Source: *Pí Wèi Lùn* (脾胃论), 1249
Literal: "Spleen, Stomach Discussion"
C&C, F&S: "Discussion of the Spleen and Stomach"
PMPH: "Treatise on the Spleen and Stomach"
Formulas:
bǔ zhōng yì qì tāng (补中益气汤) (Chapter 6A)
rùn cháng wán (润肠丸) (Chapter 6D)
bàn xià bái zhú tiān má tang (半夏白术天麻汤) –1 (Chapter 7B)

Author: Yáng Shì-Yíng (杨士瀛) *aka* Yáng Rén-Zhāi (杨仁斋)
Source: *Rén Zhāi Zhí Zhǐ Fāng* (仁斋直指方), 1264
Literal: "Ren-Zhai's Straight Indications Formula Discussion"
C&C: "Straight Directions of Benevolent Aid"
F&S: "Straight Direction from [Yang] Ren-Zhai"
PMPH: "[Yang] Ren-zhai's Direct Guidance on Formulas"
Formula: *yù quán wán* (玉泉丸) (Chapter 15A)

Author: Lǐ Gǎo (李杲) *aka* Lǐ Dōng-Yuán (李东垣), edited by Luō Tān-Yì (罗天益)
Source: *Dōng Yuán Shì Xiào Fāng* (东垣试效方), 1266
Literal: "Dong-Yuan's Tested, Effective Formulas"
F&S: "Dong-Yuan's Tried and Tested Formulas"
PMPH: "[Li] Dong-yuan's Proven Formulas"
also as:
Dōng Héng Shì Xiào Fāng (东恒试效方), 1266
Literal: "Dong-Heng's Tested, Effective Formulas"
C&C: "Tested and Effective Formulas by Dong Heng"
Formula: *pǔ jì xiāo dú yǐn* (普济消毒饮) (Chapter 2A)

Author: Lǐ Gǎo (李杲) *aka* Lǐ Dōng-Yuán (李东垣)
Source: *Lán Shì Mì Cáng* (兰室秘藏), date unknown, published 1276
Literal: "Orchid Chamber's Secrets Concealed"
C&C, F&S, PMPH: "Secrets from the Orchid Chamber"
Formula: *qīng wèi sǎn* (清胃散) (Chapter 2B)

YUAN DYNASTY

yuán (元), 1271–1368 CE
8 books, 11 formulas

Author: Anonymous
Source: *Mì Chuán Yǎn Kē Lóng Mù Lùn* (秘传眼科龙木论), 13th century
Literal: "Secret Transmission (on) Eye (Diseases), Long-Mu's Discussion"
PMPH: "The Secret Transmission of Long-mu's Ophthalmology"

Author: Yán Yòng-Hé (严用和)
Source: *Jì Shēng Fāng* (济生方), 1253
Literal: "Aid (the) Living Formulas"
C&C, F&S, PMPH: "Formulas to Aid the Living"
Formulas:
cāng ěr zǐ sǎn (苍耳子散) (Chapter 1C)
xīn yí wán (辛夷丸) (Chapter 1C)
guī pí tāng (归脾汤) (Chapter 9)
dāng guī yǐn zǐ (当归饮子) (Chapter 13A)

Author: Luó Tiā-Yì (羅天益)
Source: *Wèi Shēng Bǎo Jiàn* (卫生宝鉴), 1281
Literal: "Protect Life Precious Mirror"
C&C, F&S, PMPH: "Precious Mirror of Health"
Formula: *lóng dǎn xiè gān tāng* (龙胆泻肝汤)

Author: Wáng Hào-Gǔ (王好古)
Source: *Yī Lêi Yuán Róng* (医垒元戎), 1291
Literal: "Medical Ramparts Supreme Commanders"
F&S: "Supreme Commanders of the Medical Ramparts"
Formula: *táo hóng sì wù tāng* (桃红四物汤) (Chapter 8C)

Author: Lǐ Zhòng-Nán (李仲南)
Source: *Yông Lèi Qián Fāng* (永类钤方), 1331
Literal: "Eternal Categories Inscribed Formulas"
C&C: "Everlasting Categorization of Seal Formulas"
F&S: "Everlasting Categorization of Inscribed Formulas"
Formula: *bǔ fèi tāng* (补肺汤) (Chapter 3F)

Author: Wēi Yì-Lín (危亦林)
Source: *Shì Yī Dé Xiào Fāng* (世医得效方), 1345
Literal: "Generations (of) Physicians Obtained Effective Formulas"
C&C, F&S, PMPH: "Effective Formulas from Generations of Physicians"
Formulas:
wǔ rén wán (五仁丸) (Chapter 6E)
qǐ jú dì huáng wán (杞菊地黄丸) (Chapter 14)

Author: Gé Kě–Jiǔ (葛可久) *aka* Gé Qián–Sūn (葛乾孙)
Source: *Shí Yào Shén Shū* (十药神书), 1348
C&C: "Miraculous Book of Ten Remedies"
F&S: "Miraculous Book of Ten Remedies for Consumption"
PMPH: "Divine Book of Ten Medicinal Formulas"

as: *Láo Zhèng Shí Yào Shén Shū* (劳症十药神书), 1348
Literal: "Consumption Disease Ten Medicines Divine Book"
F&S: "Miraculous Book of Ten Remedies for Consumption"
PMPH: "Deficiency Taxation Divine Book of Ten Medicinal Formulas"
Formula: *shí huī sǎn* (十灰散) (Chapter 5D)

Author: Huá Shòu (滑寿)
Source: *Má Zhěn Quán Shū* (麻疹全书), circa 1350
Literal: "Measles Complete Treatise"
F&S: "Complete Treatise on Measles"
Formula: *qǐ jú dì huáng wán* (杞菊地黄丸) (Chapter 14)

MING DYNASTY

míng (明), 1368–1644 or 1662 CE
21 books, 36 formulas

Author: Táo Huá (陶华)
Source: *Shāng Hán Liù Shū* (伤寒六书), 1445
Literal: "Injury (by) Cold, Six Books"
C&C: "Six Texts on Cold-Induced Disorders"
F&S, PMPH: "Six Texts on Cold Damage"
Formula: *chái gé jiě jī tāng* (柴葛解肌汤) (Chapter 1B)

Author: Anonymous (probably Táo Huá, 陶华)
Source: *Shāng Hán Quán Shēng Jí* (伤寒全生集), 1445
Literal: "Injury (by) Cold, Complete Life Collection"
C&C: "All-New Collection of Cold Induced Disorders"
F&S: "Complete Compendium of Cold Damage"
Formula: *lián qiào bài dú piān* (连翘败毒片) (Chapter 13A)

Author: Zhū Zhèn-Hěng (朱震亨) *aka* Zhū Dān-Xī (朱丹溪)
Source: *Dān Xī Xīn Fǎ* (丹溪心法), 1481
Literal: "Dan-Xi's Heart Method" (eg, "Personal Insights")
C&C, PMPH: "Teachings of [Zhu] Dan-xi"
F&S: "Essential Teachings of [Zhu] Dan-Xi"

Formulas:

èr miào săn (二妙散) (Chapter 4E)
băo hé wán (保和丸) (Chapter 6C)
tòng xiè yào fāng (痛泻药方) (Chapter 6D)
dà bŭ yīn wán (大补阴丸) (Chapter 8E)
yù píng fēng săn (玉屏风散) (Chapter 16A)

Author: Yú Tuán (虞抟)
Source: *Yī Xué Zhèng Chuán* (医学正传), 1515
Literal: "Medical Studies Correct Transmission"
C&C: "True Lineage of Medicine"
F&S: "Correct Transmission of Medicine"
Formula: *sān miào săn* (三妙散) (Chapter 4E)

Author: Xuē Jǐ (薛己) *aka* Xuē Xīn-Fǔ (薛新甫) *aka* Xuē Lì-Zhāi (薛立斋)
Source: *Zhèng Tǐ Lèi Yào* (正体类要), 1529
Literal: "Standardized Category Essentials"
C&C: "Catalogued Essentials for Correcting the Body"
F&S: "Categorized Essentials for Normalizing the Structure"
PMPH: "Categorized Synopsis of the Whole"
Formula: *bā zhēn tāng* (八珍汤) (Chapter 15C)

Author: Xuē Jǐ (薛己) *aka* Xuē Xīn-Fǔ (薛新甫) *aka* Xuē Lì-Zhāi (薛立斋)
Source: *Nèi Kē Zhāi Yào* (内科摘要), circa 1530
Literal: "Internal (Medicine) Department Selected Essentials"
C&C, F&S, PMPH: "Summary of Internal Medicine"
Formula: *jiā wèi xiāo yáo săn* (加味逍遥散) (Chapter 8B)

Author: Xuē Jǐ (薛己) *aka* Xuē Xīn-Fǔ (薛新甫) *aka* Xuē Lì-Zhāi (薛立斋)
Source: *Jiào Zhù Fù Rén Liáng Fāng* (校注妇人良方), mid-16th c.
Literal: "Corrections (and) Annotations (to) Women's Fine Formulas"
C&C: "Revised Fine Formulas for Women"
F&S: "Fine Formulas for Women with Annotations and Commentary"
PMPH: "Corrections and Annotations to Fine Formulas for Women"

Formulas:

sān bì tāng (三痹汤) (Chapter 4C)
liù jūn zǐ tāng (六君子汤) (Chapter 6A)
tiān wáng bǔ xīn dān (天王补心丹) (Chapter 9)

Author: Péng Yòng-Guāng (彭用光)
Source: *Tǐ Rén Huì Biān* (体仁汇编), 1549
Literal: "Body Benevolent Collection-Compilation"
C&C, F&S: "Compilation of Materials of Benevolence for the Body"
PMPH: "A Compilation of Benevolent Formulas"
Formula: *bǎi zǐ yǎng xīn tāng* (柏子养心汤) (Chapter 9)

Author: Zhāng Shí-Chè (张时彻)
Source: *Shè Shēng Zhòng Miào Fāng* (摄生众妙方), 1550
Literal: "Conserve Life Multitude (of) Marvelous Formulas"
C&C: "Marvelous Formulas for the Health of Multitudes"
F&S: "Multitude of Marvelous Formulas for Sustaining Life"
PMPH: "Numerous Miraculous Prescriptions for Health Cultivation"
Formulas:

jīng fáng bài dú sǎn (荆防败毒散) (Chapter 1A)
dìng chuǎn wán (定喘丸) (Chapter 3F)

Author: Zhōu Zhī-Gān (周之干) *aka* Zhōu Shèn-Zhāi (周慎斋)
Source: *Shèn Zhāi Yí Shū* (慎斋遗书), 1573
Literal: "Shen-Zhai's Dying Testament"
F&S: "Writings for Posterity of (Zhou) Shen-Zhai"
Formula: *bǎi hé gù jīn tāng* (百合固金汤) (Chapter 3E)

Author: Li Chān (李梴) *aka* Lǐ Tǐng (李挺) *aka* Lǐ Jiàn-Zhāi (李健齋)
Source: *Yī Xué Rù Mén* (医学入门), 1575
Literal: "Medical Studies Introduction"
C&C, F&S, PMPH: "Introduction to Medicine"
Formula: *wǔ zǐ yǎn zōng wán* (五子衍宗丸)

Author: Wú Kūn (吴昆)
Source: *Yī Fāng Kǎo* (医方考), 1584
Literal: "Medical Formula Investigations"
C&C, F&S, PMPH: "Investigations of Medical Formulas"
Formulas:
qīng qì huà tán wán (清气化痰丸) (Chapter 3B)
zhī bǎi dì huáng wán (知柏地黄丸) (Chapter 8E)

Author: Gōng Tíng-Xián (龚廷贤)
Source: *Wàn Bìng Huí Chūn* (万病回春), 1587
Literal: "Thousand Diseases Returned to Spring" (eg, "Restored to Health")
C&C, F&S, PMPH: "Restoration of Health from the Myriad Diseases"
Formulas:
shū jīng huó xuè tang (舒经活血汤) (Chapter 4A)
xiāng shā yǎng wèi tāng (香砂养胃汤) (Chapter 6C)
shū gān tāng (疏肝汤) (Chapter 7A) – older version

Author: Lǐ Shí-Zhēn (李时珍) *aka* Lǐ Dōng-Bì (李东壁)
Source: *Běn Cǎo Gāng Mù* (本草纲目), 1578 or 1590
Literal: "Materia Medica Guiding Outline"
C&C: "Materia Medica"
F&S: "Comprehensive Outline of the Materia Medica"
PMPH: "The Grand Compendium of Materia Medica"
Formula: *qī bǎo měi rán dān* (七宝美髯丹) (Chapter 13B)

Author: Wáng Kěn-Tāng (王肯堂)
Source: *Zhèng Zhì Zhǔn Shéng* (证治准绳), 1602
Literal: "Pattern Treatment Standards"
C&C: "Standards of Patterns and Treatment"
F&S: "Indispensible Tools for Pattern Treatment"
PMPH: "Standards for Diagnosis and Treatment"
Formula: *qīng gǔ sǎn* (清骨散) (Chapter 8E)

Author: Miào Xī-Yōng (缪希雍)
Source: *Xiān Xǐng Zhāi Yī Xué Guǎng Bǐ Jì* (先醒斋医学广笔记), 1613
Literal: "First Awakened Studio Medical Studies Extensive Short Notes"
C&C: "Wide Ranging Medical Notes from the First-Awakened Studio"
F&S: "Extensive Notes on Medicine [from the First-Awakened Studio]"
PMPH: "Extensive Notes on Medicine from Xian Xing Studio"
Formula: *zī shēng wán* (资生丸) (Chapter 6C)

Author: Gōng Tíng-Xián (龚廷贤)
Source: *Shòu Shì Bǎo Yuán* (寿世保元), 1615
Literal: "Long Life Protect (the) Source"
C&C, F&S: "Achieving Longevity by Guarding the Source"
PMPH: "Prolonging Life and Preserving the Origin"
Formulas:
bā xīan cháng shōu wán (八仙长寿丸) (Chapter 3E)
mài wèi dì huáng wán (麦味地黄丸) (Chapter 3E)
wū jī bái fèng wán (乌鸡白凤丸) (Chapter 8A)

Author: Chén Shí-Gōng (陈实功)
Source: *Wài Kē Zhèng Zōng* (外科正宗), 1617
Literal: "External Medicine True Lineage"
C&C: "True Lineage of External Medicine"
F&S, PMPH: "Orthodox Lineage of External Medicine"
Formula: *xiāo fēng sǎn* (消风散) (Chapter 13A)

Author: Wǔ Zhī-Wàng (武之望) *aka* Shū Qīng (叔卿)
Source: *Jì Yīn Gāng Mù* (济阴纲目), 1620
Literal: "Benefit *Yin* (Women) General Outline"
C&C: "Materia Medica to Aid Yin"
F&S: "Comprehensive Outline on Benefiting Yin"
PMPH: "A Compendium of Female Disorders"
Formula: *qiān jīn zhǐ dài wán* (千金止带丸) (Chapter 8D)

Author: Zhāng Jiè-Bīn (张介宾) *aka* Zhāng Jǐng-Yuè (张景岳)
Source: *Jǐng Yuè Quán Shū* (景岳全书), 1624
Literal: "Jing-Yue's Complete Writings"
C&C: "Collected Treatises of [Zhang] Jing-Yue"
F&S: "Collected Treatises of [Zhang] Jing-Yue - 1624"
PMPH: "The Complete Works of [Zhang] Jing-yue"
Formulas:
tòng xiè yào fāng (痛泻药方) (Chapter 6D)
chái hú shū gān sǎn (Chapter 7A)
zuǒ guī wán (左归丸) (Chapter 16A)
yòu guī wán (右归丸) (Chapter 17B)

Author: Hóng Jī (洪基) *aka* Hóng Jiǔ-Yǒu (洪九有)
Source: *Shè Shēng Mì Pōu* (摄生秘剖), 1638
Literal: "Sustaining Life Secrets, Explanation"
C&C: "Secrets Investigations into Obtaining Health"
F&S: "Dissecting the Secrets of Sustaining Life"
PMPH: "Penetrating the Secrets of Health Cultivation"
Formula: *tiān wáng bǔ xīn dān* (天王补心丹)

QING DYNASTY

qīng (清) 1644–1911 CE
18 books, 35 formulas

Author: Fù Rén-Yǔ (傅仁宇)
Source: *Fù Shì Yǎn Kē Shěn Shì Yáo Hán* (傅氏眼科审视瑶函), 1644
Literal: "Master Fu's Ophthalmology Examination Inspection (of the) Jade Case"
PMPH: "A Close Examination of the Precious Classic [on Ophthalmology]"
also as:
Shěn Shì Yáo Hán (审视瑶函), 1642
Literal: "Examination Inspection (of the) Jade Case"
C&C: "Scrutiny of the Priceless Jade Case"
F&S: "Scrutiny of the Precious Jade Case"

Author: Yù Chāng (喻昌) *aka* Yù Jiā-Yán (喻嘉言)
Source: *Yī Mén Fǎ Lǜ* (医门法律), 1658
Literal: "Physicians' Door (to) Methods (and) Rules",
C&C, F&S, PMPH: "Precepts for Physicians"
Formula: *qīng zào jiù fèi wán* (清燥救肺丸) (Chapter 3A)

Author: Luō Měi (罗美)
Source: *Míng Yī Fāng Lùn* (名医方论), 1675
Literal: "Famous Physicians' Formulas Discussion"
F&S: "Discussion of Famous Physicians' Formulas Past and Present"
PMPH: "Discussion on Famous Physicians' Formulas"
aka:
Gǔ Jīn Míng Fāng (古今名方), 1675
Literal: "Ancient, Modern Famous Formulas"
C&C: "Famous Classic and Contemporary Formulas"
Formula: *xiāng shā liù jūn zǐ tāng* (香砂六君子汤) (Chapter 6A)

Author: Wāng Áng (汪昂)
Source: *Yī Fāng Jí Jiě* (医方集解), 1682
Literal: "Medical Formulas Collected, Explained"
C&C: "Analytic Collection of Medical Formulas"
F&S, PMPH: "Medical Formulas Collected and Analyzed"
Formulas:
jiàn pí wán (健脾丸) (Chapter 6C)
lóng dǎn xiè gān tāng (龙胆泻肝汤) (Chapter 7C)
bì xiè fēn qīng yǐn (萆薢分清饮) (Chapter 11A)
jīn suǒ gù jīng wán (金锁固精丸) (Chapter 11C)

Author: Chéng Guó-Péng (程国彭)
Source: *Yī Xué Xīn Wù* (医学心悟), 1732
Literal: "Medical Studies Mind Awakening (eg, Insights)"
C&C: "Medical Revelations"
F&S: "Awakening of the Mind in Medical Studies"
PMPH: "Easy Access to Medicine"
Formulas:
juān bì tāng (蠲痹汤) – 2 (Chapter 4A)
bàn xià bái zhú tiān má tang (半夏白术天麻汤) -2 (Chapter 7B)

Author: Wú Qiān (吴谦)
Source: *Yī Zōng Jīn Jiàn* (医宗金鉴), 1742
Literal: "Medical Tradition Golden Mirror"
C&C, F&S, PMPH: "Golden Mirror of the Medical Tradition"
Formulas:
wǔ wèi xiāo dú yǐn (五味消毒饮) (Chapter 2A)
táo hóng sì wù tāng (桃红四物汤) (Chapter 8C)
zhī bǎi dì huáng wán (知柏地黄丸) (Chapter 8E)
dān shēn yǐn (丹参饮) (Chapter 10)

Author: Fāng Zhào-Quán (方肇权)
Source: *Fāng Shì Mài Zhèng Zhèng Zōng* (方氏脉症正宗), 1749
Literal: "Fang's Pulse (and) Disease Orthodox Lineage"
F&S, PMPH: "Fang's Orthodox Lineage of Pulse and Symptoms"
Formula: *sān miào sǎn* (三妙散) (Chapter 4E)

Author: Wú Yí-Luò (吴仪洛) *aka* Wú Zūn-Chéng (吴遵程)
Source: *Běn Cǎo Cóng Xīn* (本草从新), 1751
Literal: "Materia Medica From (the) New"
C&C, F&S, PMPH: "Thoroughly Revised Materia Medica"
Herbs:
xī yáng shēn (西洋参), Radix Panacis Quinquefolii (Chapter 16A)
dōng chóng xià cǎo (冬虫夏草), Cordyceps (Chapter 18B)

Author: Gù Shì-Chéng (顾世澄)
Source: *Yáng Yī Dà Quán* (疡医大全), 1760
Literal: "Sores Medicine Great Compendium"
F&S: "Great Compendium of Medicine for Sores"
Formulas:
nèi xiāo luǒ lì wán (内消瘰疬丸) (Chapter 2A)
xī guā shuāng (西瓜霜) (Chapter 2A)

Author: Xiāng Tiān-Ruì (项天瑞)
Source: *Tóng Shòu Lù* (同寿录), 1762
Literal: "Common Longevity Records"
F&S: "Collection for the Common Pursuit of Longevity"
Formula: *fù kē zhǒng zǐ wán* (妇科种子丸) (Chapter 8A)

Author: Wèi Zhī-Xiù (魏之琇)
Source: *Xù Míng Yī Lèi Àn* (续名医类案), 1770
Literal: "Continuation (of) Famous Doctors' Categorized Cases"
C&C, F&S: "Continuation of Famous Physicians' Cases Organized by Categories"
PMPH: "Supplement to 'Classified Case Records of Famous Physicians'"
Formula: *yī guàn jiān* (一贯煎) (Chapter 7A)

Author: Shěn Jīn-Ào (沈金鳌)
Source: *Shěn Shì Zūn Shēng Shū* (沈氏尊生书), 1773
Literal: "Shen Shi's Venerate Life Books"
PMPH: "Shen's Books on Respecting Life"
F&S: "Shen's Book for Revering Life"
Formula: *yù quán wán* (玉泉丸) (Chapter 15A)

Author: Dài Tiān-Zhāng (戴天章)
Source: *Guǎng Wēn Yì Lùn* (广瘟疫论), 1774
Literal: "Widespread Warm Epidemic Discussion"
C&C, F&S: "Discussion of Widespread Warm Epidemics"
PMPH: "Treatise on Widespread Warm Pestilence"
Formula: *ěr lóng zuǒ cí wán* (耳聋左慈丸) (Chapter 7B)

Author: Wú Táng (吴瑭) *aka* Wú Jū-Tōng (吴鞠通)
Source: *Wēn Bìng Tiáo Biàn* (温病条辨), 1798
Literal: "Warm Diseases Systematic Differentiation"
C&C, PMPH: "Systematic Differentiation of Warm Diseases"
F&S: "Systematic Differentiation of Warm Pathogen Diseases – 1798"
Formulas:
sāng jú yǐn (桑菊饮) (Chapter 1B)
yín qiào sǎn (银翘散) (Chapter 1B)
xìng sū sǎn (杏蘇丸) (Chapter 3C)
shā shēn mài dōng tāng (沙参麦冬汤) (Chapter 3E)
xuān bì tāng (宣痹汤) (Chapter 4E)

Author: Chén Niàn-Zǔ *aka* Chén Xiū-Yuán (陈念祖 / 陈修园)
Source: *Shí Fāng Gē Kuò* (时方歌括), 1801
Literal: "Contemporary Formulas (as a) Song Collection"
C&C: "Collected Songs About Contemporary Formulas"
F&S: "Compendium of Songs on Modern Formulas"
PMPH: "Summary Verses of Post-Classical Formulas"
Formula: *dān shēn yǐn* (丹参饮) (Chapter 10)

Author: Wáng Qīng-Rèn (王清任)
Source: *Yī Lín Gǎi Cuò* (医林改错), 1830
Literal: "Physicians' Circle, Correction (of) Errors"
C&C, F&S: "Correction Of Errors Among Physicians"
PMPH: "Correction of Errors in Medical Works"
Formulas:
shēn tòng zhú yū tāng (身痛逐瘀丸) (Chapter 4B)
bǔ yáng huán wǔ tāng (补阳还五湯) (Chapter 4C)
shào fǔ zhú yū tāng (少腹逐瘀汤) (Chapter 8C)
gé xià zhú yū tāng (膈下逐瘀汤) (Chapter 7A)
tōng qiào huó xuè tāng (通窍活血汤) (Chapter 10)
xuè fǔ zhú yū tāng (血府逐瘀汤) (Chapter 10)

Author: Xiè Yuán-Qìng (谢元庆)
Source: *Liáng Fāng Jí Yè* (良方集腋), 1842
Literal: "Fine Formulas Collection Small"
C&C, F&S: "Small Collection of Fine Formulas"
PMPH: "A Collection of Fine Formulas from Various Sources"
Formula: *qī lí sǎn* (七厘散) (Chapter 5A)

Author: Zhāng Bǐng-Chéng (张秉成)
Source: *Chéng Fāng Biàn Dú* (成方便读), 1904
Literal: "Established Formulas Convenient Reader"
C&C, F&S: "Convenient Reader of Established Formulas"
PMPH: "Convenient Reader on Established Formulas"
Formula: *sì miào wán* (四妙丸) (Chapter 4E)

NATIONALIST REPUBLIC OF CHINA

zhōng guó mín zú zhǔ yì gòng hé guó (中国民族主义共和国), 1911-1949
1 book, 2 formulas

Author: Zhāng Xī-Chún (张锡纯)
Source: *Yī Xué Zhōng Zhōng Cān Xī Lù* (医学衷中参西录), 1918-1934
Literal: "Medical Studies Heartfelt (towards) Chinese, Respecting Western, Records"
C&C: "Records of Heart-Felt Experiences in Medicine with Reference to the West"
F&S: "Essays on Medicine Esteeming the Chinese and Respecting the Western – 1918-1934"
PMPH: "Records of Chinese Medicine with Reference to Western Medicine"
Formulas:
huó luò xiào líng dān (活络效灵丹) (Chapter 5A)
zhèn gān xī fēng tāng (镇肝息风汤) (Chapter 7B)

PEOPLE'S REPUBLIC OF CHINA

zhōng huá rén mín gòng hé guó (中华人民共和国), 1949-present
5 books, 5 formulas

Author: Zhāng Bó-Nè (张伯讷)
Source: *Zhōng Yī Fāng Jì Lín Chuáng Shǒu Cè* (中医方剂临床手册), 1950s
Literal: "Chinese Medicine Formulas Dosing Clinical Manual"
C&C: "Clinical Handbook of Chinese Herbal Formulas"
F&S: "Clinical Handbook of Chinese Medical Formulas (1950s)"
Formula: *èr xiān tāng* (二仙汤) (Chapter 8E)

Author: Hú Guāng-Cí (胡光慈)
Source: *Zá Bìng Zhèng Zhì Xīn Yì* (杂病证治新义), 1958
Literal: "Miscellaneous Disorders Patterns (and) Treatment New Significance"
C&C: "New Significance of Patterns and Treatment in Miscellaneous Diseases"
F&S: "Deriving New Treatments for Patterns of Miscellaneous Disorders"
Formula: *tiān má gōu téng yǐn* (天麻钩藤饮) (Chapter 7B)

Author: Chinese Medicine Research Institute of China Academy of TCM (中国中医研究院中医研究所)
Source: *Quán Guó Zhōng Yào Chéng Yào Chù Fāng Jí* (全国中药成药处方集), 1962
Literal: "Nation-wide Chinese Medicine Manufactured Medicine Medical Prescription Collection"
C&C: "National Collection of Chinese Herbal Prepared Medicines"
F&S: "Nationwide Collection of TCM Patent Formulas"
Formula: *huáng lián shàng qīng wán* (黄连上清丸) (Chapter 3A)

Author: Chinese Herbal Medicine Committee, Ministry of the Interior
Source: *Zhōng Guó Guó Yào Gù Yǒu Chéng Fāng Xuǎn Jí* (中国国药故有成方选集), 1967
Literal: "China's Chinese Medicine Administration Selected Formulas Anthology"
C&C: "A Selection of Traditional Prescriptions of Chinese Medicine"
Formula: *níng sòu wán* (宁嗽丸) (Chapter 3B)

Author: Anonymous
Source: *Zhōng Huā Rén Mín Gòng Hé Guó Yào Diǎn* (中华人民共和国药典), 2005
Literal: "People's Republic of China (Herbal) Medicine Dictionary"
C&C: "Chinese Herbal Pharmacopoeia by People's Republic of China"
Formula: *míng mù dì huáng wán* (明目地黄丸) (Chapter 14)

INDEX OF FORMULAS, ALPHABETICALLY

HOW TO DOSE CHINESE HERBAL PRODUCTS

The key to effectiveness in taking Chinese herbal products is dosage. The traditional method in China boils 50-200 grams of an herbal formula 3 times to make 3 large cups of decoction. These are taken over the course of one day.

Pills, tablets and concentrated powders can be effective, even in smaller doses. Adult dosage should be 2-3 g., 2-3 x day. These work out as follows:

Extracted granules (EG) powder:	1 spoon = 1 g.
Extracted granule (EG) capsule:	1 capsule = .5 g.
Teapills (MS, PF, TL, some PM):	7 pills = 1 g.
Larger teapills (HT):	4 pills = 1 g.
Tablets (GF, HC, K, SF):	1 tablet = .7 g.
Uncoated tablets (PM):	1 tablet = .7 g.
Coated tablets (PM):	1 tablet = .5 g.

Children > 6 years: give adult doses. Children, infant to 5 years: adjust dosage.

Indications of dosing being too strong: nausea, loose stool, headache, discomfort. Reduce dosage.

Virtually all government approved herbal products for export from China meet Good Manufacturing Practice (GMP) standards and have been certified to contain no heavy metals, pharmaceuticals, or chemicals. Many American manufacturers use imported herbs that have been lab tested and independently certified in the United States.

BIBLIOGRAPHY AND RECOMMENDED READING

Cited Texts:

Chen & Chen:
Chinese Herbal Formulas and Applications, John K. Chen and Tina T. Chen, Art of Medicine Press, City of Industry, CA, 2009

Chen & Chen, *Medical Herbology*:
Chinese Medical Herbology and Pharmacology, John K. Chen and Tina T. Chen, Art of Medicine Press, City of Industry, CA, 2004

Bensky et al:
Chinese Herbal Medicine Formulas & Strategies, 2nd Edition, Volker Scheid, Dan Bensky, Andrew Ellis and Randall Barolet, Eastland Press, Seattle, WA, 2009

Bensky, Clavey, Ströger, *Materia Medica*:
Chinese Herbal Medicine Materia Medica, 3rd Edition, Dan Bensky, Steven Clavey, Erich Ströger with Andrew Gamble, Eastland Press, Seattle, WA, 2004

Ellis:
Notes From South Mountain, Andrew Ellis, Thin Moon Publishing, Berkeley, CA, 2003

OTHER BIBLIOGRAPHY:

Chinese Herbal Formulas, Treatment Principles and Composition Strategies, Yifan Yang, Churchill Livingstone Elsevier, 2010

Chinese Herbal Patent Formulas, The Clinical Desk Reference, Jake Fratkin, Shya Publications, Boulder, CO, 2001

Formulas of Traditional Chinese Medicine, Long Zhixian, Chief Editor, Beijing University of TCM, Academy Press, Beijing, 1998.

Pharmacology of Traditional Chinese Medical Formulae, The English-Chinese Encyclopedia of Practical Chinese Medicine, Higher Education Press, Beijing, 1989

A Practitioner's Formula Guide, A Comprehensive Guide to Plum Flower and Min Shan Brand Formula, Alisa Wrinkle, Laura Stropes & Teo Potts, Elemental Essentials Press, Oakland, CA, 2008

WEBINAR / MP3 LECTURES

The contents of this book are available as 22 recorded lectures, each at two hours. Available as video webinar or MP3 audio presentations. Go to:

http://drjakefratkin.com/teaching/webinars/
the-most-important-chinese-herbal-formulas

or

http://www.easterncurrents.ca/learning/earn-ceus/recorded-courses/
the-most-important-chinese-herbal-formulas

For a Complete Listing of Herbal Products by Therapeutic Category, See:

"WHO'S GOT WHAT"

For free download, go to:
www.drjakefratkin.com/whos-got-what

BIOGRAPHY

JAKE PAUL FRATKIN, OMD, L.Ac., Dipl. Ac., C.H. (NCCAOM) trained in Korean, Japanese and Chinese styles of acupuncture since 1975, and Chinese herbal medicine since 1982, and has studied and taught *qi gong* and Yang family *Taijiquan* since 1974. His training includes one year advanced hospital training in Beijing. He is the author of *Chinese Herbal Patent Medicines, The Clinical Desk Reference,* a compendium of 1250 Chinese herbal products available in the United States, and the editor-organizer of Wu and Fischer's *Practical Therapeutics of Traditional Chinese Medicine*, Paradigm Publications, 1997. He is the recipient of *Acupuncturist of the Year*, 1999, by the AAAOM and *Teacher of the Year,* 2006, American Association of Teachers of Acupuncture and Oriental Medicine (AATAOM). Dr. Fratkin lives and practices in Boulder, Colorado, USA.

Books by Jake Paul Frakin:

Chinese Herbal Patent Formulas, Shya Publications, 1986.

Practical Therapeutics of Traditional Chinese Medicine, Paradigm Publications, 1997. Wu Yan and Warren Fischer, edited and orgnaized by Jake Fratkin.

Chinese Herbal Patent Medicines, The Clinical Desk Reference, Shya Publications, 2001.

A Calligrapher's Yi Jing, Xinshi Harrison Tu (calligraphy) and Jake Fratkin (translations), Shya Publications, 2004.

Essential Chinese Formulas, 225 Classical and Modern Prescriptions Organized by Clinical Category, Shya Publications, 2014.

TCM Case Studies in Autoimmune Disorders. Zeng Shengping and Jake Fratkin, People's Medical Publishing House, 2014.

A collection of various articles on TCM can be found at:
http://drjakefratkin.com/articles

CODE LETTERS OF HERBAL COMPANIES

AL	Alembic (Kan)
BP	Blue Poppy
CC	Chinese Classics
CMS	Chinese Modular Solutions (Kan)
CP	Classical Pearls
DrJ	Dr. Jake Fratkin's Herbal Formulas
DS	Dr. Shen's
EG	"Standardized" extract granules or capsules from Taiwan and China: Acuherb, E-Fong, Evergreen, Guang Ci Tang, Herbal Times, KPC, Legendary, Mintong, Nong's, Qualiherb, Sunten, etc.
EV	Evergreen
GC	Guang Ci Tang (Active Herb)
GF	Golden Flower
GN	Great Nature (People's Herbs)
GW	Gentle Warrior (Kan)
HC	Health Concerns
HS	Honso
HT	Herbal Times (Nuherbs)
JD	Jade Dragon (Nuherbs)
JW	Jade Woman's Herbals
K	Kan Herbals and Traditionals
KP	Kaiser Pharmaceutical, *aka* KPC (Taiwan)
MS	Minshan (China)
PF	Plum Flower (Mayway)
PH	People's Herbs
PiM	Pine Mountain (Institute of Traditional Medicine)
PM	Patent Medicine (various manufacturers, China)
SF	Seven Forest (Institute of Traditional Medicine)
SW	Spring Wind
TL	Tanglong (China)
TT	Three Treasures
TZ	TCMZone

Manuals for each of the product lines can be obtained from the manufacturers. These will detail ingredients and indications.